Lecture Notes
Clinical
Pharmacology
and Therapeutics

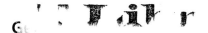

BSc
Consultant Physician and Honorary Clinical Senior Lecturer
Glasgow Royal Infirmary
Glasgow

John L. Reid

DM FRCP FRSE
Emeritus Professor of Medicine and Therapeutics
University of Glasgow

Matthew R. Walters

MD FRCP MSc
Professor of Clinical Pharmacology and Honorary Consultant Physician
Division of Cardiovascular and Medical Sciences
University of Glasgow

Eighth Edition

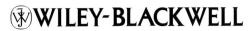 WILEY-BLACKWELL

A John Wiley & Sons, Ltd., Publication

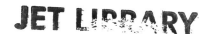

This edition first published 2010, © 2010 by Gerard McKay, John Reid and Matthew Walters
Previous editions 1982, 1985, 1989, 1992, 1996, 2001, 2006

Blackwell Publishing was acquired by John Wiley & Sons in February 2007. Blackwell's publishing program has been merged with Wiley's global Scientific, Technical and Medical business to form Wiley-Blackwell.

Registered office: John Wiley & Sons Ltd, The Atrium, Southern Gate, Chichester, West Sussex, PO19 8SQ, UK

Editorial offices: 9600 Garsington Road, Oxford, OX4 2DQ, UK
                    The Atrium, Southern Gate, Chichester, West Sussex, PO19 8SQ, UK
                    111 River Street, Hoboken, NJ 07030-5774, USA

For details of our global editorial offices, for customer services and for information about how to apply for permission to reuse the copyright material in this book please see our website at www.wiley.com/wiley-blackwell

The right of the authors to be identified as the authors of this work has been asserted in accordance with the Copyright, Designs and Patents Act 1988.

Library of Congress Cataloging-in-Publication Data

McKay, Gerard A.   Lecture notes. Clinical pharmacology and therapeutics / Gerard A. McKay, John L. Reid, Matthew R. Walters. – 8th ed.
     p. ; cm.
  Other title: Clinical pharmacology and therapeutics
  Rev. ed. of: Lecture notes. Clinical pharmacology & therapeutics / John L. Reid, Peter C. Rubin, Matthew R. Walters. 7th ed. 2006.
  Includes bibliographical references and index.
  ISBN 978-1-4051-9778-6
1. Clinical pharmacology.   I. Walters, Matthew R.   II. Reid, John L. Lecture notes. Clinical pharmacology & therapeutics.   III. Title.   IV. Title: Clinical pharmacology and therapeutics.
  [DNLM: 1. Pharmacology, Clinical. 2. Drug Therapy. QV 38 M457L 2010]
  RM301.28.R45 2010
  615'.1–dc22

                                                                                                  2010019097

A catalogue record for this book is available from the British Library.

Set in 8/12pt Stone Serif by Aptara® Inc., New Delhi, India
Printed and bound in Singapore by Fabulous Printers Pte Ltd

1   2010

Contents

Contributors

The following have contributed substantially to the writing, revision and rewriting of the chapters in the eighth edition of *Lecture Notes in Clinical Pharmacology and Therapeutics*.

Ailsa Brown Scottish Medicines Consortium, Glasgow
(Chapter 25)

Andrew Gallagher Diabetes Centre, Southern General Hospital, Glasgow
(Chapter 1)

Derek Gillen Gastroenterology unit, Gartnavel General Hospital, Glasgow
(Chapter 3)

Charles Gourlay Cancer Research Centre, University of Edinburgh
(Chapter 15)

Claire Higgins Developmental Medicine, University of Glasgow
(Chapter 13)

Shazya Huda Developmental Medicine, University of Glasgow
(Chapter 24)

Nicholas Kennedy Consultant in Infectious Disease, NHS Lanarkshire
(Chapter 10)

Hing Leung Cancer Sciences, University of Glasgow
(Chapter 14)

Alisdair Macconnachie Brownlee Centre, Gartnavel General Hospital, Glasgow
(Chapter 11)

Frances Macdonald Scottish Medicines Consortium, Glasgow
(Chapter 2)

Scott Nelson Developmental Medicine, University of Glasgow
(Chapters 13 and 24)

Edward Newman Clinical Neurosciences, University of Glasgow
(Chapter 7)

Manish Patel Respiratory Unit, Wishaw General Hospital, Glasgow
(Chapter 6)

Kenneth Paterson Scottish Medicines Consortium, Glasgow
(Chapter 25)

Prabhakar Rajan Cancer Sciences, University of Glasgow
  (Chapter 14)

Andrew Seaton Brownlee Centre, Gartnavel General Hospital, Glasgow
  (Chapter 9)

Katy Teo Cancer Sciences, University of Glasgow
  (Chapter 14)

Stephen Waring York Hospital NHS Trust, York
  (Chapter 26)

Preface

Clinical pharmacology is the science of medicine discovery, development, regulation and utilisation in the context of the effects of drugs on humans. As such, some knowledge of clinical pharmacology is essential for all professionals involved in the treatment of patients with medicines. We live in an era of intensive research which drives new discoveries and maintains the field of therapeutics in a state of constant evolution: keeping this knowledge up to date can be a challenge. The discovery of new medicines increases the complexity of drug treatment regimens, and the ability to use drugs in a safe, appropriate and effective fashion needs to be taught and maintained.

The pace of change and the growing recognition of the challenges of safe prescribing are reflected in the eighth edition of *Lecture Notes: Clinical Pharmacology and Therapeutics*. This edition sees very significant changes to the content and structure of the text. Each chapter has been revised, updated and in some cases re-written, with particular focus upon the clinical relevance of the subject matter. New clinical chapters covering the treatment of Human Immunodeficiency Virus and the management of urological disease have been added, together with an overview of medicines regulation. In each chapter we have moved away from more abstract concepts and placed greater emphasis upon the practical aspects of clinical pharmacology and the *application* of the knowledge this book contains. We have also restructured the sections to strengthen the links between the basic principles of clinical pharmacology and their use in a clinical context. Although many aspects of the book have changed, our overall goal remains as stated in the preface to the first edition: 'to describe with brevity and clarity the scientific background of rational prescribing while giving an insight into practical aspects of therapeutics'.

In the pursuit of this goal we have sought to equip the reader with skills essential for the modern healthcare professional. We hope to encourage a thoughtful and holistic approach to drug prescribing, incorporating consideration and clear understanding of the principles of the pathophysiology of disease, the molecular mechanisms of drug action in humans and an appreciation of drug therapy in the context of overall health care. We have taken steps in this edition further to instill a sense of familiarity with the emerging concepts of pharmacogenetics and personalised medicine.

In the nearly 30 years since the first edition of *Lecture Notes in Clinical Pharmacology*, there has been only one change to the editorial team. The eighth edition sees a second change: Peter Rubin has stepped down from his role as an author and editor. Peter has been replaced by Gerard McKay, a consultant in Clinical Pharmacology at the Glasgow Royal Infirmary.

We are grateful to Peter for his immeasurable contributions since the first edition, and to the expert colleagues who have reviewed and extensively revised the text of the eighth edition. In our view this new volume maintains the tradition of the lecture notes series, providing a clearly written and up-to-date review of a dynamic and evolving field. For those who use it, we hope this book will provide a clear understanding not only of how but also when to use drugs.

Gerard A. McKay
John L. Reid
Matthew R. Walters

Acknowledgements

We acknowledge the help and assistance freely given by many colleagues, commenting, reviewing and updating chapters related to their specialist interest and expertise. We particularly acknowledge the input and contribution of Jonathan Cavanagh, Derek Connolly, Gordon Lowe, David McCarey, Brian McCreath, Robert Lindsay, John McMurray, Brian Murphy, Roger Sturrock and Simon Thomas.

We are grateful to Laura McMichael for her role in collecting, collating and coordinating the text and revisions.

Part 1

Principles of Clinical Pharmacology

Chapter 1

Pharmacodynamics and pharmacokinetics

Clinical scenario

A 50-year-old obese man with type-2 diabetes, hypertension and hyperlipidaemia has made arrangements to see his general practitioner to review his medications. He is on three different drugs for his diabetes, four different antihypertensives, a statin for his cholesterol and a dispersible aspirin. These medications have been added over a period of 2 years despite him not having any symptoms and he feels that if anything they are giving him symptoms of fatigue and muscle ache. He has also read recently that aspirin may actually be bad for patients with diabetes. He is keen to know why he is on so many medications, if the way he is feeling is due to the medications and whether they are interfering with the action of each other. What knowledge might help the general practitioner deal with this?

Key points – what is pharmacodynamics and pharmacokinetics?

The variability in the relationship between dose and response is a measure of the sensitivity of a patient to a drug.

This has two components: dose – concentration and concentration – effect.

The latter is termed **pharmacodynamics**. The description of a drug concentration profile against time is termed **pharmacokinetics**.

Lecture Notes: Clinical Pharmacology and Therapeutics, 8th edition. By Gerard McKay, John Reid and Matthew Walters. Published 2010 by Blackwell Publishing Ltd.

In simple terms pharmacodynamics is what the drug does to the individual taking it and pharmacokinetics is what the individual does to the drug.

Clinical pharmacology seeks to explore the factors that underlie variability in pharmacodynamics and pharmacokinetics for the optimisation of drug therapy in individual patients.

Introduction

A basic knowledge of the mechanism of action of drugs and how the body deals with drugs allows the clinician to prescribe them safely and effectively. Prior to the twentieth century, prescribing medication was based on intelligent observation and folklore with medical practices depending largely on the administration of mixtures of natural plant or animal substances. These preparations contained a number of pharmacologically active agents in variable amounts (e.g. powdered bark from the cinchona tree, now known to contain quinine, being used by natives of Peru to treat 'fevers' caused by malaria).

During the last 100 years an increased understanding has developed for biochemical and pathophysiological factors that influence disease. The chemical synthesis of agents with well-characterised and specific actions on cellular mechanisms has led to the introduction of many powerful and effective drugs. Additionally, advances in the detection of these compounds in body fluids have facilitated investigation into the relationships between the dosage regimen, the profile of drug concentration against time in body fluids, notably the plasma, and corresponding profiles of clinical effect. Knowledge of this concentration–effect relationship, and the factors that influence drug concentrations, underpin early stages of the drug development process.

More recently the development of genomics and proteomics has provided additional insights and opportunities for drug development with new and more specific targets. Such knowledge will replace the concept of one drug and/or one dose fitting all.

Principles of drug action (pharmacodynamics)

Pharmacological agents are used in therapeutics to:
1 Alleviate symptoms, for example:
  • paracetamol for pain
  • glyceryl trinitrate spray for angina
2 Improve prognosis – this can be measured in number of different ways – usually measured as a reduction in morbidity or mortality, for example:
  • prevent or delay end-stage consequences of disease, e.g. anti-hypertensive medication and statins in cardiovascular disease, levodopa in Parkinson's disease
  • replace deficiencies, e.g. levothyroxine in hypothyroid
  • cure disease, e.g. antibiotics, chemotherapy
Some drugs will both alleviate symptoms and improve prognosis, e.g. beta-blockers in ischaemic heart disease. If a prescribed drug is doing neither, one must question the need for its use and stop it. Even if there is a clear indication for use, the potential for side effects and interactions with any other drugs the patient is on also needs to be taken into account.

Mechanism of drug action

Action on a receptor

A receptor is a specific macromolecule, usually a protein, situated either in cell membranes or within the cell, to which a specific group of ligands, drugs or naturally occurring substances (such as neurotransmitters or hormones), can bind and produce pharmacological effects. There are three types of ligands: agonists, antagonists and partial agonists.

An **agonist** is a substance that stimulates or activates the receptor to produce an effect, e.g. salbutamol at the β_2-receptor.

An **antagonist** prevents the action of an agonist but does not have any effect itself, e.g. losartan at the angiotensin II receptor.

A **partial agonist** stimulates the receptor to a limited extent, while preventing any further stimulation by naturally occurring agonists, e.g. aripiprazole at the D2 and 5-HT1A receptors.

The biochemical events that result from an agonist–receptor interaction to produce an effect are complex. There are many types of receptors and in several cases subtypes have been identified which are also of therapeutic importance, e.g. α and β adrenoceptors, nicotinic and muscarinic cholinergic receptors.

Action on an enzyme

Enzymes, like receptors, are protein macromolecules with which substrates interact to produce activation or inhibition. Drugs in common clinical use, which exert their effect through enzyme action generally do so by inhibition, for example:
1 aspirin inhibits platelet cyclo-oxygenase
2 ramipril inhibits angiotensin-converting enzyme

Drug receptor antagonists and enzyme inhibitors can act as competitive, reversible antagonists or as non-competitive, irreversible antagonists. Effects of competitive antagonists can be overcome by increasing the dose of endogenous or exogenous agonists, while effects of irreversible antagonists cannot usually be overcome resulting in a longer duration of the effect.

Action on membrane ionic channels

The conduction of impulses in nerve tissues and electromechanical coupling in muscle depend on the movement of ions, particularly sodium, calcium and potassium, through membrane channels. Several groups of drugs interfere with these processes, for example:

1 nifedipine inhibits the transport of calcium through the slow channels of active cell membranes

2 furosemide inhibits Na/K/Cl co-transport in the ascending limb of the loop of Henle

Cytotoxic actions

Drugs used in cancer or in the treatment of infections may kill malignant cells or micro-organisms. Often the mechanisms have been defined in terms of effects on specific receptors or enzymes. In other cases chemical action (alkylation) damages DNA or other macromolecules and results in cell death or failure of cell division.

Dose–response relationship

Dose–response relationships may be steep or flat. A steep relationship implies that small changes in dose will produce large changes in clinical response or adverse effects, while flat relationships imply that increasing the dose will offer little clinical advantage (Fig. 1.1).

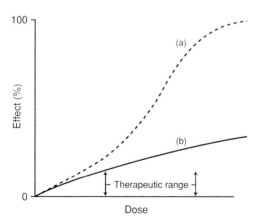

Figure 1.1 Schematic examples of a drug (a) with a steep dose– (or concentration–) response relationship in the therapeutic range, e.g. warfarin an oral anticoagulant; and (b) a flat dose– (or concentration–) response relationship within the therapeutic range, e.g. thiazide diuretics in hypertension.

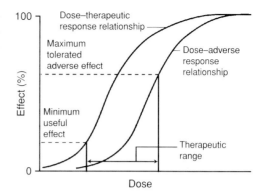

Figure 1.2 Schematic diagram of the dose–response relationship for the desired effect (dose–therapeutic response) and for an undesired adverse effect. The therapeutic index is the extent of displacement of the two curves within the normal dose range.

In clinical practice the maximum therapeutic effect may often be unobtainable because of the appearance of adverse or unwanted effects: few, if any, drugs cause a single pharmacological effect.

The concentration–adverse response relationship is often different in shape and position to that of the concentration–therapeutic response relationship. The difference between the concentration that produces the desired effect and the concentration that causes adverse effects is called the therapeutic index and is a measure of the selectivity of a drug (Fig. 1.2).

The shape and position of dose–response curves for a group of patients is variable because of genetic, environmental and disease factors. However, this variability is not solely an expression of differences in response to drugs. It has two important components: the dose–plasma concentration relationship and the plasma concentration–effect relationship.

$$\text{Dose} \rightarrow \text{Concentration} \rightarrow \text{Effect}$$

With the development of specific and sensitive chemical assays for drugs in body fluids, it has been possible to characterise dose–plasma concentration relationships so that this component of the variability in response can be taken into account when drugs are prescribed for patients with various disease states. For drugs with a narrow therapeutic index it may be necessary to measure plasma concentrations to assess the relationship between dose and concentration in individual patients (see Chapter 21, section 'Therapeutic drug monitoring').

Principles of pharmacokinetics

Absorption

Drug absorption after oral administration has two major components: absorption rate and bioavailability. Absorption rate is controlled partially by the physicochemical characteristics of the drug but in many cases it is modified by the formulation. A reduction in absorption rate can lead to a smoother concentration–time profile with a lower potential for concentration-dependent adverse effects and may allow less frequent dosing.

Bioavailability is the term used to describe the fraction of the dose that is absorbed into the systemic circulation. It can range from 0 to 100% and depends on a number of physicochemical and clinical factors. Low bioavailability may occur if the drug has low solubility or is destroyed by the acid in the stomach. Changing the formulation can affect the bioavailability of a drug and it can also be altered by food or the co-administration of other drugs. For example, antacids can reduce the absorption of quinolone antibiotics, such as ciprofloxacin, by binding them in the gut. Other factors influencing bioavailability include metabolism by gut flora, the intestinal wall or the liver.

First-pass metabolism refers to metabolism of a drug that occurs en route from the gut lumen to the systemic circulation. For the majority of drugs given orally, absorption occurs across the portion of gastrointestinal epithelium that is drained by veins forming part of the hepatoportal system. Consequently, even if they are well absorbed, drugs must pass through the liver before reaching the systemic circulation. For drugs that are susceptible to extensive hepatic metabolism, a substantial proportion of an orally administered dose can be metabolised before it ever reaches its site of pharmacological action, e.g. insulin metabolism in the gut lumen is so extensive that it renders oral therapy impossible.

The importance of first-pass metabolism is twofold:

1 It is one of the reasons for apparent differences in drug bioavailability between individuals. Even healthy people show considerable variation in liver metabolising capacity.
2 In patients with severe liver disease first-pass metabolism may be dramatically reduced, leading to the appearance of greater amounts of active drug in the systemic circulation.

Distribution

Once a drug has gained access to the bloodstream it begins to distribute to the tissues. The extent of this distribution depends on a number of factors including plasma protein binding, lipid solubility and regional blood flow. The volume of distribution, V_D, is the *apparent volume* of fluid into which a drug distributes on the basis of the *amount* of drug in the body and the *measured concentration* in the plasma or serum. If a drug was wholly confined to the plasma, V_D would equal the plasma volume – approximately 3 L in an adult. If, on the contrary, the drug was distributed throughout the body water, V_D would be approximately 42 L. In reality, drugs are rarely distributed into physiologically relevant volumes. If most of the drug is bound to tissues, the plasma concentration will be low and the apparent V_D will be high, while high plasma protein binding will tend to maintain high concentrations in the blood and a low V_D will result. For the majority of drugs, V_D depends on the balance between plasma binding and sequestration or binding by various body tissues, for example, muscle and fat. Volume of distribution can therefore vary considerably.

Clinical relevance of volume of distribution

Knowledge of volume of distribution (V_D) can be used to determine the size of a *loading dose* if an immediate response to treatment is required.

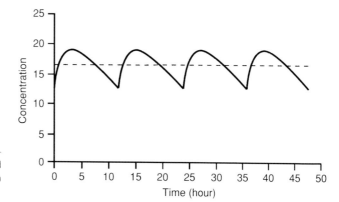

Figure 1.3 Steady-state concentration–time profile for an oral dose (—) and a constant rate intravenous infusion (- - - - -).

This assumes that therapeutic success is closely related to the plasma concentration and that there are no adverse effects if a relatively large dose is suddenly administered. It is sometimes employed when drug response would take many hours or days to develop if the regular maintenance dose was given from the outset, e.g. digoxin.

In practice, weight is the main determinant to calculating the dose of a drug where there is a narrow therapeutic index.

Plasma protein binding

In the blood, a proportion of a drug is bound to plasma proteins – mainly albumin (acidic drugs) and α_1-acid glycoprotein (basic drugs). Only the unbound, or free, fraction distributes because the protein-bound complex is too large to pass through membranes. It is the unbound portion that is generally responsible for clinical effects – both the target response and the unwanted adverse effects. Changes in protein binding (e.g. resulting from displacement interactions) generally lead to a transient increase in free concentration but are rarely clinically relevant. However, a lower total concentration will be present and the measurement might be misinterpreted if the higher free fraction is not taken into account. This is a common problem with the interpretation of phenytoin concentrations, where free fraction can range from 10% in a normal patient to 40% in a patient with hypoalbuminaemia and renal impairment.

Clearance

Clearance is the sum of all drug-eliminating processes, principally determined by hepatic metabolism and renal excretion. It can be defined as the theoretical volume of fluid from which a drug is completely removed in a given period of time.

When a drug is administered continuously by intravenous infusion or repetitively by mouth, a balance is eventually achieved between its input (dosing rate) and its output (the amount eliminated over a given period of time). This balance gives rise to a constant amount of drug in the body which depends on the dosing rate and clearance. This amount is reflected in the plasma or serum as a steady-state concentration (Css). A constant rate intravenous infusion will yield a constant Css, while a drug administered orally at regular intervals will result in fluctuation between peak and trough concentrations (Fig. 1.3).

Clearance depends critically on the efficiency with which the liver and/or kidneys can eliminate a drug; it will vary in disease states that affect these organs, or that affect the blood flow to these organs. In stable clinical conditions, clearance remains constant and is directly proportional to dose rate. The important implication is that if the dose rate is doubled, the $Css_{average}$ doubles: if dose rate is halved, the $Css_{average}$ is halved for most drugs. In pharmacokinetic terms this is referred to as a first-order or linear process, and results from the fact that the rate of elimination is proportional to the amount of drug present in the body.

Single intravenous bolus dose

A number of other important pharmacokinetic principles can be appreciated by considering the concentrations that result following a single intravenous bolus dose (see Fig. 1.4) and through a number of complex equations the time at which steady state will be achieved after starting a regular treatment schedule or after any change in dose can be predicted.

As a rule, in the absence of a loading dose, steady state is attained after four to five half-lives (Fig. 1.5).

Furthermore, when toxic drug levels have been inadvertently produced, it is very useful to estimate how long it will take for such levels to reach the therapeutic range, or how long it will take for the entire drug to be eliminated once the drug has been stopped. Usually, elimination is effectively complete after four to five half-lives (Fig. 1.6).

The elimination half-life can also be used to determine dosage intervals to achieve a target concentration–time profile. For example, in order to obtain a gentamicin peak of 8 mg/L and a trough

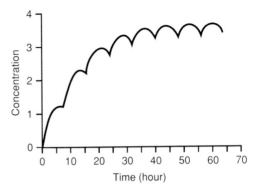

Figure 1.5 Plot of concentration versus time illustrating the accumulation to steady state when a drug is administered by regular oral doses.

of 0.5 mg/L in a patient with an elimination half-life of 3 hours, the dosage interval should be 12 hours. (The concentration will fall from 8–4 mg/L in 3 hours to 2 mg/L in 6 hours, to 1 mg/L in 9 hours and to 0.5 mg/L in 12 hours.) However, for many drugs, dosage regimens should be designed to maintain concentrations within a range

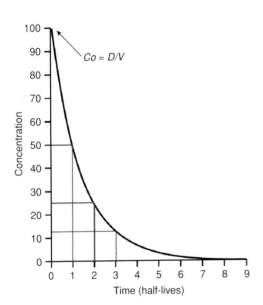

Figure 1.4 Plot of concentration versus time after a bolus intravenous injection. The intercept on the y- (concentration) axis, C_0, is the concentration resulting from the instantaneous injection of the bolus dose.

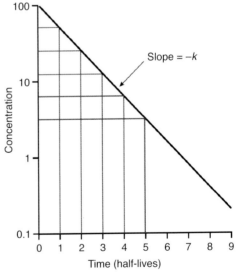

Figure 1.6 Semi-logarithmic plot of concentration versus time after a bolus intravenous injection. The slope of this line is $-k$; the elimination rate constant and the elimination half-life of the drug can be determined from such a plot by noting the time at which the concentration has fallen to half its original value.

that avoids high (potentially toxic) peaks or low, ineffective troughs. Excessive fluctuations in the concentration–time profile can be prevented by giving the drug at intervals of less than one half-life or by using a slow-release formulation.

Linear versus non-linear kinetics

In the discussion on clearance, it was pointed out that the hallmark of linear pharmacokinetics is the proportionality between dose rate and steady-state concentration. This arises because the rate of elimination is proportional to the amount of drug in the body, while the clearance remains constant. This is not, however, always the case for a few drugs such as phenytoin, alcohol and heparin. When the enzymes responsible for metabolism reach a point of saturation, the rate of elimination, in terms of amount of drug eliminated in a given period of time, does not increase in response to an increase in concentration (or an increase in the amount of drug in the body) but becomes constant. This gives rise to non-linear or zero-order kinetics.

The clinical relevance of non-linear kinetics is that a small increase in dose can lead to a large increase in concentration. This is particularly important when toxic side effects are closely related to concentration, as with phenytoin.

Principles of drug elimination

Drug metabolism

Drugs are eliminated from the body by two principal mechanisms: (i) liver metabolism and (ii) renal excretion. Drugs that are already water-soluble are generally excreted unchanged by the kidney. Lipid-soluble drugs are not easily excreted by the kidney because, following glomerular filtration, they are largely reabsorbed from the proximal tubule. The first step in the elimination of such lipid-soluble drugs is metabolism to more polar (water-soluble) compounds. This is achieved mainly in the liver, but can also occur in the gut and may contribute to first-pass elimination. Metabolism generally occurs in two phases:

Phase 1 – Mainly oxidation, but also reduction or hydrolysis to a more polar compound: **Oxidation** can occur in various ways at carbon, nitrogen or sulphur atoms and N- and O-dealkylation. These reactions are catalysed by the cytochrome P-450-dependent system of the endoplasmic reticulum. Knowledge of P-450, which exists as a superfamily of similar enzymes (isoforms), has increased greatly recently and is divided into a number of families and subfamilies. Although numerous P-450 isoforms are present in human tissue, only a few of these have a major role in the metabolism of drugs. These enzymes, which display distinct but overlapping substrate specificity, include CYP1A2, CYP2C9, CYP2C19, CYP2D6, CYP2E1 and CYP3A4. Induction or inhibition of one or more of these enzymes may form the basis of clinically relevant drug interactions. Phase 1 metabolites usually have only minor structural differences from the parent drug, but may exhibit totally different pharmacological actions. For example, the metabolism of azathioprine produces the powerful antimetabolite 6-mercaptopurine.

Phase 2 – conjugation usually by glucoronidation or sulphation to make the compound more polar: This involves the addition of small endogenous molecules to the parent drug, or to its phase 1 metabolite, and this change almost always leads to abolition of pharmacological activity. Multiple forms of conjugating enzymes are also known to exist, although these have not been investigated to the same extent as the P-450 system.

Metabolic drug interactions

The wide range of drugs metabolised by the P-450 system provides the opportunity for interactions of two types, namely enzyme induction and inhibition.

Clinical scenario

A 24-year-old woman goes to a family planning clinic for advice about contraception. The patient has a history of epilepsy which is stable on carbamazepine 200 mg twice daily. What options are available to the general practitioner?

Induction

Enzyme induction, which may be defined as the increase in amount and activity of drug-metabolising enzymes, is a consequence of new protein synthesis resulting from prolonged exposure to the inducing drug. While a drug may induce its own metabolism, it can also accelerate the metabolism and clearance of unrelated compounds. Many compounds are known to act as enzyme inducers in animals at toxicological dose levels, but relatively few drugs produce clinically significant induction in humans when used at therapeutic dose levels. For practical purposes anticonvulsants (carbamazepine, phenytoin) and rifampacin are the most potent enzyme inducers in clinical use and have produced numerous clinically significant drug interactions, related primarily to increases in the metabolism of CYP2C9, CYP2C19 and CYP3A4 substrates (including, for example, oestrogen and progesterone the constituents of a combined oral contraceptive pill). Enzyme induction is not, however, limited to administration of prescription drugs. St John's wort, a herbal remedy can also cause enzyme induction as can cigarette smoking (induction of CYP1A2 substrates, e.g. theophylline) and ethanol (induction of CYP2E1 but unlikely to be clinically relevant).

Key points – enzyme induction and inhibition

Enzyme induction produces clinical changes over days or weeks, but the effects of enzyme inhibition are usually observed immediately. In most circumstances, these changes are manifest as:
- Therapeutic failure resulting from induction
- Adverse effects resulting from inhibition

Clinical relevance occurs when drug therapy needs to be altered to avoid the consequences of the drug interaction and this is most common and most serious in compounds that have a narrow therapeutic index.

Clinical scenario

A 58-year-old man with chronic obstructive pulmonary disease is admitted to hospital with an infective exacerbation. He is on three different inhalers and additionally takes simvastatin for hypercholesterolaemia. He is allergic to penicillin. The admitting doctor prescribes nebulised salbutamol, prednisolone and clarithromycin along with the patient's usual medications. The next day the patient complains of general aches and pains. Could this be due to a drug interaction?

Inhibition

Concurrently administered drugs can also lead to inhibition of enzyme activity, with many P-450 inhibitors showing considerable isoform selectivity. Some of the most clinically relevant inhibitors are listed in Table 1.1, together with the isoform inhibited. In some cases this can lead to potentially dangerous adverse events, e.g. ketoconazole decreases the metabolism of the CYP3A4 substrate, terfenadine, leading to QT interval prolongation and torsades de pointes.

As with induction, P-450 inhibition is not limited to drug administration. Grapefruit juice is an inhibitor of CYP3A4 activity and produces clinically significant interactions with a number of drugs, including midazolam, simvastatin and terfenadine. This type of information, together with some knowledge of the enzymes involved in a particular drug's clearance, makes it much easier to understand and predict drug interactions.

Clearly, pronounced enzyme inhibition, which may result in plasma concentrations of the inhibited drug being many times higher than

Table 1.1 P-450 inhibitors involved in drug interactions.

Major human P-450s	Typical inhibitors
CYP1A2	Furafylline, fluvoxamine, ciprofloxacin
CYP2C9	Fluconazole, ketoconazole, sulfaphenazole
CYP2C19	Omeprazole, ketoconazole, cimetidine
CYP2D6	Quinidine, fluoxetine, ritonavir
CYP2E1	Disulfiram
CYP3A4	Ketoconazole, itraconazole, ritonavir, clarithromycin, diltiazem

Table 1.2 Major enzymes displaying genetic polymorphism.

Enzyme	Typical substrates	Characteristics
CYP2C19	(S)-Mephenytoin, diazepam, omeprazole	About 2–5% of white people are poor metabolisers, but 18–23% of Japanese people have this phenotype
CYP2D6	Propafenone, flecainamide, desipramine	About 7% of white people are poor metabolisers, but this frequency is only about 2% in black Americans and <1% in Japanese/Chinese
N-acetyl-transferase	Hydralazine, sulphonamides, isoniazid, procainamide	About 50% of white people are slow acetylators

intended, can be a major safety issue. For example, co-administration of ketoconazole or ritonavir with the hypnotic drug midazolam increases the midazolam plasma exposure (AUC – area under the curve) by 15–20 times, a situation which should be avoided.

Genetic factors in metabolism

The rate at which healthy people metabolise drugs is variable. Although part of this variability is a consequence of environmental factors, including the influence of inducers and inhibitors, the main factor contributing to interindividual variability in metabolism is the underlying genetic basis of the drug-metabolising enzymes. Although there is probably a genetic component in the control of most P-450 enzymes, some enzymes (e.g. CYP2C19 and CYP2D6) actually show genetic polymorphism. This results in distinct subpopulations of poor and extensive metabolisers, where the poor metabolisers are deficient in that particular enzyme. There are a number of enzymes under polymorphic control and some clinically important examples are shown in Table 1.2. As with enzyme inhibition, genetic polymorphism is primarily a concern for drugs that have a narrow therapeutic index and that are metabolised largely by a single polymorphic enzyme. In such cases, the phenotype of the patient should be determined and lower doses of the drug used, or alternative therapy should be considered.

Renal excretion

Three processes are implicated in renal excretion of drugs:

1 *Glomerular filtration*: This is the most common route of renal elimination. The free drug is cleared by filtration and the protein-bound drug remains in the circulation where some of it dissociates to restore equilibrium.

2 *Active secretion in the proximal tubule*: Both weak acids and weak bases have specific secretory sites in proximal tubular cells. Penicillins are eliminated by this route, as is about 60% of procainamide.

3 *Passive reabsorption in the distal tubule*: This occurs only with un-ionised, i.e. lipid-soluble, drugs. Urine pH determines whether or not weak acids and bases are reabsorbed, which in turn determines the degree of ionisation.

If renal function is impaired, for example, by disease or old age, then the clearance of drugs that normally undergo renal excretion is decreased.

Chapter 2

Clinical trials and drug development

Clinical scenario

A chemist in a major pharmaceutical company has been doing some research into a compound that seems to have some benefit in neuronal protection in in vitro models. This discovery has caused some excitement – if it is shown to have efficacy in humans then it might be useful in patients with acute strokes. What are the various stages that this compound has to go through in development before it can be licensed as a drug to be used in patients?

Key points

- Many compounds are screened as potential drugs but few make it through to being used in patients
- Drug development is a lengthy process with high costs, particularly in the later stages
- Rigorous regulatory requirements have to be met before a drug can be tested in humans
- To get a license a drug has to be shown to be safe and efficacious

Introduction

Drug regulation in the UK and elsewhere came about as a result of the use of thalidomide in the late 1950s and early 1960s. Thalidomide was marketed as a sedative that had little hangover

effect, and was also used in treatment of morning sickness in pregnancy. In 1961 it became clear that thalidomide use in early pregnancy resulted in the congenital defect phocomelia where the long bones of the fetus fail to develop properly. This resulted in the formation of the Committee on Safety of Drugs and the passing of the Medicines Act in 1968, providing for a system of licensing affecting manufacture, sale, supply and importation of medicinal products into the UK. Drug regulation in the UK was initially under the control of the Medicines Control Agency. This was merged in 2003 with the Medical Devices Agency to form the Medicines and Healthcare products Regulatory Agency (MHRA). Other countries in Europe had similar systems to regulate drug development and as early as 1965 there was a European directive to try and harmonise the processes within Europe. This has now evolved and European legislation now takes precedence over the Medicines Act. The MHRA contributes to the work of the European Medicines Evaluation Authority (EMEA). At a European level, new drugs can now either be reviewed and licensed across all members states simultaneously, i.e. in partnership, or the drug can get a license from one member state first, and undergo a shortened 'mutual recognition' review and approval in the other member states.

Developing a new drug takes, in general, more than 10 years from patent filing, through the development process to marketing. There are many

Lecture Notes: Clinical Pharmacology and Therapeutics, 8th edition. By Gerard McKay, John Reid and Matthew Walters. Published 2010 by Blackwell Publishing Ltd.

stages that a drug has to go through to be approved for use. Many drugs will enter development but few will reach the end of the process and gain regulatory approval. Even then approximately only one in seven new products will become a commercial success, recouping the investment in its development. Once a drug is licensed for use there are means by which the safety in the longer term can be monitored. With the increasing complexity of diseases, society and drug development the pharmaceutical companies are moving towards alternative research strategies, such as translational research, to try and improve the speed by which drugs make it from 'bench to bedside'.

Drug development and regulation

Combinatorial chemistry, involving the rapid synthesis and computer simulation of a large number of different but structurally related molecules, has allowed pharmaceutical research companies to routinely produce and screen tens of thousands of compounds each year. This library of compounds can be tested for specific activities, using high-throughput screening techniques providing the starting point for taking promising compounds forward to the more traditional preclinical and animal studies. This approach has been embraced by pharmaceutical research companies as a means of increasing the productivity of drug development. In general, this has meant a move away from a serendipitous approach to drug discovery to a more focused one.

Preclinical studies

Preclinical studies include in vitro studies and animal studies that are designed to find out if a drug is likely to be useful before any testing in humans is done.

In vitro studies

Drugs can now be assessed relatively extensively by in vitro work using cell cultures, bacteria, enzymes, isolated tissues and perfused organ systems. Additionally certain aspects of drug development

that traditionally have been tested in healthy volunteers, such as drug interactions in the liver, can now be largely tested using cell cultures, so even when a drug moves into clinical testing in vitro work still has an ongoing role.

Animal studies of efficacy and toxicity

New chemical entities are tested in animals to look for desirable pharmacological effects and to assess toxic effects. Acute and in most cases chronic toxicity studies will be carried out in animals using increasing doses, until clear toxic effects are noted, including a proportion of the animals dying. These studies provide 'pointers' to focus the safety assessments in human studies. In Europe the guidelines require that the toxic effects of the drug should be assessed in two mammalian species (one non-rodent) over 2 weeks of dosing before a single dose is administered to a human (see later). In addition, mutagenicity, carcinogenicity and the impact of drugs on reproduction will be assessed and pharmacokinetic studies in animals can be used to help predict the doses needed when the drug is first used in humans.

Clinical trials

Clinical trials have to be performed under highly regulated processes in order to minimise the risk to participants. This principle of protecting the rights of the trial subjects comes from the Declaration of Helsinki (initially agreed by the World Medical Association in 1964, with six revisions since, the last being in October 2008). The International Conference on Harmonization (ICH) is a project that brings together the regulatory authorities of the three main regions, Europe, Japan and the United States, with the aim of producing common guidelines relating to quality, e.g. manufacturing, safety and efficacy requirements. Their Good Clinical Practice Guidelines were established to provide a unified standard for the three major regions undertaking clinical trials as a means of ensuring more economical use of human, animal and material resources, and the elimination of unnecessary delay in the global development and availability of new medicines. This also ensures maintaining safeguards on quality, safety and efficacy, and regulatory obligations to protect public health. It should be noted however that ICH has not produced global harmonisation in all matters. The three main regions still have some differences in their requirements for drug development, which manufacturers must take into account in their planning.

Phase I clinical trials

These usually involve healthy volunteers. They are designed to find out how the drug affects the human body and vice versa. This will be a combination of assessing the pharmacodynamics of the drug, including detailed safety screens and the pharmacokinetics. The results of Phase I clinical studies will determine whether there is potential for the drug to move towards the next stage of development. At this stage the drug has to be shown to be relatively safe and, where feasible, for a reasonable signal of efficacy to have been established. This is easier in some disease areas (e.g. hypertension) than others (e.g. oncology). Usually less than 100 individuals are involved.

Specific types of Phase I clinical studies

1 *First-in-man studies*: A medicine may work well in the laboratory, but a clinical trial will find out if it works well in people and is safe to use. Phase I studies can only start to answer these questions, but their main benefit is the highly controlled environment, and relatively clean baseline. Studies will start with low, single doses, in just a couple of volunteers. The serious side effects experienced by volunteers taking part in the trial of TGN1412 in March 2006 at Northwick Park Hospital in London are extremely rare but highlights the need for thoroughly testing a treatment before widespread use. First-in-man studies may also provide evidence for proof of concept, for example a demonstration of inhibition of relevant enzyme systems.

2 *Dose ranging studies*: Healthy volunteer Phase I clinical studies can be used to start the process of predicting the optimal dose of a medication

before it gets tested in large clinical trials. The doses will start low and single dose, and then be escalated and move to multiple dosing with bloods taken for plasma concentrations of drug, and dose–concentration curves plotted. Pharmacodynamic responses to the drug, both desired and side effects will be noted with the aim of selecting a dose range that will give you the desired effect but with few side effects. This range will then be taken into Phase II trials. Selecting the dose is a critical part of the drug development process. Too low a dose taken into large clinical trials may mean that a good drug will fail. Too high a dose and the same good drug may fail because of unwanted side effects. In most disease areas it is difficult to select the optimal dose based on the response in healthy individuals, and Phase II studies are more valuable for this aim.

3 *Interaction studies*: There is a lot of potential for drugs to interact with other drugs or dietary factors. A lot of the potential for interaction occurs through the effect of drugs on enzymes in the liver, both induction and inhibition. A lot of these interactions can now be predicted from in vitro studies but if such studies suggest a clinically relevant interaction may exist, many regulatory authorities will require that the effect be quantified more accurately via a clinical interaction study. An example of this is when there are concerns that a drug may cause an interaction mediated through an effect on cytochrome P450 3A4. Midazolam is almost exclusively metabolised by this enzyme. If a drug in development is thought to interact through an effect on cytochrome P450 3A4 then dosing the drug with and without midazolam will allow you to quantify the effect. If the drug is an enzyme inducer then the amount of midazolam measured in the plasma will be less and if an enzyme inhibitor the amount of midazolam measured in the plasma will be greater.

4 *Safety studies*: Phase I studies can be used to look at specific safety issues in drug development. For example, based on pharmacology or toxicology results a drug may be thought to have potential to cause prolongation of the QT interval on the ECG which may predispose to cardiac arrhythmias. A simple Phase I study using an escalating dose of

drug with ECG recording can show whether there is any relationship between concentration of drug in the plasma and electrocardiographic QT interval. Such studies in healthy individuals can however only be seen as an initial screen, and cannot provide the definitive answer. Patients, who are often older and have additional co-morbidities, are likely to be more predisposed to safety issues therefore the large Phase III and IV studies are required for fully assessing safety profiles.

Phase II clinical trials

These crucial studies, often called 'proof of concept' look at whether a drug works in the patient population that might benefit from the treatment. They are usually conducted by specialists in the field, in a relatively controlled environment, and are designed to assess efficacy or markers of efficacy and the dose–response relationship, taking the dose range suggested from Phase I. A key goal is to decide whether the odds are acceptably good that the compound is effective, may have an acceptable benefit/risk ratio and, if so, to define a single dose to be taken into the Phase III trials. However some disease areas have very limited markers of efficacy which can be measured in a short, small trial, therefore in these cases dose selection is significantly more difficult and sometimes more than one dose will be taken into Phase III. In addition to looking at markers of efficacy this stage of development allows the identification of side effects in the target patient population. Phase II would normally involve designing a double blind randomised control trial against placebo and possibly also a study against a standard reference drug therapy as control. If the exploratory type II studies suggest good efficacy and acceptable safety, tolerability and pharmacokinetic profiles then the larger Phase III clinical trials can be planned. This decision has potentially huge cost implications as the costs rise exponentially once you start Phase III clinical trials. In general, pharmaceutical companies aim to balance the 'development risk' profile of their development portfolio, i.e. to have a mix of higher and lower risk products. High-risk products have a greater chance of failing before they reach patients, while the lower risk development programmes may bring less benefit to patients and face more competition.

Phase III clinical trials

These are the expensive trials, often involving many thousands of patients, more definitively quantifying the extent to which the drug is effective and in what patient groups. Given the increase in numbers of patients exposed less common side effects may be seen and the benefit/risk ratio can be more clearly estimated. These are the key regulatory studies, and as such inform the labelling and patient information for the drug when it is marketed. At the same time as these trials are underway the pharmaceutical company will be investing considerable efforts into scaling up the manufacturing process, and completing the stability studies on the dose form and packaging which will be taken to market. While various formulations can be tested in Phase II, Phase III studies must be conducted using the final formulation. A key challenge with biotechnology products, which are not manufactured using conventional chemistry, is to develop manufacturing processes and robust assay methods which can guarantee consistent levels of biological activity between batches.

During Phase III the regulatory affairs department within companies will be pulling together the large amount of manufacturing, preclinical and clinical data necessary for making a formal application to the relevant regional and national regulatory authorities for a product license. Each major regulator requires the data structured in a different way; therefore, first priority will usually be given to submissions to the Food and Drug Administration (FDA) and the EMEA. Review times by these regulators vary based on circumstances, but it usually takes approximately 1 year.

Based on the data submitted, each regulatory authority will produce a factual summary of the preclinical and clinical results, including the key safety information and dosing instructions. This document will also state whether the marketing approval is general or restricted, e.g. hospital use only. The relevant document issued by the EMEA is called the summary of product characteristics (SPC) and provides the key information required to aid a decision by the prescriber as to whether the drug is indicated. A second valuable document is the European Public Assessment report (EPAR), found on the EMEA website, which provides a more detailed summary of the Agency's review of the data submitted. Over time, the SPC will be updated by the company as key new information becomes available, but clinical publications and treatment guidelines are also invaluable in providing additional detail which will not be found in the SPC.

In the UK each new drug in the British National Formulary has an inverted triangle symbol next to it reminding doctors that it is a new product and that any suspected adverse effects should be reported to the Committee for Safety of Medicines via the yellow card scheme.

Clinical scenario

The new drug compound for neuroprotection has now been tested in Phase III clinical trials and has shown good efficacy with an acceptable benefit: risk ratio. It gets approved by the regulatory authorities and the company wants to start marketing the drug. Is there a limit to what the company can do in its marketing strategy? How is its safety monitored? What happens if concerns about side effects become apparent?

Phase IIIb and IV studies

New drugs can only be marketed on the basis of its licensed indications. Even when a new drug gets a license it does not necessarily mean that there is widespread use. In many countries, including the UK, drugs have to undergo a health economic evaluation before being available for use in patients (see Chapter 25). Companies will also have ongoing clinical studies to support their product. Phase IIIb studies, are aimed to widen the license, e.g. to populations not initially approved (e.g. children or elderly). Additionally as well as a means of looking at longer term safety of drugs some Phase IV studies are undertaken by companies to investigate

efficacy against comparators, as if better efficacy is shown for their product this might improve their market share.

Pharmacovigilance

The regulatory authorities including the EMEA have greatly increased the obligation on pharmaceutical companies to set up risk-management plans. While these were initially limited to exceptional cases where a drug was thought to have a greater risk they are becoming more common and expensive, e.g. for most of the new oncology drugs. They often require specific databases to be set up, e.g. web-based, and are run for years, with regular reports back to EMEA.

Phase IV pharmacovigilance studies are performed after marketing approval and the granting of a product license. They are usually observational studies utilising data collected on specific drugs. Sometimes these are studies run by the companies themselves who set up a database or utilise information collected elsewhere. Examples of the types of repositories used for such studies include the GP database in the UK which was used to confirm a link between the oral contraceptive and the risk of deep vein thrombosis. Other examples include registries for drugs used in certain conditions, e.g. anti-convulsant use in pregnancy. It was through this that the evidence emerged that sodium valproate was the most likely of the anti-convulsants to cause neural tube defects, in addition to causing long term neurodevelopmental side effects on the offspring of mothers taking this drug.

Sometimes observational studies or meta-analysis of randomised control trials will raise concern about a particular medication, e.g. increased cardiovascular risk with the oral hypoglycaemic agent rosiglitazone. The options in situations like this are for the company to withdraw the drug or the regulatory authorities to suspend the license until the concern is investigated further. In the UK if a drug is thought to cause concerns it is marked with a black triangle in the British National Formulary (BNF) with prescribers encouraged to report any problems through the yellow card scheme.

Yellow card scheme

In the UK all new drugs are labelled in the BNF asking prescribers to report any side effects that may be attributable to the drug. This is done by completing a yellow card which can also now be done online. The MHRA monitor all drugs through this scheme. Information is assessed by a team of medicine safety experts who study the benefits and risks of medicines. If a new side effect is identified, information is carefully considered in the context of the overall side effect profile for the medicine, and how the side effect profile compares with other medicines used to treat the same condition. The MHRA is advised by the Commission on Human Medicines (CHM), which is the Government's independent scientific advisory body on medicines safety. The CHM is made up of experts from a range of health professionals and includes lay representatives. Where necessary action is taken based on the balance of benefit and risk.

Translational research

Traditionally research is divided into basic research and applied research. Often there was delay in getting the basic research into meaningful treatments for patients. Translational research is a way of thinking about and conducting scientific research to make the results of research applicable to the population under study and in medicine is used to translate the findings in basic research more quickly and efficiently into medical practice. Translational research has been invested in by pharmaceutical companies as a means of aiding the drug development process and by governments trying to provide health care to the populations they serve.

Patient populations that require treatment are increasingly complex. The process that explores needs, develops treatments in basic laboratory research, and tests safety and efficacy in clinical trials can be thought of as translational research – the so-called 'bench to bedside' approach to research. There needs to be a means of ensuring that the findings from clinical trials are applicable in the population that is being treated requiring a move away from considering research evidence quality in a hierarchical way and a need to consider other evidence apart from randomised clinical trials in judging whether or not specific treatments work in real life. If research processes can be incorporated within this to evaluate the complex interacting factors such as environment, costs, healthcare policy, etc., this may allow, at government level, the provision of enduring evidence-based healthcare policies. All of this requires a collaborative multi-disciplinary approach.

Part 2

Aspects of Therapeutics

Chapter 3

Drugs and gastrointestinal disease

Introduction

Symptoms relating to the gastrointestinal tract are extremely common, accounting for about one in ten presentations to primary care. This chapter will review treatment of the more frequently encountered gastrointestinal conditions.

Clinical scenario

An obese 55-year-old man presents to his general practitioner (GP) with a history of retrosternal burning discomfort which tends to occur at night and occasionally wakes him from sleep. The GP makes a preliminary diagnosis of reflux disease. What treatment strategies are available?

Gastro-oesophageal reflux disease

Aims

1 To relieve symptoms
2 To heal oesophagitis
3 To prevent complications

Relevant pathophysiology

Gastro-oesophageal reflux disease (GORD) is an increasing problem in western countries, with around 20% of people in the UK experiencing symptoms at least once per week. This increase is likely to be multi-factorial, although increasing obesity is likely to be one important factor.

Most patients with GORD secrete a normal amount of gastric acid. However, they often have a functionally incompetent lower oesophageal sphincter that relaxes inappropriately at times other than during swallowing. This allows an excessive reflux of gastric contents, containing acid and pepsin, into the oesophagus. This tendency to reflux is further exacerbated if a hiatus hernia is present, since this further diminishes the barrier to reflux. Furthermore, once refluxed into the oesophagus, this acidic material often remains in contact with the mucosa for prolonged periods as a result of impaired physiological clearance mechanisms.

Drugs used in the treatment of GORD:
1 Antacids and antacid/alginate combinations
2 Drugs that inhibit gastric acid secretion:
   - H_2-receptor antagonists
   - Proton pump inhibitors: omeprazole, lansoprazole, esomeprazole, pantoprazole, rabeprazole
3 Drugs that act on oesophageal and/or gastric motility:
   - Metoclopramide, domperidone

Lecture Notes: Clinical Pharmacology and Therapeutics, 8th edition. By Gerard McKay, John Reid and Matthew Walters. Published 2010 by Blackwell Publishing Ltd.

Antacids and antacid/alginate preparations

Antacids

Mechanism

These drugs are weak alkalis, so they partly neutralise free acid in the stomach. They may also stimulate mucosal repair mechanisms around ulcers, possibly by stimulating local prostaglandin release.

Pharmacokinetics

Most antacids (principally salts of magnesium or aluminium) are not absorbed from the gut to any appreciable extent. Some, such as sodium bicarbonate, are absorbed.

Adverse effects

Antacids that contain aluminium tend to cause constipation. Those containing magnesium have the opposite effect. Sodium bicarbonate in large quantities may alter acid–base status causing metabolic alkalosis and may promote the formation of phosphate-containing renal calculi. Absorbable antacids should not be administered in the long term. Antacids with a high sodium content should be avoided in patients with impaired cardiac function or chronic liver disease.

Drug interactions

Antacids may reduce the absorption of a wide range of drugs from the gut. These include digoxin, phenothiazines and tetracyclines.

Clinical use and dosage

Antacids are mainly used for symptomatic relief in patients with GORD, peptic ulcer or non-ulcer dyspepsia.

Suitable antacids are:

Aluminium hydroxide 5–15 mL 6-hourly

Magnesium trisilicate 10–20 mL or 1–2 tablets as required.

When antacids are combined with an alginate, the latter is thought to provide an additional protective coating to the lower oesophagus, reducing mucosal contact with refluxed gastric contents.

Drugs that inhibit gastric acid secretion

Histamine H_2-receptor antagonists

These are discussed below, since they have generally been less successful in the management of GORD than in peptic ulcer. To be effective in the treatment of GORD, they may have to be given in much higher doses than in peptic ulcer (e.g. ranitidine, 300 mg 6-hourly).

Proton pump inhibitors: omeprazole, lansoprazole, pantoprazole, rabeprazole and esomeprazole

Mechanism

These drugs are irreversible inhibitors of the proton pump on the parietal cell surface. The proton pump is an enzyme (H^+/K^+-ATPase) that actively secretes hydrogen ions into the gastric lumen. It is the final common pathway in the process of acid secretion. Blocking this enzyme therefore causes a marked suppression of gastric acid secretion to any stimulus, including food.

Pharmacokinetics

These drugs are administered as delayed-release preparations. The bioavailability of omeprazole after the first dose is limited, but increases with repeated once-daily dosing to reach a plateau by around the fifth day. They have short elimination half-lives (1–2 hours) due to conversion in the liver to inactive metabolites. However, they have a prolonged pharmacological effect due to their irreversible binding to active proton pumps. As they only bind to active proton pumps, they are most effective when taken around meal times.

Adverse effects

These are generally mild and infrequent. In particular, diarrhoea, skin rash and headache have all been reported. However, an increased relative risk for both gastrointestinal and chest infections has been recognised in patients taking these drugs.

Drug interactions

Omeprazole reduces the clearance and prolongs the elimination of diazepam, phenytoin and the

R enantiomer of warfarin through inhibition of their hepatic metabolism. There is also evidence to suggest that some proton pump inhibitors (PPIs) may reduce the antiplatelet action of clopidogrel. This is of particular concern in patient with recent coronary artery stenting.

Clinical use and dosage

Although most effective in the treatment of severe, erosive oesophagitis, they have become most frequently used in the empirical therapy of symptomatic reflux disease. They are superior to H_2-receptor antagonists in controlling the symptoms of the condition and in healing oesophagitis since they are more powerful inhibitors of acid secretion.

They are also used: (a) in the short-term management of duodenal ulcers (DUs) and gastric ulcers (GUs); (b) in the treatment and prophylaxis of NSAID-induced ulcers; (c) in combination with antibiotics in the eradication of *Helicobacter pylori*; and (d) in the treatment of Zollinger–Ellison syndrome. Intravenous preparations are also used in combination with endoscopic treatment for the treatment of bleeding peptic ulcers.

Comment. Based on the pathophysiology of the condition, it should be apparent that relapse will be rapid in most patients once treatment is withdrawn. Many patients, particularly those with severe grades of the condition, will require long-term treatment with a PPI. Patients with mild GORD may obtain sufficient symptom relief from an antacid or H_2-receptor antagonist taken as required.

Drugs that act on oesophageal and/or gastric motility

Metoclopramide, domperidone

These drugs are discussed in greater detail later in this chapter. They may have some efficacy in patients with mild grades of GORD because of their actions on the motility of the upper gut: they have a weak tonic effect on the lower oesophageal sphincter; they may also improve oesophageal clearance and gastric emptying. However, they are seldom effective alone. Metoclopramide is not recommended for long-term use because of its adverse effects on the central nervous system (CNS) (see below).

Peptic ulcer

Clinical scenario

A 60-year-old man presented to his GP with upper abdominal pain which was troublesome at night and in the afternoon. The pain was felt over the epigastrium but did not radiate. The pain was worse when hungry but there were no other exacerbating factors. On examination there was some tenderness over the epigastrium. An endoscopy was arranged which revealed a small duodenal ulcer. A biopsy taken at endoscopy revealed the presence of H. pylori. What treatment should be offered?

Aims

1 To relieve pain
2 To heal the ulcer
3 To prevent ulcer recurrence

Relevant pathophysiology

It is traditional to regard peptic ulceration as the result of an imbalance between aggressive and protective factors in the upper gastrointestinal tract. The principal aggressive forces are gastric acid and pepsin. The two most important factors disrupting the balance between acid/peptic attack and mucosal resistance are *H. pylori* infection and non-steroidal anti-inflammatory drugs (NSAIDs). *H. pylori* stimulates increased gastrin release and thereby increased acid secretion in genetically susceptible individuals. In addition, it causes direct damage to the mucosa, thus further disrupting the physiological balance. NSAIDs impair mucosal resistance but do not alter acid secretion.

Almost all patients with DUs, and most patients with GUs have *H. pylori* infection. It is now clear that eradication of *H. pylori* infection is associated with prolonged remission from peptic ulceration and indeed usually with permanent cure. Recognition of the role of *H. pylori* infection in peptic ulcer and the development of effective eradication treatments for it have had enormous impact on our approach to the patient with peptic ulceration.

Drugs used in the treatment of peptic ulcer

1 Antacids
2 Drugs that inhibit gastric acid secretion:
- H$_2$-receptor antagonists
- PPIs
- Synthetic prostaglandin analogues
3 Drugs that do not directly inhibit gastric acid secretion:
- Chelated salts of bismuth
- Sucralfate
4 Drug combinations to eradicate *H. pylori*.

H$_2$-receptor antagonists

There are four such agents available (cimetidine, ranitidine, nizatidine and famotidine). They are all competitive antagonists for histamine at the H$_2$-receptor found on parietal cells.

Mechanism
By competing with histamine at the H$_2$-receptor, these drugs reduce acid secretion by the parietal cells, especially at night and in the fasting state. They are less effective in reducing food-stimulated acid secretion.

Pharmacokinetics
They are well absorbed following oral administration. They have relatively short half-lives and are excreted largely unchanged by the kidneys.

Adverse effects
These are rare and are usually of a minor nature. Cimetidine is weakly anti-androgenic in humans. It may therefore cause impotence or gynaecomastia. Either cimetidine or ranitidine may cause reversible mental confusion, particularly in frail, elderly patients. Some potentially serious cardiac dysrhythmias have occurred following intravenous injections of H$_2$-receptor antagonists.

Drug interactions
Cimetidine inhibits oxidative drug metabolism by the liver. It interacts with many drugs but only three are of clinical importance. These are phenytoin, theophylline and warfarin. These three drugs are metabolised in the liver and have narrow therapeutic indices; cimetidine will slow their metabolism and may induce toxicity.

No clinically relevant drug interactions have been reported with the other H$_2$-receptor antagonists.

Clinical use and dosage
H$_2$-receptor antagonists can heal DUs and benign GUs. Patients with GUs should have endoscopy and biopsy to exclude gastric carcinoma. Healing of GUs should also be documented endoscopically. The H$_2$-receptor antagonists can be effective in some patients with GORD, especially in milder grades of severity. For patients with erosive or ulcerative oesophagitis complicating GORD, the H$_2$-receptor antagonists are unlikely to be effective unless higher doses are given (see above).

H$_2$-receptor antagonist doses

Recommended doses for DU and GU are:

Ranitidine 150 mg twice daily or 300 mg in the evening

Cimetidine 400 mg twice daily or 800 mg in the evening

Nizatidine 300 mg in the evening

Famotidine 40 mg in the evening

Seventy-five to eighty per cent of DUs will heal within 4 weeks, increasing to around 90% by 8 weeks. GUs tend to be slower to heal, but over 80% should have healed by 8 weeks. If single evening doses are used, it is important that patients are advised to have nothing further by mouth after the dose. Eating food will stimulate gastric acid secretion through gastrin release and vagal activity and can reduce the pharmacological effect of the H$_2$-receptor antagonist.

Higher doses are recommended for GORD. Single evening dosage regimens are not appropriate. In GORD, H_2-receptor antagonists should be given at least twice daily. For ranitidine, a dose of up to 300 mg four times daily may be required.

H_2-receptor antagonists are of no proven value in the management of patients with upper gastrointestinal haemorrhage, whether from peptic ulceration or other sources. They may be used prophylactically in some critically ill patients in an effort to prevent stress-related gastric mucosal bleeding. However, this should not be a major problem in countries where high standards of intensive care are available, particularly where early nasogastric feeding is employed.

Comment. Although H_2-receptor antagonists can heal peptic ulcers, relapse is common after stopping treatment. These drugs can be continued as long-term maintenance treatment, typically in half of their initial dose. However, the role of such treatment has become markedly reduced since the importance of eradication of *H. pylori* has been appreciated (see below).

Although often tried, H_2-receptor antagonists are of no proven value in non-ulcer dyspepsia. Some of the H_2-receptor antagonists are now available in low doses 'over the counter'. They are likely to be used in this way by patients with mild dyspepsia or GORD for symptomatic relief.

Proton pump inhibitors

For DU, omeprazole 20 mg daily or lansoprazole 30 mg daily will heal around 90% of ulcers within 4 weeks. In patients with GU, the same doses are used, but treatment for 8 weeks is recommended.

Similar doses of PPI have been shown to have a protective effect against ulcer development in patients taking long-term NSAIDs ('gastroprotection'). Their use in this role is particularly important in patients with an increased risk of NSAID-related ulcer, such as older patients or those with a past history of peptic ulcer.

Synthetic prostaglandins: misoprostol

Mechanism

Prostaglandins are weak inhibitors of gastric acid secretion when given in pharmacological doses. Their mechanism of action is not fully understood. In addition, prostaglandins have a series of properties loosely referred to as 'cytoprotection'. This means that they have been shown in animal studies to prevent or limit experimental damage to the gastric or duodenal mucosa from a variety of noxious stimuli. It is unclear whether or not this is an important property regarding their clinical use. Cytoprotection can be demonstrated at doses below those required for inhibition of gastric acid secretion.

Pharmacokinetics

Misoprostol has a short plasma half-life. It may act on the stomach both locally and systemically.

Adverse effects

There is diarrhoea in up to 40% of patients, but this is usually mild and self-limiting. Misoprostol and other prostaglandins are potentially abortifacient and so should not be given to women of childbearing age.

Clinical use and dose

The main indication is to prevent gastric mucosal damage and GUs in patients who are taking NSAIDs. The dose is 200 µg twice to four times daily.

Comment. Misoprostol can be considered as an alternative to PPIs for those patients who genuinely require to take NSAIDs and who have a past history of peptic ulcer or upper gastrointestinal bleeding.

For patients already on NSAIDs who are found to have a peptic ulcer, the NSAID should be stopped if possible. However, even if the NSAID has to be continued (in a patient with rheumatoid arthritis, for example) the ulcer can be healed with any type of anti-ulcer drug. There is no specific indication for misoprostol in this situation.

Drugs that do not directly inhibit gastric acid secretion

Chelated salts of bismuth: tripotassium dicitrato bismuthate

Mechanism
The mechanisms through which bismuth salts heal ulcers are not fully understood. They do not directly inhibit acid secretion. However, they do suppress *H. pylori* infection and thus reduce the hypersecretion of acid induced by the infection. In addition, they may form an insoluble protective layer over the ulcer base, preventing further damage by acid and pepsin. They may also stimulate local prostaglandin production.

Pharmacokinetics
A small quantity of bismuth is absorbed following oral administration. Urinary excretion of bismuth continues for over 2 weeks after stopping a course of treatment.

Adverse effects
The liquid preparation should be avoided because of an unpleasant smell and taste and the fact that it discolours the tongue. The liquid or tablet preparation may colour the faeces black. The long-term consequences of bismuth absorption are unknown, so this drug is not recommended for continuous or repeated administration.

Comment. In the management of patients with peptic ulcer, the main use of a bismuth-containing compound is as part of a drug combination against *H. pylori*. This compound, when combined with metronidazole and another antibiotic, such as tetracycline, can eradicate the infection in 80–90% of patients within 2 weeks. However, since frequent doses are necessary and compliance may be a problem, PPIs have largely replaced bismuth in the eradication of *H. pylori*.

Sucralfate (sucrose aluminium octasulphate)

Mechanism
The exact mechanism of ulcer healing by sucralfate is unknown. It may act by coating ulcer bases or by stimulating local prostaglandin release. It does not directly affect acid secretion. However, like the bismuth salts it suppresses *H. pylori* infection and thus reduces the acid hypersecretion stimulated by the infection. It probably suppresses *H. pylori* by interfering with the ability of the organism to bind to the mucosal epithelial cells.

Clinical use and dosage
Sucralfate is indicated for the treatment of DU and benign GU. The usual dose is 1 g four times daily or 2 g twice daily. Healing rates are comparable to those obtained with H_2-receptor antagonists. Sucralfate should not be used in patients with chronic renal failure because of the risk of aluminium absorption and toxicity.

Pharmacokinetics
Sucralfate acts locally; only small amounts of aluminium are absorbed.

Adverse effects
Constipation.

Drug interactions
Sucralfate can reduce the absorption of a number of different drugs, including phenytoin and tetracyclines.

Drug combinations to eradicate *H. pylori*

Almost all patients with DU, and many patients with GU, are chronically infected with *H. pylori*. Successful eradication of this bacterium is usually associated with permanent cure of ulcer recurrence. Re-infection with *H. pylori* after eradication appears to be rare, at least in developed countries.

Eradication of *H. pylori* usually requires both acid suppression and antibiotic treatment. The most widely used regimen combines a PPI with clarithromycin and amoxicillin for 1 week. Metronidazole can replace amoxicillin in patients who have a penicillin allergy.

Nausea and vomiting

Aims

1 To establish an underlying cause and give specific treatment if possible
2 To give symptomatic treatment

Relevant pathophysiology

Vomiting is controlled by two separate brainstem centres: the chemoreceptor trigger zone and the vomiting centre. The trigger zone may be activated endogenously or exogenously by toxins or drugs such as opiates. It is rich in dopaminergic receptors. Activation of the trigger zone stimulates the vomiting centre. The act of vomiting is controlled by the vomiting centre, mainly through vagal action. The vomiting centre has afferent input from the gut, higher cortical centres and the vestibular apparatus. Muscarinic and histamine H_1-receptors are highly concentrated around the area of the vomiting centre.

Drugs used in treatment of vomiting

Anticholinergic drugs: hyoscine

Mechanism
They compete with acetylcholine at muscarinic receptors in the gut and CNS and have antispasmodic action in the gut wall. They may be successful in motion sickness because of their central action.

Adverse effects
Adverse effects are drowsiness plus typical anticholinergic effects of dry mouth, blurred vision and difficulty in micturition.

Clinical use
A 0.3–0.6 mg dose of hyoscine is usually adequate prophylaxis for motion sickness.

Antihistamines: promethazine

Mechanism
Antihistamines are competitive antagonists of histamine at H_1-receptors, acting mainly on the vomiting centre rather than on the chemoreceptor trigger zone. They have weak anticholinergic effects.

Adverse effects
Adverse effects are drowsiness, occasional insomnia and euphoria. Central effects are accentuated by alcohol.

Clinical use
Antihistamines are used in motion sickness or in vestibular disorders. They are widely used in the treatment of allergic rhinitis and other allergic reactions (see Chapter 16, 'Immunopharmacology').

Promethazine is given at a dose of 25 mg 8-hourly.

Dopamine antagonists

Phenothiazines: chlorpromazine and prochlorperazine

Mechanism
The general clinical pharmacology of phenothiazines is described in Chapter 8. These drugs act mainly on the chemoreceptor trigger zone. They have dopamine receptor antagonist properties as well as anticholinergic and other actions.

Adverse effects
Prolonged use may produce Parkinsonian-type tremor or other dyskinesias.

Clinical use and dose
Phenothiazines are effective in a variety of situations, including the vomiting of chronic renal failure and neoplastic disease, and drug-induced vomiting.

Recommended doses are:
Chlorpromazine 25–50 mg 8-hourly
Prochlorperazine 5–25 mg orally or 12.5 mg i.m.
  (tablets and suppositories, for buccal and rectal administration respectively, are also available).

Metoclopramide

Mechanism

Metoclopramide is a central dopamine receptor antagonist, effective at blocking stimuli to the chemoreceptor trigger zone. It also has effects on upper gastrointestinal tract motility, as described above.

Adverse effects

Metoclopramide may cause acute extrapyramidal reactions, such as opisthotonous, oculogyric crisis or other dystonias. These are particularly a hazard when metoclopramide is used in the treatment of children and young adults. They can be treated with an intravenous anticholinergic agent, such as benzotropine.

Metoclopramide raises serum prolactin levels and may cause gynaecomastia by virtue of its antidopaminergic effects.

Drug interactions

Metoclopramide potentiates the extrapyramidal side effects of phenothiazines.

Clinical use and dose

Metoclopramide is effective in most causes of vomiting, apart from motion sickness. The usual dose is 10 mg 8-hourly, orally or parenterally.

Domperidone

Mechanism

Domperidone is a dopamine antagonist, effective at the chemoreceptor trigger zone.

Adverse effects

Domperidone is less likely to cause extrapyramidal reactions than metoclopramide. It raises prolactin levels and may produce cardiac dysrhythmias following rapid intravenous injection.

Clinical use and dose

Domperidone is effective in most situations, especially nausea and vomiting related to cytotoxic drug therapy. The usual oral dose is 10–20 mg

4- to 8-hourly. It can also be administered rectally via suppository.

Cannabinoids: nabilone

Mechanism

Tetrahydrocannabinol is one of the active constituents of marijuana. Nabilone is a synthetic cannabinoid used in the treatment of nausea and vomiting during cytotoxic therapy. Its mode of action is unclear.

Adverse effects

Nabilone causes drowsiness, dizziness and dryness of the mouth. Euphoria and hallucinations are rare.

Clinical use and dose

Nabilone at a dose of 1–2 mg twice daily is of value in treating patients receiving cytotoxic agents. Prolonged use may produce toxic effects on CNS.

Serotonin antagonists: ondansetron

Mechanism

Ondansetron is a selective antagonist of serotonin at $5\text{-}HT_3$-receptors. Its exact mode of action in controlling nausea and vomiting is unclear but it has both CNS and peripheral actions.

Adverse effects

Ondansetron causes constipation and headache; flushing may occur.

Clinical use and dose

Ondansetron is indicated for the treatment of nausea and vomiting associated with cytotoxic therapy or radiotherapy. The dose and rate of administration depends on the severity of the problem and on the chemotherapy used.

Diarrhoea and constipation

Diarrhoea

In all patients presenting with diarrhoea it is important to identify and eliminate a cause where possible. If the cause is unclear, symptomatic relief may be helpful. The drugs used will depend upon the cause of the diarrhoea and are discussed below under the conditions that cause diarrhoea.

Irritable bowel syndrome

This common condition is the most frequent cause of chronic, recurrent abdominal pain. It may also cause bloating and upset of bowel habit (with diarrhoea, constipation or both).

The pathophysiology is poorly understood. There are abnormal motility patterns in the bowel, and patients may be unduly sensitive to distension or contraction of visceral smooth muscle. The diets of patients who do not have diarrhoea are sometimes deficient in fibre. There is a relationship between psychological stress and symptoms in some patients.

Mebeverine is an antispasmodic agent which does not have significant anticholinergic effects. It is useful in relieving symptoms in some patients in a dose of 135 mg three times daily.

Enteric-coated capsules of peppermint oil are useful in relieving gut spasm in some patients. The capsules may cause heartburn if bitten into.

Visceral analgesia with tricyclic antidepressant drugs can be an effective therapeutic strategy. These are started at low doses, such as 10 mgs of amitriptyline, then escalated to effect. Anticholinergic side effects (discussed in Chapter 14) are often the limiting factor in this dose escalation. There is also some evidence to support the use of the SSRI drug citalopram in this fashion.

Non-pharmacological measures, such as dietary wheat or dairy reduction, probiotics and cognitive behavioural therapy, are adjuncts which can be considered in parallel with the above treatments.

Pancreatic insufficiency

A preparation of exogenous pancreatic enzymes containing trypsin, lipase and amylase is taken with meals by patients with chronic pancreatic exocrine insufficiency, such as in chronic pancreatitis or cystic fibrosis. These allow intraluminal digestion to occur in the small bowel.

H_2-receptor antagonists or PPIs may also be given. These prevent both denaturation of the pancreatic enzymes by gastric acid and also reduce the demand for pancreatic bicarbonate secretion, which may reduce pain.

Drugs used in non-specific diarrhoea

Codeine phosphate
This is a useful agent for symptomatic control of diarrhoea. It raises intracolonic pressure and sphincter tone. It should not be given to patients with colonic diverticular disease and should be used only cautiously in patients with inflammatory bowel disease, and only under careful supervision.

Morphine
Kaolin and morphine mixture British Pharmaceutical Codex (BPC) is a time-honoured remedy containing only small quantities of morphine. It is unpalatable and so is taken as a liquid.

Diphenoxylate
This is an opiate derivative. It is combined with atropine in the preparation Lomotil. It is more expensive than codeine phosphate and is probably not more effective.

Loperamide
Loperamide is a synthetic opiate with some anticholinergic activity. It may cause dizziness or dryness of the mouth. The usual dose is 2 mg three or four times daily.

Constipation

There is a wide variation in normal bowel habit. It is therefore important to establish exactly what the patient means by constipation before embarking on treatment.

Drugs used in non-specific constipation

Drugs that increase faecal bulk
These consist of non-absorbable polysaccharides as in bran, ispaghula or sterculia. They are generally

effective in simple constipation, particularly where the intake of dietary fibre is poor. They are the agents of choice where treatment is likely to be prolonged, but may be slow to act and therefore require a degree of persistence.

Stimulant laxatives

These agents stimulate intestinal motility, probably through an effect on the myenteric nerve plexus. Examples are senna and bisacodyl. They should be avoided when intestinal obstruction is suspected. Prolonged use leads to hypotonicity of the bowel and thereby eventually may exacerbate chronic constipation.

Stool softeners

The best known agent in this group is liquid paraffin. It acts by lubricating the faeces, which aids passage along the bowel. It may cause slight perianal irritation. Long-term use can lead to malabsorption of fat-soluble vitamins. It is not indicated for infants as inhalation of the liquid may produce lipoid pneumonia.

Osmotic laxatives

These agents retain and/or draw water into in the bowel. They increase faecal bulk and moisten faeces. Commonly used examples are the non-absorbable disaccharide lactulose and salts of magnesium. Polyethylene glycol-based medications have also been increasingly used in recent years.

Comment. The commonest cause of constipation is lack of dietary fibre and most cases will respond to a high-fibre diet.

Inflammatory bowel disease

Clinical scenario

A 30-year-old woman is referred to a gastroenterology clinic with a 3-month history of lower abdominal discomfort, malaise, anorexia and intermittent bloody diarrhoea. During exacerbations she passed up to 10 liquid stools per day with blood and mucous. The gastroenterologist suspects inflammatory bowel disease and arranges colonoscopy. What treatment strategies are available?

Aims

1 To obtain remission in periods of relapse
2 To maintain periods of remission
3 To reduce long-term risk of bowel cancer

Relevant pathophysiology

Ulcerative colitis and Crohn's disease are chronic inflammatory conditions of unknown aetiology. However, there is an increasing appreciation of important roles for both host genetics and also for alterations in the mucosal immune response to resident luminal bacteria. Both diseases are characterised by episodes of remission and relapse. Drug treatment is aimed at controlling inflammation and bringing about remission. Treatment of these conditions is not only pharmacological but also depends on psychological support, correction of nutritional deficiencies and appropriate use of surgery.

Drugs used in the treatment of inflammatory bowel disease

Corticosteroids

These agents are discussed in detail in Chapter 17.

Steroids are of proven value in the treatment of acute relapses of ulcerative colitis and Crohn's disease. They may be given rectally, orally or intravenously depending on the extent and severity of the condition.

Budesonide is a synthetic corticosteroid with potentially less systemic side effects as it undergoes extensive first-pass metabolism in the liver. An oral controlled release formulation of budesonide is used for the treatment of terminal Crohn's disease and for microscopic colitis.

Steroids are of no value for either ulcerative colitis or Crohn's disease in remission and should be withdrawn once clinical remission is achieved.

Aminosalicylates

Preparations are designed to deliver the drug to the colon: Mesalazine (a controlled release preparation of 5-aminosalicylic acid (5-ASA)), olsalazine (two molecules of 5-ASA linked by an azo bond that is split by colonic bacteria to release 5-ASA within the colon) and balsalazide (a prodrug of 5-ASA). Sulphasalazine consists of 5-ASA linked to sulphapyridine by an azo bond that is split in the colon by bacterial azo-reductases.

Mechanism

It is thought that 5-ASA exerts a local anti-inflammatory effect.

Adverse effects

Blood dyscrasias, renal damage and (with olsalazine) watery diarrhoea (if not taken with food).

Clinical use

These drugs can be used alone in the management of mild–moderate ulcerative colitis and as adjuncts to corticosteroids in severer disease. They have a key role in the maintenance of remission in ulcerative colitis. However, there is little evidence for a role for them in Crohn's disease. There is also accumulating evidence that they have a chemoprotective effect, reducing the risk of future bowel cancer in patients with ulcerative colitis.

Thiopurines (azathioprine, 6-mercaptopurine)

Mechanism

These are immunosuppressive agents which may be useful in improving control in patients with severe inflammatory bowel disease proving difficult to control on steroids and aminosalicylates.

Side effects

They may cause bone marrow suppression. They also may reduce the immune response particularly to viral infections. Drug-induced hepatitis and acute pancreatitis are other rare, but important side effects of thiopurines. The risk of these side effects can be reduced, but not eliminated by the measurement before treatment of the activity of one of their metabolising enzymes, thiopurine methyl transferase (TPMT). Patients with low activity of this enzyme should not receive a thiop-

urine, whilst they should only be used cautiously in those with intermediate activity.

Clinical use

Patients on azathioprine should be told to report to their doctor immediately if they develop symptoms such as sore throat, a bleeding tendency or epigastric pain. In addition, their blood count and liver function must be checked regularly.

Other immunosuppressants

The use of these drugs is restricted to physicians with expertise in their use.

Ciclosporin is used in patients with severe ulcerative colitis that has not responded to parenteral corticosteroids. The modern evidence-based dose of 2 mg/kg/day is as efficacious as the previously used dose of 4 mg/kg/day, but is thought to be associated with a lesser risk of significant side effects.

Methotrexate may induce remission in patients with Crohn's disease that have either not been able to tolerate or are unresponsive to thiopurines.

Infliximab is a monoclonal antibody against tumour necrosis factor-α. It is administered by intravenous infusion for the treatment of severely active Crohn's disease that has not responded to corticosteroids, azathioprine or methotrexate. It has a murine component and may therefore generate antibodies which can be responsible for both loss of efficacy and also infusion reactions. More recently, adalumimab, a humanised antibody which is administered by subcutaneous injection has also become available. Unfortunately, patients may also develop antibodies to this agent.

Drugs adversely affecting gastrointestinal function

Virtually any drug may cause nausea, vomiting or diarrhoea and a detailed drug history is essential in patients with such complaints. Some specific drug-induced gastrointestinal problems are listed in Table 3.1, and a list of common drug-related gastrointestinal symptoms is given in Table 3.2.

Table 3.1 Drugs that may adversely affect gastrointestinal function.

Drug	Comment
Antacids containing aluminium sucralfate	Constipation
Antacids containing magnesium	Diarrhoea
Oral iron salts	Nausea; constipation or diarrhoea (only nausea is dose-related); darkens stools as does bismuth
Bisphosphonates	Severe oesophagitis, oesophageal ulcers and erosions
Antibiotics	Oral *and/or* oesophageal candidiasis; diarrhoea
Aspirin/NSAID	Dyspepsia; gastric erosions (with or without significant bleeding); GUs; increased risk of perforation or bleeding of existing GUs or DUs; NSAIDs may cause ulceration, stricture or perforation of small intestine; NSAIDs may promote relapse of inflammatory bowel disease
Oral potassium supplements	Ulceration or perforation at sites of stasis (e.g. oesophageal or intestinal stricture)
Nicorandil	Gastrointestinal ulceration (especially oral/anal)

NSAID, non-steroidal anti-inflammatory drug; DUs, duodenal ulcers; GUs, gastric ulcers.

Diarrhoea is common in patients receiving antibiotics. This is usually attributed to an alteration in the intracolonic bacterial flora. In some patients a colitis may result from antibiotic therapy: antibiotic-associated colitis or pseudomembranous colitis. This is a result of the proliferation of *Clostridium difficile* in the bowel and the secretion of an endotoxin. Prevention is of this is achieved by the limited, judicious use of antibiotics and good hygiene in clinical areas. Treatment depends on the prescription of an antibiotic, which is poorly absorbed when given orally. Two suitable agents are vancomycin and metronidazole.

Table 3.2 Common drug-related gastrointestinal symptoms.

Nausea and vomiting	Iron; thiopurines; metformin; antimuscarinics
Diarrhoea	Antibiotics (some are associated with *C. difficile* diarrhoea); iron; magnesium-containing antacids; PPIs; NSAIDs
Constipation	Aluminium-containing antacids; iron; verapamil; opiates
Gastrointestinal ulceration	Bisphosphonates (oesophageal); aspirin and NSAIDs; nicorandil; oral potassium salts (at strictures/sites of stasis)
Black stool	Iron; bismuth

NSAIDs, non-steroidal anti-inflammatory drugs; PPIs, Proton pump inhibitors.

Key points

- Gastrointestinal symptoms are very common.
- Treatments for GORD are effective but relapse is frequent following cessation of therapy
- Antibiotic therapy to eradicate *H. pylori* is a crucial part of pharmacotherapy for peptic ulcer disease
- Treatment of inflammatory bowel disease involves a variety of immunosuppressive and anti-inflammatory agents; surgery may be required in severe cases

Chapter 4

Management of coronary artery disease and its complications

Clinical scenario

A 63-year-old man is admitted to hospital with central, crushing chest pain radiating to his left arm. He is breathless and has associated nausea. On examination he is sweaty, tachycardic and hypotensive. An electrocardiogram *(ECG) shows anterolateral ST depression and T wave inversion. Chest x-ray (CXR) is clear. What is the diagnosis and how should he be managed?*

Key points

- Drugs used in ischaemic heart disease can be for symptomatic relief, prognostic benefit or both
- Diagnosing acute coronary syndromes (ACS) is important as early therapeutic intervention can improve outcome
- Cardiovascular risk factor identification and treatment improves outcomes in patients with established coronary artery disease

Introduction

Ischaemic heart disease is usually due to coronary atheroma. Chapter 5 described the pharmacological approaches that have been proven to

Lecture Notes: Clinical Pharmacology and Therapeutics, 8th edition. By Gerard McKay, John Reid and Matthew Walters. Published 2010 by Blackwell Publishing Ltd.

modify risk factors of hypertension and hyperlipidaemia and thus prevent or slow the progression of atherosclerosis and cardiac target organ damage. Where these primary prevention approaches are unsuccessful or introduced too late, patients will present with complications and symptoms ranging from angina pectoris to acute myocardial infarction in addition to cardiac arrhythmias and cardiac failure. Heart failure is most commonly a consequence of ischaemic heart disease with myocardial infarction. The prevalence of complications of coronary artery disease, particularly heart failure, increases markedly with advancing age.

The risk of cardiovascular events in an individual patient is greatly increased by pre-existing heart disease whether symptomatic, such as angina or myocardial infarction, or asymptomatic (left ventricular hypertrophy or dysfunction). Therapeutic strategies were previously directed to relieve symptoms including relief of pain, breathlessness or peripheral oedema. This remains an important aspect of management. In recent years, randomised clinical trials have confirmed therapeutic approaches that also improve outcome by reducing further cardiovascular events. Aggressive management of risk factors such as blood pressure and cholesterol is increasingly recognised as an important aspect of secondary prevention of cardiovascular disease (see Chapter 5).

Angina pectoris, myocardial infarction and ACS

Aims

- Symptom relief
- Prevention of worsening or recurrent angina and myocardial infarction
- Prevention of non-coronary atherosclerotic problems, e.g. stroke
- Improved survival

Relevant pathophysiology

Angina is the symptom experienced when myocardial oxygen delivery is insufficient to meet myocardial energy requirements. The major determinants of myocardial oxygen consumption are heart rate and the force of myocardial contraction. Angina occurs in two forms:

1 *Stable angina*: Attacks are predictably provoked by exertion or excitement and recede when the increased energy demand is withdrawn. The underlying pathology is usually chronic coronary artery disease, with moderate to severe fixed stenosis of the coronary arteries with super-added variation in coronary tone. Anaemia and thyrotoxicosis can precipitate or aggravate angina by reducing oxygen delivery and increasing energy requirements, respectively. Treatment can be directed at increasing myocardial oxygen supply (coronary vasodilatation) or reducing myocardial oxygen consumption (reduce heart rate, contractility, preload and afterload). Drugs that reduce heart rate also increase the duration of diastole, the time when most myocardial blood flow occurs.

2 *Unstable angina*: In unstable angina, which is one type of ACS (see below), attacks occur with increasing frequency and severity and on lesser exertion or at rest and are unpredictable. The underlying pathology is usually rupture or dissection of an atheromatous plaque with thrombus formation or extension in the coronary arteries. Spasm may be an additional mechanism. Acute changes in coronary artery pathology are presumed and therapeutic attention directed to halting, reversing or bypassing the coronary arterial occlusive

process in the hope of avoiding myocardial infarction. Given the nature of the pathophysiological process, antithrombotic therapy is the key. At the same time, treatment is aimed at reducing myocardial energy requirements. Severe unstable angina can progress to myocardial infarction or death.

In recent years unstable angina and non-ST segment elevation myocardial infarction (non-STEMI), along with ST segment elevation myocardial infarction (STEMI) have, collectively, become known as ACS. This categorisation reflects how the treatment of ACS is determined by the way in which the patient presents. Unstable angina and non-STEMI may be indistinguishable at presentation (with confirmation of infarction depending on an increase in a cardiac biomarker such as troponin T or tropinin I) and are managed similarly with anti-platelet therapy, antithrombotic therapy (e.g. heparin), anti-ischaemic drugs and, increasingly, early percutaneous coronary intervention (PCI) or coronary artery bypass surgery. There is evidence that early 'revascularisation' for non-STEMI ACS reduces recurrent angina and myocardial infarction. STEMI is managed differently and should be treated by thrombolysis (see Chapter 18) or primary PCI.

Drugs used in angina

Glyceryl trinitrate

Mechanism
A potent, direct, short-acting, smooth muscle relaxant with widespread vasodilator activity. Whether the predominant effect is a direct action on the coronary arteries to increase flow or a peripheral (systemic) reduction in pre- and afterload is disputed.

Pharmacokinetics
Virtually 100% first-pass metabolism and it is therefore given sublingually, buccally, transdermally as a patch or paste, or intravenously. Very rapid clearance by liver metabolism: half-life about 2 minutes.

Adverse effects

These are dose related and result from vasodilatation and hypotension: headache, flushing and postural dizziness. These symptoms can be terminated by swallowing the tablet or spitting it out or by removing the patch.

Clinical use and dose

Glyceryl trinitrate

This is generally kept as a 'rescue' treatment for 'breakthrough' angina. Ideally, glyceryl trinitrate (GTN) should be taken to prevent angina. For example, it can be taken sublingually by the patient before carrying out a task known to produce angina. The total daily dose may be determined individually as that required to control symptoms. GTN is also available in patch form. The shelf life of sublingual GTN is only 6 months. For patients with infrequent angina, GTN by sublingual spray or chewable isosorbide dinitrate have a much longer shelf life and are more appropriate.

Isosorbide dinitrate and isosorbide mononitrate

The clinical pharmacology of isosorbide dinitrate is similar to GTN, but it is also effective orally and has a longer half-life of 40 minutes. Isosorbide mononitrate has an even longer half-life. It is the active metabolite of isosorbide dinitrate and is claimed to have more consistent pharmacokinetics and longer duration of action. Early trials demonstrated loss of efficacy with long-acting nitrates after several weeks, especially with high doses. This was shown to be a result of tolerance and drug effect could be restored by a short break of treatment. Subsequently it has been shown that a 6- to 8-hours nitrate-free interval in every 24 hours allows restoration of nitrate efficacy. A long-acting formulation of isosorbide mononitrate can be used once daily, while short-acting formulations of isosorbide dinitrate should be prescribed two to three times per day but with no doses given between 6 p.m. and 8 a.m. (i.e. an eccentric dosing regimen to give a nitrate-free interval). It must be realised that the patient has no anti-anginal cover over this period and, hence, is most vulnerable to a coronary event. If nocturnal angina is troublesome then the nitrate-free interval can be switched to the daytime.

Doses

Isosorbide dinitrate: 30–120 mg daily in two to three doses.

Isosorbide mononitrate: 20–120 mg daily in one dose (or two doses not more than 8 hours apart).

Transdermal GTN: 5–15 mg.

Comment. Nitrate patches should be removed at night to ensure efficacy during the day.

Potassium channel activators

Nicorandil, a compound that has several mechanisms of action including activation of potassium channels and nitrate-like activity, is available for the management of angina. Nicorandil's pharmacodynamic profile is very similar to that of nitrates although tolerance may be less of a problem. In an outcome trial nicorandil reduced major coronary events, but this was driven by a reduction in hospitalisation for chest pain rather than hard end points such as myocardial infarction (MI) or death.

Beta-receptor blockers

The detailed clinical pharmacology of these drugs is described in Chapter 5. Their role in angina depends mainly on decreasing myocardial oxygen consumption by:

1 Limiting the increased heart rate associated with exercise and anxiety

2 Limiting the increased force of contraction associated with the same stimuli

3 Increasing the length of diastole, the period during which coronary blood flow occurs

Beta-blockers have been shown to reduce sudden death and reinfarction following a myocardial infarct.

Adverse effects

Lethargy, fatigue, bradycardia and bronchospasm are common side effects. Rebound worsening of angina, myocardial infarction or tachycardia has been reported when beta-blockers are suddenly withdrawn. Reduce dose over 24–48 hours if beta-blockers are being withdrawn in such patients.

Clinical use

There are no reliable data to say whether β_1 selective or non-selective beta-blockers should be preferred in stable and unstable angina. The major post-myocardial infarction trials showing beta-blocker benefit used non-selective agents. The only absolute contraindication for a beta-blocker is asthma.

Doses

Atenolol: 50–200 mg daily in two divided doses.
Metoprolol: 100–400 mg daily in two or three divided doses.
Bisoprolol: 5–20 mg once daily.
Carvedilol 25–50 mg in two divided doses.
These drugs must all be given in an individually titrated dose to control symptoms and attenuate postural and exercise-induced tachycardia.

Calcium antagonists

There are two major groups:
1 Dihydropyridines including nifedipine, nicardipine, nitrendipine, felodipine and amlodipine
2 Heart rate limiting ones including verapamil and diltiazem

Calcium antagonists are further described in Chapter 5. Their principal action is inhibition of the slow calcium-ion channel component of the smooth muscle action potential leading to:
1 Reduction in afterload.
2 Decreased tone in vascular smooth muscle cells including coronary arteries.
3 Decreased contractility in myocardial cells.
4 Depressant effects by verapamil and diltiazem on sinus node and atrioventricular node function and therefore slow heart rate. These drugs have additional anti-arrhythmic activity.

Pharmacokinetics

All drugs are well absorbed following oral administration. They are cleared by liver metabolism.
All undergo extensive first-pass metabolism. Active metabolites may contribute to their effects.

Adverse effects

Headache, nausea, flushing and ankle swelling with nifedipine and other dihydropyridines. The side effects of nifedipine appear to be diminished markedly by combination with a beta-blocker. Constipation occurs with verapamil.

Short-acting formulations of calcium antagonists, particularly dihydropyridines, should be avoided, especially in patients not treated with a beta-blocker as there is some evidence that rapid onset vasodilatation, leading to a fall in blood pressure and reflex tachycardia, can worsen angina or even precipitate myocardial infarction. Slow-release formulations of nifedipine have a smoother pharmacodynamic profile, as do long-acting calcium antagonists like amlodipine. They have no effect on cardiovascular survival but may reduce the need for intervention.

There is a general perception that beta-blockers may be more effective anti-anginal agents than calcium channel blockers and should be the first choice agent for angina prophylaxis.

Drug interactions

Verapamil or diltiazem should not be given routinely with beta-blockers since the combined negative inotropic and chronotropic effects can cause bradyarrhythmias and heart block and can rarely precipitate heart failure. Bradycardia may also follow use of these agents with digoxin or amiodarone.

Clinical use

They may be used in stable or unstable angina. Verapamil and diltiazem are alternative first-line agents to a beta-blocker in intolerant patients in stable or unstable angina. Nifedipine and other dihydropyridines are used to best effect in combination with beta-blockers in severe angina.

Doses

Verapamil: 40 mg two or three times daily up to 360 mg daily in divided doses or as a single dose of a slow-release preparation.
Nifedipine: up to 120 mg daily as a long-acting preparation.
Amlodipine: 5–10 mg once a day.

Diltiazem: 60 mg two or three times daily up to 480 mg daily in divided doses or as a slow-release formulation once or twice daily.

General principles of management of angina

There are three major components to the treatment of angina:

1 Management of the risk factors for coronary atherosclerosis (e.g. lipid lowering, aspirin, anti-hypertensive drugs, cessation of smoking)

2 Treatment of symptoms

3 Preventing or delaying myocardial infarction and death

There is considerable evidence that treating the first two goals will achieve the third goal by default. There is also evidence that surgical revascularisation of patients with angina and severe coronary artery disease improves prognosis in certain patients, but the studies showing this are old and predate the modern medical treatment of patients with severe coronary disease and left ventricular dysfunction.

Where possible, objective evidence of coronary disease should be sought using electrocardiography and exercise testing. This provides diagnostic confirmation and, importantly, objective evidence of the severity of the underlying ischaemia, providing the indication for coronary angiography.

Stable angina

1 Modify cardiovascular risk factors such as cigarette smoking, treat hypertension and prescribe a statin to lower LDL cholesterol.

2 Prescribe prophylactic aspirin; clopidogrel is an alternative in aspirin-intolerant patients.

3 Angiotensin-converting enzyme (ACE) inhibitors such as ramipril or perindopril may prevent cardiovascular events and death in patients with angina or post-infarction.

4 Treat any underlying precipitating cause such as anaemia, thyrotoxicosis or arrhythmias.

5 Prescribe prophylactic therapy with a beta-blocker or a rate-limiting calcium antagonist if a beta-blocker is contraindicated.

6 Prescribe treatment with GTN for breakthrough attacks of angina or to be taken before undertaking the effort or activity that provokes pain.

7 If prophylaxis with a beta-blocker is unsuccessful add a dihydropyridine calcium antagonist, long-acting nitrate or nicorandil.

8 Coronary angiography is indicated under three circumstances:

- The diagnosis of angina is in doubt.
- Symptoms are not controlled with medical therapy, i.e. revascularisation by coronary artery bypass graft (CABG) or PCI is indicated on symptomatic grounds. Patients who fail to respond to the combination of two anti-anginal drugs should be considered for revascularisation.
- Stress testing suggests the presence of severe coronary artery disease, i.e. surgical revascularisation might be indicated on prognostic grounds.

Unstable angina

Once the diagnosis is established, for example by symptoms accompanied by ST segment or T wave changes on the ECG, the patient should be treated with aspirin and low-molecular-weight heparin; clopidogrel should be added in higher risk patients. A beta-blocker (or verapamil or diltiazem if contraindicated) and an intravenous nitrate should be used to relieve symptoms. A high dose of atorvastatin (80 mg daily) has been shown to improve outcome in patients with ACS. If symptoms persist, coronary revascularisation is indicated though addition of a dihydropyridine calcium antagonist may also be considered. Platelet glycoprotein receptor (GPIIb/IIIa) antagonists improve outcome in severe unstable angina and are frequently used in patients requiring emergency revascularisation who should also receive clopidogrel. It is recommended that clopidogrel is continued for 6 to 12 months. Thereafter, patients should be treated as for stable angina.

Cardiac arrhythmia

Not all electrocardiographically documented arrhythmias require treatment. In each instance, the physician must consider the balance between the symptomatic or prognostic significance of the arrhythmia and the potential side effects of therapy. The indications for active treatment in certain circumstances are clear, such as in the termination or prophylaxis of arrhythmias that are life threatening, producing major haemodynamic sequelae or troublesome symptoms. Treatment of arrhythmias may involve either pharmacological or non-pharmacological therapy. Where pharmacological therapy is indicated, the choice of the most appropriate anti-arrhythmic drug depends on several factors:

1 Patient-related:
 • Electrocardiographic diagnosis
 • Possible mechanism of the arrhythmia
 • Nature of underlying cardiac disease (if any), especially coronary artery disease and/or left ventricular dysfunction
 • Requirement for acute or long-term therapy
2 Drug-related:
 • Mechanism of drug action – primary and secondary
 • Pharmacokinetics
 • Haemodynamic effects of the drug
 • Electrophysiological effects of the drug, e.g. effects on conduction, QT interval, etc.

Under different circumstances, the aim of the therapy may be termination of a tachycardia with restoration of sinus rhythm (e.g. supraventricular tachycardia), control of ventricular rate without restoration of sinus rhythm (e.g. atrial fibrillation) or prevention of recurrent episodes of tachycardia.

Relevant pathophysiology

Normal electrophysiology

Cardiac muscle may be divided into three electrophysiologically distinct types:
1 Tissue with spontaneous pacemaker activity, i.e. the sinoatrial (SA) and atrioventricular (AV) nodes
2 Specialised high-velocity conducting tissue – the His–Purkinje system
3 'Working' atrial and ventricular myocardium

The action potentials of SA and AV nodal cells undergo diastolic depolarisation, which results in the generation of spontaneous action potentials. The upstroke of the cardiac action potential in these cells is dependent on the 'slow' inward calcium current. Conduction velocity in nodal tissue, e.g. AV node, is slow, accounting for the delay between atrial and ventricular systole. The refractoriness of the AV node (i.e. the failure to conduct impulses at short intervals) limits the rate at which atrial impulses are transmitted to the ventricles, of particular importance in atrial fibrillation.

Depolarisation in His–Purkinje tissue and atrial and ventricular myocardium depends on the rapid inward sodium current. The action potential upstroke and conduction velocity are much faster than those in nodal tissue, allowing electrical activation of the atria or ventricles in a short period of time, permitting coordinated contraction. Under normal circumstances, atrial and ventricular myocardium has no intrinsic automaticity, while that of the His–Purkinje network is slow (30 beats/minute).

Mechanisms of arrhythmias

Arrhythmias may arise either from abnormal automaticity triggered after depolarisation or from disorders of impulse conduction. Most clinically important arrhythmias depend on the latter mechanism, and are examples of the 're-entry' phenomenon. Re-entry can occur when an advancing wave of depolarisation from a premature impulse finds one pathway temporarily inexcitable (refractory) as a result of prematurity, resulting in conduction block. Depolarisation may proceed by another route and reach the distal part of the refractory area after a long enough period to allow partial excitability to have recovered. The impulse can then travel in a retrograde direction through the area of previous conduction block. If the time taken for the impulse to pass around such a circuit exceeds the refractory period of the normal tissue at the site proximal to the area of conduction block, this tissue will be re-excited, and the potential for a continuous 'circus' movement will exist. Atrial flutter, supraventricular tachycardias, ventricular tachycardia secondary to previous

Table 4.1 Classification of anti-arrhythmic drug actions.

Class	Drugs
I: Fast sodium channel inhibitors	Ia: Quinidine, procainamide, disopyramide
	Ib: Lidocaine, phenytoin, mexiletine, tocainide
	Ic: Flecainide
II: Antisympathetic agents	Beta-blockers
III: Prolongation of action potential duration	Amiodarone, bretylium, sotalol
IV: Slow calcium channel antagonists	Verapamil, diltiazem
Not classified	Digoxin, adenine nucleotides

myocardial infarction and ventricular fibrillation are all examples of re-entry.

Triggered activity is the likely basis for the arrhythmias of digitalis toxicity as a consequence of intracellular calcium overload.

Classification of anti-arrhythmic drugs

The most commonly used classification of anti-arrhythmic drug action was proposed by Singh and Vaughan Williams, following observations on the electrophysiological effects of drugs on isolated tissues. Four principal modes of action have been identified (Table 4.1). However, individual drugs may have actions in more than one category, and their effects in abnormal myocardium (e.g. during ischaemia) differ from those under normal physiological conditions. The anti-arrhythmic actions of digitalis and adenosine are not included in the Vaughan Williams classification, and are considered separately.

Class I action

Agents with class I activity block sodium channels and reduce the rapid inward sodium current, resulting in slowing of conduction, an increase in refractory period, or both. This action is sometimes termed 'local anaesthetic' or 'membrane stabilising'. Class I drugs are subdivided according to their subsidiary properties. Class Ia agents lengthen action potential duration moderately and cause minor slowing of intracardiac conduction and widening of the QRS complex in therapeutic concentrations. Class 1b drugs shorten action poten-

tial duration and have no effect on intracardiac conduction or the QRS complex in sinus rhythm. Class Ic drugs have no net effect on action potential duration, but slow intracardiac conduction, and widen the QRS complex.

Class II action

Drugs with class II action decrease the arrhythmogenic effects of catecholamines. This may occur by competitive antagonism at β-adrenoceptors (e.g. beta-blockers), by non-competitive adrenoceptor antagonism (e.g. amiodarone) or by inhibition of noradrenaline release at sympathetic nerve terminals (e.g. bretylium).

Class III action

Class III activity involves inhibition of outward (repolarising) currents, resulting in lengthening of action potential duration and effective refractory period without interference with the inward sodium current. The basis of this action in clinically available drugs in this category is inhibition of the rapid component of the delayed rectifier current I_{kr}. The action of class Ia drugs in lengthening action potential duration is also mediated by I_{kr} inhibition. Currently available drugs in this category possess additional class II (e.g. bretylium, sotalol) or both class I, II and IV activity (e.g. amiodarone), but drugs with 'pure' class III activity are under development and are likely to be licensed shortly.

Class IV action

Inhibition of the slow inward Ca^{2+} current by this class of drugs results in slowed conduction and

Table 4.2 Non-pharmacological therapy of arrhythmias.

Arrhythmia	Indication	Technique
Atrial fibrillation	Termination	DC cardioversion
	Rate control	AV nodal ablation/pacemaker
	Prophylaxis	Catheter ablation
Atrial flutter	Termination	DC cardioversion
	Prophylaxis	Catheter ablation
Supraventricular tachycardia (AV nodal and AV re-entry)	Termination	Valsalva manoeuvre
	Prophylaxis	Catheter ablation
Ventricular tachycardia	Termination	DC cardioversion, overdrive pacing
		Implantable cardioverter-defibrillator
	Prophylaxis	Catheter ablation, surgery
Ventricular fibrillation	Termination	DC cardioversion Implantable cardioverter-defibrillator

DC, direct current.

increased refractoriness in the AV node. This action is of value in blocking supraventricular tachycardia involving the AV node as one limb of a re-entry circuit, or in slowing the ventricular response to atrial fibrillation.

Pharmacological versus non-pharmacological therapy

Anti-arrhythmic drugs exert powerful electrophysiological effects on the heart. While these may be beneficial, it is increasingly recognised that potentially lethal arrhythmias may be provoked by drug action. This phenomenon, termed proarrhythmia, has been identified increasingly in recent years as a result of randomised clinical trials that demonstrated an increased mortality in patients receiving certain anti-arrhythmic drugs compared with placebo. As a result of this problem, and the limited efficacy of drug therapy in many instances, a non-pharmacological approach is now used for the definitive treatment of arrhythmias, e.g. catheter ablation. However, drug treatment, by virtue of its ease of administration and widespread availability, is still the commonest initial therapeutic approach. Full discussion of the indications for drug versus non-pharmacological treatment is beyond the scope of this chapter, but an indication of the arrhythmias in which non-pharmacological approaches are used is given in Table 4.2.

Class I agents

General

Although class I drugs have been the mainstay of anti-arrhythmic drug therapy for many years, results from several recent clinical trials have shown them to be inferior to other (class III) agents in terms of efficacy and safety in the prophylaxis of symptomatic arrhythmias. Class I drugs increase the risk of death in patients with asymptomatic ventricular premature beats after myocardial infarction. Overall, the benefit/risk margin for class I agents is narrow, the risks of producing conduction block or exacerbating arrhythmias are considerable and use of these drugs is declining. They should only be used under expert supervision. All class I agents interfere with sodium channel activity, and reduce Na^+ influx. This may reduce intracellular Na^+ concentrations and, by Na^+/Ca^{2+} exchange, result in a reduced intracellular Ca^{2+} concentration. Thus, all class I agents have a potentially negative inotropic effect and need to be used with great caution in patients with overt or incipient heart failure. In some instances (e.g. quinidine) the negative inotropic effect may be balanced by peripheral vasodilation. Of the subgroups, group Ib agents have the least negative inotropic action, and group Ia the most.

Class Ia agents

Quinidine
Mechanism
Quinidine reduces the maximal rate of depolarisation, depresses spontaneous phase 4 diastolic depolarisation in automatic cells, slows conduction and also prolongs the effective refractory period of atrial, ventricular and Purkinje fibres.

Pharmacokinetics
Seventy per cent of the drug is absorbed from the gut. With conventional preparations measurable levels are obtained within 15 minutes and the peak effect occurs between 1 and 3 hours. However, because the average half-life is of the order of 6 hours, slow-release preparations are more commonly used. It is 80–90% bound to plasma proteins and is metabolised by hydroxylation; the inactive metabolites are excreted in the urine. Anti-arrhythmic effects are seen with drug levels of 2.3–5.0 mg/L. In cirrhosis the clearance of quinidine is reduced. There is also less binding to plasma proteins and hence lower plasma levels are effective.

Adverse effects
Quinidine has a vagolytic action, which increases AV conduction. This may lead to acceleration in ventricular rate in patients with atrial flutter or fibrillation. Progressive QRS and QT prolongation may occur, the latter leading to polymorphic ventricular tachycardia (torsades de pointes). Higher concentrations are associated with decreased myocardial contractility, hypotension or electrophysiological effects with possible sinus arrest, SA or AV block. Other adverse effects include gastrointestinal symptoms with nausea, vomiting and diarrhoea; cinchonism (symptoms of headache, deafness and tinnitus described initially on overdose of cinchona bark); hypersensitivity reactions with fever, purpura, thrombocytopaenia and hepatic dysfunction.

Drug interactions
Quinidine increases digoxin plasma levels and may precipitate digoxin toxicity if the dose of digoxin is not reduced to compensate.

Clinical use and dose
Quinidine now has limited use. The dose is 200–600 mg orally 6-hourly after an initial test dose.

Procainamide
Mechanism
Procainamide has similar electrophysiological properties to quinidine.

Pharmacokinetics
Procainamide can be administered either intravenously or orally (being 75% bioavailable). However, because it has a relatively short half-life of the order of 3.5 hours, it is usually given as a slow-release preparation. The compound is metabolised to *N*-acetyl procainamide (NAPA), which has class III anti-arrhythmic activity in its own right. Anti-arrhythmic activity of procainamide occurs at blood levels of 4–10 mg/L and toxic effects are likely with blood levels of 16 mg/L. Relatively high plasma levels of both parent drug and NAPA occur in renal impairment and cardiac failure.

The drug is metabolised by acetylation in the liver by an enzyme that also metabolises isoniazid and hydralazine. The enzyme is bimodally distributed in the population; slow acetylators theoretically require smaller doses for anti-arrhythmic activity than fast acetylators.

Adverse effects
Rapid intravenous administration may cause hypotension with vasodilatation and reduced cardiac output. ECG changes include QRS and QT prolongation. In toxic doses PR prolongation may occur, leading ultimately to AV block. On chronic oral therapy at high dosage many patients develop a drug-induced lupus erythematosus syndrome with a positive antinuclear factor.

Drug interactions

Procainamide reduces the antimicrobial effect of sulphonamides. The mechanism appears to be formation of *p*-aminobenzoic acid from procaine.

Clinical use and dose

Procainamide is used predominantly in the termination or prophylaxis of ventricular tachycardias, including lidocaine-resistant arrhythmias. It is administered intravenously, 50–100 mg every 5 minutes to a total dose of 1000 mg or until hypotension or QRS widening occurs. It is rarely used in chronic oral form.

Disopyramide

Mechanism

Disopyramide has electrophysiological properties similar to quinidine.

Pharmacokinetics

Disopyramide is 70–80% bioavailable. The half-life in normal subjects is 6–8 hours. Fifty per cent is excreted unchanged in the urine; a further 25% is excreted in the form of the main metabolite – the N-dealkylated form of disopyramide. The dose should be reduced in severe renal failure when creatinine clearance levels are less than 25 mL/minute. The therapeutic range is 2–5 mg/L.

Adverse effects

Disopyramide has marked negative inotropic actions and should be avoided in patients with left ventricular dysfunction. Other adverse effects are related primarily to anticholinergic activity, with urinary retention, glaucoma and blurred vision. QT prolongation occurs with increasing plasma concentrations, and may predispose to torsades de pointes. Contraindications to therapy include sick sinus syndrome and prostatic hypertrophy.

Clinical use and dose

Disopyramide is occasionally used for atrial and ventricular arrhythmias, including those resistant to lidocaine. The dose is 100–200 mg 6-hourly orally or by slow-release preparation. It is also available for slow intravenous injection 2 mg/kg over 20 minutes.

Class Ib agents

Lidocaine (formerly lignocaine)

Mechanism

Lidocaine causes only marginal slowing of conduction velocity in Purkinje fibres and in ventricular muscle, but is selectively active in suppressing ventricular premature beats and ventricular tachycardia. Like other class Ib agents, it has no useful action against supraventricular tachycardias.

Pharmacokinetics

Lidocaine is not given orally because it is hydrolysed in the gastrointestinal tract and is subjected to extensive first-pass metabolism in the liver so that adequate blood levels are not achieved. Following intravenous administration, the elimination half-life is about 100 minutes. The clearance of lidocaine is reduced in cardiac failure and lower rates of infusion are required.

Adverse effects

Although therapeutic concentrations have little haemodynamic effect, high levels of lidocaine cause bradycardia, hypotension and even asystole. Nausea and vomiting may also occur. At levels ≥ 5 mg/L, central nervous system adverse effects may occur with paraesthesiae, twitching and even grand mal seizures.

Clinical use and dose

Lidocaine has no action on atrial arrhythmias, but it is used in the termination of haemodynamically stable ventricular tachycardia and the short-term prevention of recurrent ventricular tachycardia or fibrillation after myocardial infarction. Lidocaine is given by the intravenous route, with a loading dose of 1–2 mg/kg body weight by rapid injection followed by an infusion of 1–2 mg/min to maintain arrhythmia suppression. The dose requires reduction in the presence of cardiac failure or liver disease. Therapeutic blood levels are 1.5–5.0 mg/lL.

Mexiletine

Mechanism

This primary amine has similar electrophysiological action to lidocaine.

Pharmacokinetics

Mexiletine is active after both oral and intravenous administration. It is extensively metabolised to *p*-hydroxy- and hydroxymethylmexiletine and to their corresponding deaminated alcohols by hepatic metabolism. The half-life in normal subjects is 9–12 hours. However, this may be increased, particularly following acute myocardial infarction. Oral absorption is reduced when given with morphine or diamorphine.

Adverse effects

Toxic effects include nausea, dizziness, drowsiness, tremor and hypotension, common at plasma levels above 2.0 mg/L.

Clinical use and dose

Mexiletine is occasionally used in the treatment of ventricular arrhythmias but therapy is commonly limited by patient intolerance. Mexiletine is given initially as a 1–3 mg/kg i.v. bolus injection, then 20–45 µg/kg per min by i.v. infusion, followed by 0.6–1.2 g orally in 24 hours. Effective plasma levels are 0.75–2.0 mg/L; the therapeutic range is narrow.

Phenytoin

Phenytoin has class Ib activity similar to lidocaine. Haemodynamic adverse effects include dose-related impairment of myocardial contractility following intravenous use. Adverse effects are reviewed in the chapter on anticonvulsants. It finds occasional use as an alternative to lidocaine or in digoxin-induced arrhythmias, given in 50–100 mg rapid intravenous doses over 5 minutes, up to 1000 mg.

Class Ic agents

Flecainide

Mechanism

Flecainide slows conduction in the atria, His–Purkinje system, accessory pathways and ventricles. In therapeutic concentration it causes lengthening of the PR and QRS intervals. Flecainide is effective against atrial arrhythmias and tachycardias involving accessory pathways (Wolff–Parkinson–White syndrome).

Pharmacokinetics

Flecainide is well absorbed orally, and about 27% is excreted unchanged in the urine. The remainder undergoes biotransformation to active metabolites, but the plasma concentrations of the unconjugated, pharmacologically active forms are considerably less than those of the parent drug. Flecainide is not extensively protein-bound. The average elimination half-life in normal subjects is 14 hours, permitting twice daily administration. The half-life is increased in cardiac and renal failure.

Adverse effects

Flecainide may exacerbate pre-existing conduction disorders and should be used with great care in patients with SA disease, AV nodal disease or bundle branch block. In patients with permanent pacemakers, it may cause an acute increase in the ventricular stimulation threshold, with a risk of asystole in pacemaker-dependent patients. Exacerbation of ventricular arrhythmias may occur. These are not normally of the torsades de pointes type, but rather a sustained (often incessant) monomorphic ventricular tachycardia with gross widening of the QRS complex and a relatively slow rate (120–140/minutes). Neurological disturbances such as ataxia and taste disturbance may occur at higher doses.

Clinical use and dose

Flecainide is effective in the chemical cardioversion of recent-onset atrial fibrillation, and in the maintenance of sinus rhythm after cardioversion or in paroxysmal atrial fibrillation. The drug is also used in the prophylaxis of AV re-entry tachycardia in the Wolff–Parkinson–White syndrome. Flecainide should not be used in patients with prior myocardial infarction or left ventricular dysfunction. It is a potentially hazardous drug, and its use should be restricted to arrhythmia specialists.

Chronic oral doses range from 50 to 150 mg twice daily with target therapeutic plasma concentrations of 0.2–1.0 mg/L. There is also a modified release preparation now available. Intravenous flecainide (up to 2 mg/kg) may be given by slow infusion over 30 minutes.

Propafenone

This class Ic agent has additional minor beta-blocking and calcium antagonist properties.

Pharmacokinetics

Propafenone undergoes variable metabolism. Fast acetylators metabolise the drug rapidly to an active metabolite, in contrast to slow acetylators. There is therefore a marked variability in the plasma half-life of the native drug, but the overall pharmacodynamic properties of the active drug and metabolite are similar. Propafenone exhibits non-linear kinetics as a result of saturation of hepatic metabolism. For this reason, an increase in the daily dose from 300 to 600 mg daily results in doubling of the plasma concentration, while a further doubling in plasma concentration occurs when the dose is increased from 600 to 900 mg per day.

Adverse effects

The cardiac and non-cardiac adverse effects of propafenone are similar to those of flecainide. In addition, the weak beta-blocking action may be of significance in patients with asthma in whom the drug is contraindicated. The calcium antagonist properties also render the drug unsuitable for patients with myasthenia gravis.

Clinical use and dose

Propafenone is indicated for the prophylaxis of paroxysmal atrial fibrillation or supraventricular tachycardia. As with flecainide, its use should be avoided in patients with prior myocardial infarction or impaired left ventricular function The dosage ranges from 450 to 900 mg daily in two or three divided doses.

Class II agents

β-Adrenoceptor antagonists

The pharmacokinetics, adverse effects and mechanisms of action are discussed in Chapter 5.

Clinical use

These compounds are useful in anti-arrhythmic therapy in view of their freedom from significant pro-arrhythmic effects. They may be used for the control of inappropriate sinus tachycardia, or the prophylaxis of paroxysmal atrial fibrillation or supraventricular tachycardia. Beta-blockers are ineffective in restoring sinus rhythm in atrial fibrillation. However, they are used either singly or in conjunction with digoxin to control the ventricular rate in permanent atrial fibrillation by virtue of their slowing effect on AV nodal conduction. β-adrenoceptor antagonists reduce the risk of sudden death in long-term therapy after myocardial infarction and in congestive heart failure. Other clinical situations in which the beta-blockers have useful anti-arrhythmic action include mitral valve prolapse, and the congenital long QT syndromes.

Bretylium

This agent has adrenergic neurone blocking activity and suppresses noradrenaline release. It is eliminated by the kidney with a half-life of 7–12 hours. Bretylium also has class III action on Purkinje fibres and is effective in ventricular arrhythmias, particularly ventricular fibrillation refractory to lidocaine or procainamide, and repeated electrical defibrillation. Adverse effects include hypotension. It is administered by the intravenous route, 5–10 mg/kg, or by the intramuscular route, 5 mg/kg.

Class III agents

Amiodarone

Mechanism

Amiodarone prolongs the action potential duration and effective refractory period in all cardiac tissues. It is a non-competitive α- and β-adrenoceptor antagonist, and also has class I, II and IV activity.

Pharmacokinetics

After oral administration, considerable accumulation occurs in muscle and fat, and the therapeutic action may take several weeks to develop fully. Amiodarone is metabolised in the liver to desethylamiodarone, which is also electrophysiologically active. The steady-state therapeutic plasma

concentrations of amiodarone and desethylamiodarone are in the range of 1–2 mg/L. Elimination of amiodarone is complex, with an initial relatively rapid (1–2 days) and extremely slow terminal half-life (more than 30 days).

Adverse effects

Amiodarone has little negative inotropic effect, and is the best tolerated of all the anti-arrhythmic agents in heart failure. Amiodarone depresses sinus node automaticity and intracardiac conduction; therefore, it should be used with caution in the presence of SA or AV nodal disease. In common with all drugs that prolong ventricular repolarisation, amiodarone may provoke torsades de pointes ventricular tachycardia, but this occurs less frequently than with other class III agents. The use of amiodarone is limited principally by its non-cardiac side effects, of which the most important are pulmonary (alveolitis), hepatic (hepatitis), neurological (tremor, ataxia), thyroid (hyper- or hypothyroidism), testicular (orchitis) and cutaneous (photosensitivity). The last effect occurs in a high percentage of patients, of whom a small minority develop a slate-grey discoloration of light-exposed areas, especially the nose and cheeks. Corneal micro-deposits occur in almost all patients, but do not interfere with vision.

Clinical use and dose

Amiodarone is effective in a wide variety of supraventricular and ventricular arrhythmias. In view of its adverse effects, chronic amiodarone therapy should be used only in life-threatening or severely disabling arrhythmias, when other anti-arrhythmic agents have failed or are contraindicated, and non-pharmacological therapy is not appropriate. An oral loading dose of 600–1200 mg daily is given for 2 weeks, and then reduced to 100–400 mg daily. Intravenous amiodarone may be effective in the acute conversion or control of troublesome supraventricular and ventricular arrhythmias, including recent-onset atrial flutter and fibrillation. It has a relatively slow onset of action, which makes its use suitable only for haemodynamically stable arrhythmias. The initial dose is 300 mg i.v. given over 30 minutes to avoid hypotension, followed by up to 1200 mg/24 hours. The intravenous preparation is irritant and should be given via a central vein.

Drug interactions

Amiodarone potentiates the effect of warfarin and increases plasma digoxin levels. Dose reduction is required in both cases.

Sotalol

Mechanism

Sotalol is a non-selective beta-blocker, which also possesses class III activity and thus prolongs atrial and ventricular action potential duration and refractory period. It has no class I activity at therapeutic concentrations.

Clinical use

Sotalol appears to be more effective than other beta-blockers, particularly in supraventricular tachycardias involving accessory pathways and in ventricular arrhythmias. It may be used in the prophylaxis of recurrent ventricular tachycardia. The side effects are those of other beta-blockers (see Chapter 5) with the additional predisposition to torsades de pointes. The principal risk factors for this are female gender, bradycardia, left ventricular hypertrophy or dysfunction, high plasma concentrations, co-existing potassium depletion and co-administration of other drugs that lengthen QT interval. The dosage of sotalol in anti-arrhythmic therapy ranges from 80 to 320 mg twice daily.

Class IV agents

Verapamil

Mechanism

Verapamil inhibits the slow inward Ca^{2+} current. Its anti-arrhythmic actions stem from decreasing AV conduction.

Pharmacokinetics

Bioavailability is only 10–20% owing to extensive first-pass metabolism. It is eliminated by the kidneys.

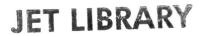

Adverse effects

The commonest side effect is constipation. In view of its depressant effects on the SA and AV nodes, verapamil is contraindicated in heart block or SA disease. Verapamil has significant negative inotropic action, and is contraindicated in heart failure. Additional effects include nausea, dizziness and facial flushing.

Drug interactions

Verapamil potentiates the negative effects of digoxin and beta-blockers on AV nodal conduction. Verapamil and beta-blockers in combination may cause high-grade AV block or asystole, particularly if either is administered intravenously. Beta-blockers also enhance the negative inotropic action of verapamil.

Clinical use and dose

Verapamil is ineffective in restoring sinus rhythm in atrial flutter and atrial fibrillation, but its effect on increasing AV block allows control of the ventricular rate. Verapamil given intravenously is useful in terminating re-entry supraventricular arrhythmias by transient block of AV nodal conduction and is useful when adenosine is ineffective or contraindicated in cardioversion of supraventricular tachycardia. It should not be used in the termination of undiagnosed wide-complex tachycardias where ventricular tachycardia cannot be excluded. Verapamil can also be used orally. Intravenous verapamil is administered by infusion or slow injections over 2–3 minutes. Oral dosage is 80–120 mg three times daily.

Diltiazem

This calcium channel blocker has similar anti-arrhythmic properties to verapamil. Dosage is 60–120 mg thrice daily of conventional release diltiazem. Sustained-release preparations may be taken once or twice daily.

Comment. Calcium channel blockers of the dihydropyridine class (e.g. nifedipine) do not interfere with AV nodal conduction and have no anti-arrhythmic action.

Digitalis glycosides

The term digitalis or digitalis glycoside refers to any of the cardioactive steroids that share an aglycone ring structure and have positive inotropic and electrophysiological effects. In the United Kingdom, the vast majority of clinicians use the cardiac glycoside, digoxin.

Mechanism

A major effect is to decrease sodium transport out of the cardiac cell by inhibiting Na^+/K^+ ATPase (the sodium pump). The resulting accumulation of sodium results in an increase of intracellular calcium ions by Na^+/Ca^{2+} exchange, which is responsible for the positive inotropic effects of digitalis glycosides. These drugs exert their anti-arrhythmic effect by virtue of enhancing vagal inhibition of sinus node automaticity and AV nodal conduction. At high concentrations, digitalis glycosides increase myocardial automaticity as a result of intracellular calcium overload.

The three major effects of digitalis glycosides on the heart are:

1 Positive inotropy
2 Decreased ventricular rate in atrial fibrillation or flutter, by decreasing AV conduction. This effect is diminished on exercise as a result of withdrawal of underlying vagal tone
3 Increased myocardial automaticity in high (toxic) concentrations, or at 'therapeutic' concentrations if other factors such as hypokalaemia are present.

Digoxin
Pharmacokinetics

Digoxin can be given orally or intravenously. The average volume of distribution is approximately 7.3 L/kg; this is decreased in patients with renal disease, hypothyroidism and in patients taking quinidine. It is increased in thyrotoxicosis. Clearance varies from individual to individual and is the result of both renal and metabolic elimination mechanisms. In healthy adults, the metabolic component is of the order of 40–60 mL/min per

70 kg, and the renal component approximates creatinine clearance. Metabolic clearance is reduced in congestive cardiac failure. Clearance in any individual can be calculated by the equations discussed elsewhere (Chapter 21). In patients with normal renal function, the elimination half-life is approximately 2 days. This is increased to approximately 4–6 days in severe renal disease.

Adverse effects
Adverse effects are determined in part by plasma concentration (>2.5 μg/L for digoxin) and in part by electrolyte balance. Digoxin and potassium compete for cardiac receptor sites and hypokalaemia can precipitate digitalis adverse effects. Hypercalcaemia also potentiates toxicity.

The common extracardiac adverse effects are anorexia, nausea, diarrhoea, vomiting, fatigue or weakness. Less commonly, neurological symptoms occur, including difficulty in reading, confusion or even psychosis. Abdominal pain is another less common manifestation.

The cardiac adverse effects may include depression of automaticity or conduction resulting in sinus bradycardia, sinus arrest, junctional rhythm or various degrees of AV block, including complete heart block. Additionally, digoxin may produce excitatory effects, resulting in ventricular ectopic beats, atrial or ventricular tachycardia, or ventricular fibrillation. The typical effects of digitalis glycosides on the ECG, i.e. prolonged PR interval and ST segment depression, do not indicate toxicity. Cardiac signs precede extracardiac signs in about 50% of cases of toxicity.

Drug interactions
Digoxin absorption is decreased by drugs that increase intestinal motility (e.g. metoclopramide), and increased by drugs that decrease motility (e.g. propantheline). Many antacids, particularly magnesium trisilicate, reduce digoxin absorption. Digoxin levels increase if quinidine or amiodarone is co-administered and toxicity can occur. The potential for toxicity is enhanced for all cardiac glycosides when diuretics are co-administered because of hypokalaemia.

Digitoxin and ouabain
Digitoxin is more lipid-soluble than digoxin and is practically 100% absorbed from the gastrointestinal tract. It is given orally and intravenously. It is extensively metabolised by the liver, and the elimination half-life is 5–7 days. Renal impairment does not appreciably alter digitoxin kinetics, but binding to plasma proteins, normally of the order of 90–97%, may be slightly decreased in uraemia.

It seems likely that digitoxin is excreted in the bile and is then reabsorbed to some extent, i.e. it has an enterohepatic circulation. Colestyramine (cholestyramine), which can bind cardiac glycosides in the gut, can interrupt the enterohepatic circulation; whether it can shorten the duration of digitoxin toxicity is still a matter for speculation.

Ouabain is poorly absorbed from the gut and is administered exclusively by the intravenous route. Its onset of action is rapid, and it has a somewhat shorter half-life than digoxin, approximately 1 day. Elimination is mainly renal.

Clinical use and doses
The principal use of cardiac glycosides is in the control of ventricular rate in atrial fibrillation, particularly when a return to sinus rhythm is not expected (e.g. chronic mitral valve disease). Combination therapy with verapamil or beta-blockers provides better control of exercise heart rate with a lower risk of toxicity than high-dose glycosides. The onset of action even after intravenous administration is delayed for several hours. Thus if clinical circumstances require urgent control of ventricular rate, other approaches such as cardioversion or intravenous amiodarone may be more appropriate. Acute digitalisation has been superseded by the use of intravenous adenosine or verapamil in the termination of supraventricular tachycardias. The use of digoxin in patients with heart failure in sinus rhythm is discussed elsewhere.

The dosing schedules used with the cardiac glycosides depend not only on the pharmacokinetic properties of the drug, but also on factors that determine individual susceptibility. The loading dose is determined by the volume of distribution and the desired plasma concentration; the maintenance dose by clearance (Chapter 1). Nomograms and simple equations are available for dose calculation. However, these must remain approximations and the patient's clinical response must influence long-term management. If a maintenance dose is employed without a loading dose, drug accumulation and activity develop slowly because steady state is not reached for 4–5 half-lives. The major determinant of digoxin clearance is renal function and the maintenance dose for this glycoside must be reduced if renal function is impaired. The average loading dose of digoxin is 1.0–1.5 mg orally, or 0.3–1.0 mg intravenously. The usual oral maintenance dose in the presence of normal renal function is 0.125–0.250 mg daily.

The use of drug monitoring of the glycoside plasma levels has been useful, particularly in renal impairment and toxicity. The normal therapeutic range of digoxin is 1–2 μg/L. Venous sampling should be performed 3–4 hours after an i.v. dose or 6–8 hours after an oral dose. If blood levels are low then compliance should be checked, and possible causes of malabsorption considered.

Treatment of digitalis-induced toxicity

Treatment of digitalis-induced arrhythmias is often difficult. The glycoside should be withdrawn, and if hypokalaemia is present, potassium chloride should be administered by infusion at a rate of 20 mmol/h (not exceeding 100 mmol total) with electrocardiographic and biochemical monitoring. Severe digitalis intoxication is treated with specific Fab antidigoxin antibodies, which bind and inactivate digoxin.

Ventricular arrhythmias may require lidocaine or phenytoin administration. Supraventricular arrhythmias may respond to beta blockade or phenytoin. Care must be observed when using verapamil and procainamide, as increased degrees of heart block may occur. Temporary pacing may be required for heart block with haemodynamic effects or in the rare instance of SA node arrest. Intra-venous amiodarone infusion has shown promise in digitoxic arrhythmias.

Adenine nucleotides

Adenosine

Mechanism

The adenine nucleoside, adenosine, acts via purinergic receptors situated in the SA and AV nodes. Stimulation of these receptors causes hyperpolarisation of the cells resulting in suppression of automaticity and conduction. This results in transient sinus bradycardia and AV block. Adenosine transiently interrupts the re-entrant circuit in AV nodal re-entry tachycardia or in AV re-entry tachycardia involving an accessory pathway, while increasing the degree of AV block in atrial flutter or fibrillation. Adenosine triphosphate (ATP) has similar actions and is used as an anti-arrhythmic in Europe. ATP is rapidly metabolised to adenosine in the plasma and probably exerts its anti-arrhythmic effects as adenosine.

Pharmacokinetics

Adenosine is metabolised to the inactive inosine. The plasma half-life of adenosine is less than 10s. Both adenosine and ATP are inactive orally.

Adverse effects

Adenosine is a vasodilator and produces marked flushing. Bolus injection causes a transient increase followed by a small fall in blood pressure, but the duration of action of a bolus dose is normally insufficient to cause clinically significant hypotension. A feeling of chest tightness or sometimes chest pain is experienced, which may be very unpleasant but is transient. Transient complete heart block lasting a few seconds may occur. Adenosine may precipitate bronchoconstriction in asthmatics.

Clinical use and dose

Adenosine is the drug of choice for the termination of regular supraventricular tachycardias. Tachycardias involving the AV node as an integral part of the re-entry circuit will be terminated, while atrial tachycardias will demonstrate transient slowing of the ventricular rate, which allows identification of the underlying rhythm, e.g. atrial flutter. Dosing of adenosine is by rapid intravenous bolus injection, using a large or central vein, starting with a bolus of 3 mg, followed by saline. The anti-arrhythmic effect occurs shortly after the onset of flushing, usually 20–30 seconds after injection. Continuous electrocardiographic recording should be made during the administration and until symptoms have passed, since diagnostic information may be lost otherwise. If the initial dose is ineffective, boluses of 6 mg, followed by 12 mg if necessary, are given at the 2- to 3-minutes intervals. If a dose of 12 mg is unsuccessful, it may be repeated once. Some patients will respond to 18 mg (although this dose is not licensed in the United Kingdom). The dose may be limited by patient intolerance. Supraventricular tachycardia may recur within minutes, once the action of adenosine has passed. The same previously effective dose can be repeated but if supraventricular tachycardia recurs, verapamil should be considered as an alternative treatment.

Drug interactions
The effects of adenosine are inhibited by purinoceptor antagonists (methylxanthines, e.g. theophylline and its derivatives) and accentuated by dipyridamole. Adenosine may be given safely to patients already receiving β-adrenoceptor antagonists or calcium channel blockers.

Heart failure

Clinical scenario

A 56-year-old man with previous anterior myocardial infarction presents with increasing shortness of breath. He has a tachycardia, is hypotensive, has a raised JVP and bibasal crepitations at he lung bases. ECG shows an old anterior MI and CXR a large heart with pulmonary oedema. The diagnosis is acute pulmonary oedema secondary to left ventricular dysfunction (subsequently confirmed by ECHO). What drugs should be used to treat this patient acutely and what treatments should he be on long term to improve prognosis?

Introduction

Definition

Physiological: An inability of the heart to maintain a cardiac output sufficient to meet the requirements of the metabolising tissues despite a normal filling pressure.

Clinical: Symptoms suggestive of heart failure (e.g. exertional breathlessness, ankle swelling, etc.) accompanied by objective evidence (usually by echocardiography) of cardiac dysfunction of sufficient severity to account for these. Most patients with heart failure have left ventricular systolic dysfunction and it is for these patients for which there is evidence-based treatment. The treatment of other causes of heart failure is less evidence-based and empirical. In patients who do not respond to appropriate therapy the diagnosis should be reviewed. The causes of heart failure are summarised in Table 4.3 and the principles of management in Table 4.4.

There is a poor relationship between haemodynamic abnormalities (the physiological definition

Table 4.3 Aetiology/management of heart failure.

Principal aims
Improve quality of life by:
- improving symptoms
- avoiding side effects
- preventing major morbid events such as myocardial infarction or stroke
- delaying death

Secondary aims
Improve cardiac performance
Improve exercise capacity
Reduce arrhythmias (ventricular and supraventricular)
Maintain renal function
Prevent electrolyte disturbance

Aetiology
In westernised countries heart failure is usually caused by one of the following:
- ischaemic heart disease
- hypertension (Chapter 5)
- heart muscle disorders
- valvular heart disease

Table 4.4 Drugs used to treat heart failure.

---

1 Diuretics: thiazides, loop diuretics
- Decrease peripheral and pulmonary oedema
- Decrease preload by reduction in circulatory volume

2 Neuroendocrine antagonists
- ACE inhibitors
- β-receptor antagonists
- ARBs
- Aldosterone antagonists

3 Drugs with a positive inotropic effect
Cardiac glycosides (mainly chronic heart failure)
β-adrenoceptor agonists (acute heart failure only)

4 Vasodilator agents
- Mainly decrease preload: nitrates (GTN, isosorbide dinitrate and isosorbide mononitrate)
- Mainly decrease afterload: hydralazine
- Decrease preload and afterload: sodium nitroprusside (acute HF only)

ARB, angiotensin receptor blocker; GTN, glyceryl trinitrate; HF, heart failure.

of heart failure; see above) and symptoms and signs of heart failure (the clinical definition of heart failure).

Relevant pathophysiology

There is a poor relationship between symptoms and cardiac performance in chronic heart failure. Treatment that improves cardiac function does not necessarily improve symptoms or prognosis and many treatments that have only modest beneficial effects on cardiac function may have clear beneficial effects on symptoms and prognosis.

In contrast, there may be a relationship between haemodynamics, symptoms and prognosis in patients with acute pulmonary oedema or cardiogenic shock.

Cardiac performance is influenced by:

1 *Preload*: This determines ventricular end-diastolic pressure and volume. In normal hearts an increased preload leads to increased end-diastolic fibre length, which, in turn, causes increased force of contraction. In heart failure this response is reduced or even reversed.

2 *Force of cardiac contraction*: This is determined largely by the intrinsic strength and integrity of the muscle cells. Force of contraction is decreased by:
- Ischaemic heart disease (myocardial infarction or chronic severe ischaemia)
- Specific disorders affecting heart muscle, such as hypertension and myocarditis
- Disorders of heart muscle of unknown cause, e.g. idiopathic dilated cardiomyopathy.

3 *Myocardial compliance*: This is an important determinant of ventricular filling and therefore of cardiac output. Compliance is decreased by:
- Fibrosis
- Hypertrophy
- Ischaemia.

4 *Afterload*: This is the ventricular wall tension developed during ejection. Afterload is increased by:
- Systemic arterial vasoconstriction
- Increased arterial pressure
- Obstruction to outflow, e.g. aortic stenosis.

5 *Neuroendocrine activation*: After an acute cardiac insult plasma concentrations of renin, angiotensin II, aldosterone, noradrenaline, endothelin, antidiuretic hormone (arginine vasopressin) and the natriuretic peptides are increased. If the patient survives and does not require treatment, then activity of the renin – angiotensin – aldosterone system (RAAS) returns to normal, probably a consequence of compensatory salt and water retention, but plasma concentrations of other neuroendocrine systems remain elevated. Once diuretics have been administered, RAAS activity increases, as do the concentrations of other neuro-hormones with the exception of the natriuretic peptides, which may decline. However, as heart failure progresses, all the above neuroendocrine systems become markedly activated. Increased sympathetic activation via arterial baroreflexes (and possibly a down-regulation of inhibitory activity of baroreceptors) leads to sympathetically mediated increases in renal renin secretion and further increases in angiotensin II and aldosterone. Local haemodynamic factors probably play an important role in activation of other systems.

Neuroendocrine activation may be responsible for many of the characteristic features of heart failure. Examples include:

Angiotensin II: vasoconstriction (especially renal), sodium retention, continuing cardiac myocyte damage causing progressive ventricular dilatation (remodelling); stimulates aldosterone secretion.

Aldosterone: sodium retention; potassium loss and myocardial fibrosis (both may lead to arrhythmias).

Sympathetic activation: vasoconstriction, arrhythmias, hypokalaemia, sodium retention. May initially increase cardiac contractility but has adverse effects on long-term cardiac function as for angiotensin II by progression remodelling following myocardial damage.

Diuretics

These drugs are first-line treatment for patients with heart failure. In mild failure a thiazide (Chapter 5) may suffice. Moderate or severe failure requires a loop diuretic.

Loop diuretics

Furosemide (frusemide), bumetanide, torasemide.

Mechanism

Inhibition of active chloride reabsorption and also of Na^+/K^+ ATPase in the ascending limb of the loop of Henle with increased salt and water loss. The increased delivery of sodium to the distal tubule encourages Na^+/K^+ exchange with a tendency to hypokalaemic alkalosis.

Pharmacokinetics

Both drugs are well absorbed following oral administration and are also available in intravenous formulations. Elimination is largely by renal excretion with a small contribution by liver metabolism. These drugs have a rapid onset and short duration of action.

Adverse effects

Salt and water depletion can occur. May cause pre-renal uraemia (increase in blood urea and creatinine concentrations). Regular monitoring of serum potassium is required. Urate retention can occur as with thiazides. Rapid intravenous injection of large doses can cause deafness.

Drug interactions

These include potentiation of nephrotoxic effects of gentamicin and cephaloridine. Hypokalaemia enhances the risk of digoxin toxicity. A loop diuretic may be combined usefully with a thiazide diuretic (or thiazide-like diuretic, e.g. metolazone 5–20 mg daily) resulting in an extremely potent diuretic combination. This combination should be used with caution and close monitoring of electrolytes. It is not clear if this combination is superior to the use of large doses of loop diuretic alone. Non-steroidal anti-inflammatory drugs (NSAIDs) may impair diuresis and provoke hyperkalaemia and renal failure. There is an increased risk of ototoxicity when used with an aminoglycoside, decreased excretion of lithium and increased risk of lithium toxicity.

Doses

Furosemide: Oral – 20 mg each morning up to 1 or 2 g each day in very resistant oedema or cardiac failure. Intravenous –20–40 mg slowly. In resistant cases up to 1 g can be infused over 2–4 hours.

Bumetanide: Oral – 0.5–5.0 mg each day. Intravenous – 0.5–2.0 mg or infusion up to 5 mg slowly.

Torasemide: 5 mg each morning up to 40 mg each day in very resistant oedema or cardiac failure.

Prevention and treatment of hypokalaemia

There is no evidence that potassium supplements (other than intravenous) are effective in preventing or treating hypokalaemia in patients with heart failure. Hypokalaemia is much less of a problem in patients with heart failure treated with ACE inhibitors or an angiotensin receptor blocker (ARB) but may still occur in patients taking very large doses of diuretics. There are three occasions where hypokalaemia is likely to be a problem:

1 Administration of high doses of loop diuretics in treating heart failure without an ACE inhibitor

2 Co-administration of digoxin since hypokalaemia potentiates digoxin toxicity

3 Administration of a thiazide diuretic to a patient with a low potassium intake, e.g. the older patient.

In general, persistent serum potassium below 3.5 mmol/L is an indication for potassium correction usually by co-administration of a potassium-sparing diuretic, the most appropriate of which is spironolactone.

Potassium-sparing diuretics

Amiloride, triamterene, spironolactone: These drugs are all diuretics themselves, but their effect is weak and they are rarely used alone. They act mainly on the distal tubule, inhibiting sodium/potassium exchange. Spironolactone acts by inhibiting the effect of aldosterone on the distal tubule and is discussed further under the section Neuroendocrine antagonists. Eplerenone is a more selective mineralocorticoid receptor antagonist and causes less gynaecomastia than spironolactone.

The adverse effect common to all of these drugs is hyperkalaemia and is particularly likely in patients with impaired renal function. Potassium supplements should rarely be required with potassium-sparing diuretics. If they are used, close monitoring of serum potassium is necessary. Potassium-sparing drugs (with the exception of spironolactone – see below) should generally be avoided in patients taking ACE inhibitors, as both agents raise potassium and severe hyperkalaemia may occur especially in the presence of renal failure. Note that there are proprietary formulations available which contain the combination of a thiazide or loop diuretic and a potassium-sparing diuretic. Spironolactone should be used only in a low dose and with caution in patients prescribed an ACE inhibitor (see below).

Doses

Amiloride: 5–20 mg/day.

Triamterene: 100–200 mg/day.

Spironolactone: 12.5–50.0 mg/day for severe heart failure. Higher doses may be used for refractory oedema.

Eplerenone: 25–50 mg/day.

Comment. Potassium-sparing diuretics are available in proprietary formulations combined with a thiazide or furosemide. Combination tablets are more expensive but may improve compliance by reducing the number of tablets to be taken.

Neuroendocrine antagonists

ACE inhibitors

ACE inhibitors not only improve symptoms, but also reduce mortality and morbidity including hospital admissions in all grades of heart failure resulting from left ventricular systolic dysfunction treated with diuretics.

Mechanism

The precise mechanism of action of ACE inhibitors has yet to be elucidated. The ACE not only converts angiotensin I to angiotensin II, but also degrades bradykinin. Angiotensin II is a powerful vasoconstrictor. It stimulates aldosterone and antidiuretic hormone release, enhances sympathetic activity, causes renal sodium retention and can cause direct damage to cardiac myocytes, increase myocardial fibrosis and stimulate vascular and myocardial hypertrophy. Bradykinin is a powerful vasodilator and also has anti-proliferative effects on smooth muscle and stimulates the production of vasodilator prostaglandins and nitric oxide.

ACE inhibitors produce both arterial and venous dilatation. The latter may be mediated through increased bradykinin or reduced sympathetic activation. ACE inhibitors increase serum and total body potassium by reducing aldosterone and should not, generally, be used with potassium-sparing drugs. (One exception is spironolactone – see below).

Adverse effects

Profound hypotension may rarely occur after the first dose in patients on diuretics or with hyponatraemia. The magnitude and duration differ between different ACE inhibitors. Other adverse reactions include postural hypotension, renal dysfunction, hyperkalaemia, cough and angioneurotic oedema.

Drug interactions

These include hyperkalaemia when combined with a potassium-sparing diuretic or an ARB and renal failure when combined with an NSAID or an ARB.

Doses

Captopril was the first orally active ACE inhibitor and has a short duration of action and has to be given two or three times a day. Enalapril, which is a prodrug for the active constituent enalaprilat, is longer acting. Several ACE inhibitors are licensed for heart failure and their long-term benefits are likely to be a class effect.

Agents used include:

Enalapril: 2.5–20.0 mg twice daily.
Lisinopril: 2.5–20.0 mg once daily.
Perindopril: 2–8 mg daily.
Ramipril: 1.25–10.00 mg once daily.

The prospective outcome trials showing benefit used high doses of ACE inhibitors. Dose-ranging studies have not shown a convincing difference between doses on symptoms or prognosis. It would however seem advisable to use in practice the same doses shown to be of benefit in large clinical trials.

β-Adrenoceptor antagonists

For the last 30 years heart failure has generally been regarded as a contraindication to beta-blockade, although a series of small studies in heart failure consistently suggested benefit. Recent large trials suggest not only that beta-blockers are safe, but also that they reduce symptoms and mortality, as well as progression of heart failure and hospital re-admission. The reduction in morbidity and mortality is substantial and additional to that of ACE inhibitors. About 5–10% of patients will deteriorate within the first few days of receiving a beta-blocker and it may take 2–6 months for benefits to become obvious. The mechanism of action of beta-blockers in heart failure seems to involve retarding or even reversing progressive ventricular dysfunction due to excessive sympathetic activity. Currently, the most promising results have been achieved with bisoprolol, carvedilol and extended release metoprolol; nebivolol may also be beneficial. Beta-blockers must be used very carefully

by those experienced in the management of heart failure. In heart failure, beta-blockers are initiated in a very low dose and the dose is up-titrated slowly over 2–3 months.

Bisoprolol: Initially 1.25 mg once daily; target dose 10 mg once daily.

Carvedilol: Initially 3.125 twice daily; target dose 25 mg twice daily orally for heart failure.

Angiotensin II antagonists

There is evidence that angiotensin II receptor antagonists or blockers (ARBs) have comparable haemodynamic and neurohumoral effects to those of ACE inhibitors in congestive heart failure (CHF). These drugs also improve symptoms. Angiotensin II antagonists have the advantage of not causing troublesome cough and can be used as an alternative to ACE inhibitors if the latter cannot be tolerated. While ARBs do improve outcome in heart failure, there is no good evidence that they are superior to ACE inhibitors.

Recent outcome trials also showed that adding an ARB in patients who remain symptomatic despite treatment with an ACE inhibitor and beta-blocker improved symptoms, lessened the risk of hospital admission for worsening heart failure and, in one trial, reduced cardiovascular mortality.

An ARB should be used like an ACE inhibitor, i.e. initiated at a low dose which should be increased gradually over a week's period with appropriate monitoring of renal function, potassium and for symptoms of hypotension.

Candesartan: Initially 4 mg once daily; target dose 32 mg once daily.

Aldosterone antagonists

Spironolactone competitively inhibits the effects of aldosterone. It is useful in treating the resistant oedema of conditions associated with excess aldosterone including nephrotic syndrome and cirrhosis. In one trial, spironolactone 25–50 mg daily reduced mortality in patients with New York Heart Association (NYHA) class III and IV heart failure already treated with a diuretic, digoxin and an ACE inhibitor (but not a beta-blocker in most cases).

Spironolactone can cause nausea, gynaecomastia in men and menstrual irregularities in women.

It may decrease the renal secretion of digoxin. There is a risk of hyperkalaemia when given with other potassium-sparing diuretics or an ACE inhibitor. Eplerenome is a newer selective mineralocorticoid antagonist which causes less gynaecomastia.

Hydralazine and isosorbide dinitrate

The combination of hydralazine and isosorbide dinitrate was shown to reduce mortality in patients with heart failure in a relatively small trial conducted before the widespread use of ACE inhibitors and beta-blockers. Recently, the same combination was shown to improve symptoms, reduce admission to hospital for worsening heart failure and increase survival in African-Americans treated with an ACE inhibitor, beta-blocker and, in many cases, spironolactone. The main role of hydralazine and isosorbide dinitrate in non – African-Americans is as an alternative in patients with renal intolerance of an ACE inhibitor or ARB.

Drugs with a positive inotropic effect

Digoxin

Digoxin now has a limited role in patients with heart failure in sinus rhythm, usually reserved for those remaining symptomatic despite an ACE inhibitor, beta-blocker and either an ARB or aldosterone antagonist. It remains a more important treatment in patients with heart failure and atrial fibrillation. The pharmacodynamics and pharmacokinetics of digoxin together with clinical uses and doses are discussed in full earlier in this chapter. Digoxin improves cardiac performance in patients with atrial fibrillation by slowing the ventricular rate. In patients with sinus rhythm, digoxin has a positive inotropic effect when given acutely. There has been controversy as to whether this effect is maintained during long-term therapy. Digoxin has autonomic actions that may be useful in heart failure. Double-blind studies have confirmed the long-term beneficial effect of digoxin on symptoms and morbidity (but not mortality) in sinus rhythm, an effect best seen in patients with severe heart failure. If digoxin is used, the dose should be adjusted to take account of renal function.

Monitoring of plasma drug levels is of limited use as there is a poor relationship between therapeutic effect (in terms of symptoms) and plasma level. Toxicity may be best judged by the occurrence of side effects (anorexia, nausea). However, in elderly patients the symptoms of digoxin toxicity are protean and the first evidence may be serious arrhythmia which is increased with hypokalaemia. Monitoring for toxicity may be warranted in this group.

Adrenoceptor agonists: dopamine and dobutamine

These drugs are currently used only in acute heart failure accompanied by hypotension and poor tissue perfusion. They have established short-term effects when given intravenously.

Mechanism

Both drugs produce their inotropic effect by β_1-adrenoceptor stimulation of the myocardium. The effects of dopamine are dose dependent and result partly from direct action and partly from indirect effects through increased noradrenaline release. Below 5 μg/kg per min the major effect is to increase renal blood flow by stimulation of dopamine receptors. As the dose is increased in the 5–20 μg/kg per min range both β_1- and α-adrenoceptor stimulant effects are seen with increased cardiac output and a modest rise in blood pressure. Above this dose range, α-receptor effects are more marked, with a further rise in blood pressure. This tends to increase afterload and is undesirable. Dobutamine has no renal vasodilator effect, less vasoconstrictor (alpha) effect and a similar inotropic effect to dopamine.

Pharmacokinetics

These drugs undergo rapid clearance. Dopamine and dobutamine must be given intravenously.

Adverse effects

Mainly tachyarrhythmias from β_1-receptor stimulation when used in excessive doses. Stimulation of β-receptors in skeletal muscle can cause hypokalaemia.

Dose

Dopamine: 5 µg/kg per min initially, increasing as required by the clinical response.

Dobutamine: 2.5 µg/kg per min initially, increasing as necessary.

Levosimendan

Levosimendan is believed to act by sensitising the cardiomyocyte contractile proteins to calcium, thus exerting a positive inotropic effect without increasing intracellular calcium or cAMP concentration, undesirable properties of adrenoceptor agonists and phosphodiesterase inhibitors. Levosimendan also causes arterial vasodilatation, possibly by opening ATP-dependent K^+ channels in vascular smooth muscle. For this reason, levosimendan has been described as an 'inodilator'. Preliminary clinical studies have confirmed that levosimendan has favourable haemodynamic effects and may improve symptoms and survival in patients with severe heart failure. These early observations require substantiation in larger trials.

Drugs affecting preload

Glyceryl trinitrate

Sublingual nitroglycerin leads to direct relaxation of smooth muscle of the systemic venous system, although such treatment is rarely adequate for acute pulmonary oedema. Subsequent venous pooling in cardiac failure leads to a reduction in left ventricular end diastolic pressure and volume, reducing pulmonary congestion. There is usually no associated rise in cardiac output. Intravenous GTN can be used acutely until oral agents can be introduced.

Isosorbide dinitrate and mononitrate

The combination of intravenous isosorbide dinitrate and intravenous diuretic has been shown to be a better treatment for acute heart failure than high-dose diuretic alone.

Drugs affecting afterload

Hydralazine

This has a direct vasodilator effect confined to the arterial bed. Reduction in systemic vascular resistance leads to a considerable rise in cardiac output. Changes in arterial blood pressure, as a consequence of the rise in cardiac output and heart rate resulting from blunting of baroreflexes, are smaller than in patients with hypertension. Its use may be of benefit in chronic heart failure when used in combination with oral nitrates. Doses up to 200 mg daily are used in heart failure. Slow acetylators are at increased risk of a drug-induced lupus syndrome.

Calcium antagonists

Until recently, heart failure was considered a contraindication to calcium antagonist use with evidence that nifedipine, diltiazem and verapamil could have adverse effects on prognosis after myocardial infarction in patients with heart failure. Recent studies with long-acting dihydropyridine calcium antagonists (amlodipine, felodipine) suggest that these agents may be safe in heart failure.

Drugs affecting preload and afterload

Sodium nitroprusside

This is a mixed venous and arteriolar dilator also used for acute reduction of blood pressure (Chapter 5). It must be given intravenously by continuous infusion in a dose range of 25–125 µg/min. Blood pressure falls rapidly and the effects wear off over 1–2 minutes after stopping the infusion. This agent is particularly useful in acute valvular insufficiency, such as mitral incompetence following an acute infarct or aortic incompetence in bacterial endocarditis. However, randomised controlled trials show a trend to increased mortality in patients with post-infarction heart failure treated routinely with this agent. It should not be used for more than 24–48 hours because of accumulation of thiocyanate.

Nesiritide

Nesiritide is recombinant human b-type natriuretic peptide which acts as an arterial and venous dilator by increasing intracellular cGMP. Intravenous administration of nesiritide reduces pulmonary capillary wedge pressure, increases cardiac output and has been shown to reduce breathlessness in patients with acute decompensated heart failure. Diuresis has not been convincingly demonstrated and there are limited safety data on this agent.

Comment: Nitrates (GTN or isosorbide dinitrate) are the only commonly used intravenous vasodilator used to treat acute heart failure. Oral vasodilators are generally reserved for patients who are intolerant of, or who have contraindications to, ACE inhibitors or ARBs. As discussed above, the combination of hydralazine and isosorbide dinitrate may be an alternative treatment if ACE inhibitor or ARB cannot be used in patients with renal intolerance.

General principles of management of heart failure

Acute left ventricular failure or pulmonary oedema

This presents with severe breathlessness, orthopnoea or nocturnal dyspnoea.

1 Sit the patient up.

2 Give high-flow oxygen.

3 Establish an i.v. line.

4 Give 5 mg diamorphine or 10 mg morphine i.v. (with an antiemetic) because:
- It has a venodilator effect reducing preload.
- It reduces the intense distress of the patient.

5 Give furosemide 40 mg i.v., more if the patient is already receiving a loop diuretic, because:
- It has a rapid off-loading effect resulting from venous dilatation.
- It has a slower off-loading effect resulting from diuresis and natriuresis.

6 If the systolic blood pressure is ≥100 mmHg and obstructive valve disease has been excluded, start on intravenous GTN or isosorbide dinitrate infusion:
- It has a venodilator effect, reducing preload.
- It has an arterial vasodilator effect, reducing afterload.
- It reduces myocardial ischaemia which is often a co-existent problem in patients with acute heart failure.

7 Correct precipitating or aggravating factors, especially arrhythmias, anaemia and ischaemia.

8 Exclude mechanical problems requiring surgery by echocardiography, e.g. valvular lesions, ruptured ventricular septum.

9 In resistant patients, appropriate therapy with an i.v. vasodilator (e.g. sodium nitroprusside) and/or inotropic agent (e.g. dobutamine or levosimendan) should be considered and the choice of drugs may be aided by invasive haemodynamic monitoring. In selected cases, placement of an intra-aortic balloon pump or a left ventricular assist device may also be considered.

Cardiogenic shock consists of hypotension and oliguria with clinical signs of poor tissue perfusion. It is usually caused by recent extensive myocardial infarction.

1 Where possible monitor both arterial and pulmonary wedge pressure.

2 Give high flow oxygen.

3 Improve cardiac performance with dobutamine or a similar inotropic drug.

4 Low-dose dopamine intravenously may improve renal function.

5 If this fails, then depending on the haemodynamic features consider placement of an intra-aortic balloon pump and try reduction of afterload with sodium nitroprusside or GTN and/or use of dobutamine, dopamine or levosimendan. In selected cases, placement of a left ventricular assist device may also be considered.

Long-term management of chronic heart failure

1 Modify cardiovascular risk factor profile, e.g. cigarette smoking, obesity. Arrange once only pneumococcal vaccination and regular immunisation against influenza.

2 Underlying causes should be treated, e.g. anaemia, hypertension, valvular disease.

3 If this proves inadequate or when there is no treatable underlying cause, diuretics should be given. The type of diuretic and dose depends on severity of failure.

4 All patients without contraindication who have heart failure resulting from left ventricular

systolic dysfunction should be treated with an ACE inhibitor, to improve symptoms further (if still present), to delay worsening heart failure and to reduce major morbidity and mortality.

5 All patients without contraindication who have heart failure due to left ventricular systolic dysfunction should be treated with a beta-blocker, to improve symptoms, to delay worsening heart failure and to reduce major morbidity and mortality.

6 In patients with persisting symptoms and/or signs of congestion, add either an ARB or spironolactone to improve symptoms and reduce major morbidity and mortality.

7 Digoxin currently remains the drug of choice for the control of ventricular rate in patients with atrial fibrillation and heart failure (these patients should usually be treated with warfarin as well).

8 In patients with persisting symptoms several strategies can be adopted:

- If evidence of cardiac dys-synchrony (e.g. broad QRS on ECG) consider cardiac resynchronisation therapy.
- Add digoxin.
- An increase in diuretic dose.
- Ensure that the patient is on the maximally tolerated dose of ACE inhibitors.

- If arterial pressure is still elevated add hydralazine and an oral nitrate or a long-acting dihydropyridine calcium antagonist (amlodipine, felodipine).
- If angina is present add a nitrate, nicorandil or a long-acting dihydropyridine calcium antagonist (amlodipine, felodipine).
- If marked oedema is present increase loop diuretic or add a thiazide diuretic or metolazone (careful monitoring of blood chemistry required).
- In resistant cases patients may be admitted for intravenous diuretic therapy. If this fails, haemodynamic monitoring may be considered. Although empirical vasodilator therapy is not of proven benefit, observational experience suggests that vasodilator therapy tailored to optimise haemodynamics may be beneficial. Haemodynamic investigation often reveals over-zealous diuretic therapy with too low a filling pressure to be the cause of the patient's symptoms.

9 Patients with atrial fibrillation should be considered for warfarin therapy.

10 Consider specialist referral for comment for cardiac support or transplantation.

Chapter 5

Primary and secondary prevention of cardiovascular disease

Clinical scenario

A 50-year-old man has been diagnosed with hypertension picked up at a routine medical at work. He attends his general practitioner (GP) for assessment of his cardiovascular risk. He has no past medical history of note, has a strong family history of ischaemic heart disease (his father had a myocardial infarction at aged 38 years) and he has a 30-year pack history of smoking. On examination he is obese and his blood pressure measurement is consistently >160/90. What are the factors that contribute to his cardiovascular risk and how should he be managed?

Key points

- A number of factors contribute to an individual's risk of cardiovascular disease
- Some risk factors are not modifiable such as age and sex but others are including smoking, hypertension, raised cholesterol and diabetes
- Non-pharmacological interventions are important in reducing an individuals risk of cardiovascular disease including smoking cessation, weight loss and increased exercise although drug treatment for blood pressure and lipid lowering is often required

Introduction

Cardiovascular diseases, particularly myocardial infarction and stroke, are not only an important cause of death and disability worldwide but are major contributors to health care costs. While genetic factors contribute to the risk of cardiovascular diseases, reversible environmental factors also play a major role. These include cigarette smoking and obesity in addition to other established risk factors such as high blood pressure, raised low-density cholesterol (and other lipids), diabetes and a pro-thrombotic state. Non-pharmacological approaches including exercise, diet and smoking cessation can make important contributions to prevention of cardiovascular disease. These should be actively pursued in all patients. However, in a large number non-pharmacological approaches will need to be augmented and supplemented with specific drug therapy. The target of such treatment is the reduction of blood pressure and/or cholesterol but the aim is long-term prevention of progression of atherosclerosis and avoidance of cardiac and vascular (cerebral and renal) complications (primary prevention). In patients presenting with heart disease or stroke, prevention of further events by reversal of plaque instability or delaying if not halting progression of atheroma (secondary prevention) is the objective. There is now good evidence from prospective randomised controlled trials of the benefits and safety of

Lecture Notes: Clinical Pharmacology and Therapeutics, 8th edition. By Gerard McKay, John Reid and Matthew Walters. Published 2010 by Blackwell Publishing Ltd.

lowering blood pressure and cholesterol in both primary and secondary prevention. Patients with diabetes and other high-risk groups appear to show proportionately more benefit from the reduction of blood pressure and cholesterol. In recent years national and international guidelines have recommended that those individuals at moderate or high risk of cardiovascular disease be identified and treated actively. High risk of cardiovascular disease (greater than 15% 10-year risk), which includes heart disease and stroke, is used as a guide for the need for treatment of cholesterol and hypertension. Increasing age is an important component of the calculation of cardiovascular risk. A substantial proportion of the population over the age of 55 are candidates for reduction of blood pressure, cholesterol or both.

Hypertension

Aim

The aim of treatment is to reduce blood pressure in order to reduce the risk of death or disability from cardiovascular disease, especially stroke, coronary artery disease and cardiac failure. However, because hypertension is often an asymptomatic condition, the treatment should control blood pressure without inducing adverse effects or otherwise interfering with the well-being of the patient. A target blood pressure of $\leq 140/85$ mmHg is generally advocated, although this may be modified for particular patients, e.g. those with co-existent diabetes (target blood pressure $<130/80$) and patients at the highest risk of cardiovascular disease (Figure 5.1).

Relevant pathophysiology

Blood pressure is the hydrostatic pressure within the systemic arteries and is determined by total peripheral resistance and cardiac output. Total peripheral resistance is invariably increased in established hypertension, although the causative mechanism is not well understood. Increases in heart rate or cardiac output are not found consistently.

Blood pressure values are not normally distributed (there is a skew to the right) in the population and there is no clear cut-off between normotensive and hypertensive values. Long-term prospective epidemiological studies indicate that, for both systolic and diastolic blood pressure, the higher the blood pressure the greater the risk of cardiovascular disease. Hypertension can be defined as a blood pressure above which treatment produces benefits in excess of risks. In practical terms this is dependent upon the selection of an arbitrary value for normal blood pressure and the frequency of hypertension varies according to the age, sex and ethnic origin in the population studied.

Primary and secondary hypertension

Hypertension is either primary or secondary. No underlying cause can be identified in about 95% of cases and the terminology of primary, idiopathic or essential is applied. There is a strong polygenic familial trend and environmental factors such as salt, obesity and alcohol consumption also contribute. Secondary types of hypertension are rare, even in younger age groups, and usually have an endocrine or renal basis.

Causes of secondary hypertension

Causes of secondary hypertension are as follows:
1 Renal diseases: Renovascular disease, particularly renal artery stenosis (as a result of fibromuscular hyperplasia in young patients and atheroma in older patients)
2 Endocrine disease
   • Hyperaldosteronism (Conn's syndrome)
   • Phaeochromocytoma
   • Hypercorticism (Cushing's syndrome)
   • Acromegaly
   • Hypothyroidism
3 Coarctation of the aorta
4 Drugs, e.g. oral contraceptives, corticosteroids, NSAIDs, ciclosporin

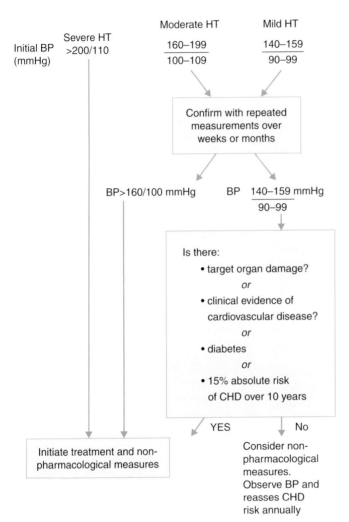

Figure 5.1 Treatment decisions based on observed blood pressure. BP, blood pressure; HT, hypertension; CHD, coronary heart disease.

Benefits of treatment

There is now unequivocal evidence that antihypertensive treatment significantly reduces stroke and coronary arterial events, together with the progression of renal and cardiac failure. These benefits have been clearly established in moderate hypertension (systolic 160–199 mmHg and/or diastolic 100–109 mmHg), in severe hypertension (systolic greater than 200 mmHg and/or diastolic greater than 110 mmHg) and in malignant or accelerated phase hypertension. In the treatment of mild hypertension (systolic 140–159 mmHg and/or diastolic blood pressure 90–99 mmHg) there again have been substantial reductions in stroke and also benefits in respect of coronary artery disease. The benefits of treatment in mild hypertension are greatest among those patients who have evidence of target organ damage (e.g. left ventricular hypertrophy (LVH), retinopathy or proteinuria), diabetes, pre-existing cardiovascular disease (e.g. prior myocardial infarction) or a high risk of cardiovascular disease (≥20% over 10 years) by virtue of other risk factors. Age and systolic hypertension increase risk and benefit. Meta-analysis of randomised trials does not show any convincing benefit of individual drugs or classes but supports the view that in terms of outcome of the treatment, 'the lower the achieved blood pressure the better'.

Antihypertensive treatment

1 Hypertension should be confirmed by several measurements of blood pressure over several days, weeks or months.

2 Patients should be counselled about hypertension, and its risk, and the relevance of other risk factors. The reason for long-term treatment should be carefully explained.

3 Hypertension should be treated as part of a management plan for reducing all identifiable cardiovascular risk factors. Mild to moderate hypertension should seldom be treated in isolation and it is important to attempt to modify all of the individual risk factors of the patient including cigarette smoking, hyperlipidaemia and diabetes mellitus and to take account of other factors such as a family history of premature cardiovascular disease.

4 Non-pharmacological approaches should always be considered although long-term compliance is low; For example,

- For the obese patient, weight reduction of 10 kg may lower blood pressure by about 20/10 mmHg.
- If salt intake is very high (more than 200 mEq per day), a modest reduction by the simple avoidance of excessively salty foods and the use of table salt may aid blood pressure control.
- Regular physical exercise.

5 Arrangements should be made for regular and convenient long-term follow-up with blood pressure measurements.

6 As required, a simple and well-tolerated antihypertensive drug regimen should be established.

Principles of antihypertensive treatment

Drugs may be given alone or in rational combinations. With newer treatment targets, patients will often require more than one drug. The simplest regimen is likely to be the most successful. Adherence with treatment is likely to be maintained best if drugs are administered once daily. A wide range of suitable first-line antihypertensive drugs is now available and the classes of drug that are currently in widespread use are thiazide diuretics, calcium antagonists, angiotensin-converting enzyme

(ACE) inhibitors and angiotensin II (AT_1) receptor blockers. Beta-blockers are no longer regarded as routine first line treatment of hypertension due to relatively poor long-term outcomes in comparison with other antihypertensive agents. The response to treatment can then be evaluated over a period of weeks or months and, if the effect is insufficient and if there are no side effects, the dosage can be increased. If side effects occur or if there is clearly no useful blood pressure response to treatment, then it is appropriate to change to another type of therapy. Where blood pressure response is inadequate despite full-dose, well-tolerated monotherapy, combination treatment with more than one drug is advocated. A fixed-dose combination may be useful for certain individual patients, not only for blood pressure control and adherence but also for satisfying the requirements of the individual patient in terms of other coronary heart disease (CHD) risk factors, or concomitant disease states. However fixed dose combinations are not without their problems and should not be used as first line treatment.

Key points

- The management of hypertension is a long-term undertaking often in asymptomatic patients
- The simplest and most effective treatment should be determined for each individual
- Reduction of blood pressure and control of other risk factors is designed to reduce cardiovascular morbidity and mortality without impairing the quality of life
- Most patients are started on single drug treatment but more than half will require a second or third drug from different classes to achieve targets of <140/85 mmHg (<130/80 if the patient has diabetes or renal disease)

Antihypertensive drugs

The most commonly used antihypertensive drug classes are listed in Table 5.1.

Diuretics

Mechanism of action

These drugs increase sodium excretion and urine volume by interfering with sodium, chloride and

Table 5.1 Indications and contraindications for the major classes of antihypertensive drugs.

	Indications		Contraindications	
	Good	Consider	Relative	Absolute
Thiazide diuretics	Old age	—	Dyslipidaemia	Gout
Beta-blockers	Myocardial infarction	Heart failure*	Heart failure*	Asthma or COPD heart block
Calcium antagonists I (dihydropyridine)	Isolated systolic HT in elderly subjects	Angina in elderly patients	—	—
Calcium antagonists II (rate-limiting drugs)	Angina	Myocardial infarction	Combination with beta-blockers	Heart block Heart failure
ACE inhibitors	Heart failure LV dysfunction in type I diabetic nephropathy	Chronic renal disease[†]	Renal impairment Peripheral vascular disease	Pregnancy Reno-vascular HT
ANGII antagonists	ACE inhibitor induced cough	Heart failure, intolerance of other antihyper-tensives	Peripheral vascular disease	Pregnancy Reno-vascular HT

*Beta-blockers may worsen heart failure, but may be used to treat heart failure.
[†]ACE inhibitors may be beneficial in chronic renal failure but should be used with caution under specialist supervision.
ACE, angiotensin-converting enzyme; COPD, chronic obstructive pulmonary disease; HT, hypertension; LV, left ventricular; ANGII, angiotensin II.

water transport across renal tubular cell membranes (Table 5.2). Diuretics are used in states of salt and water overload such as congestive heart failure (see Chapter 4), nephrotic syndrome and hepatic failure with ascites. The antihypertensive action is not related directly to diuretic efficacy, but upon more subtle alterations to the contractile responses of vascular smooth muscle. Thiazide diuretics are the preferred drugs for the treatment of hypertension. Loop diuretics, such

Table 5.2 Classification and site of action of diuretics.

	Site of action	Comment
Thiazides		
Bendroflumethiazide (bendrofluazide) Hydrochlorothiazide Chlortalidone (chlorthalidone)	Proximal part of the distal tubule	All have an antihypertensive effect. Little evidence that newer agents have any advantages over older established agents
Loop diuretics		
Furosemide (frusemide) Bumetanide	Ascending limb of loop of Henle	Effective diuretic and saliuretic but less useful for the treatment of hypertension
Potassium sparing diuretics		
Spironolactone	Distal tubule aldosterone antagonist	May be used in combination with loop diuretics in refractory oedema and can be useful for resistant hypertension
Triamterene	Sodium potassium exchange	May cause hyperkalaemia in renal failure or in the elderly

as furosemide, have greater diuretic efficacy but their effects on blood pressure are relatively short-acting and liable to provoke reflex stimulation of the renin–angiotensin system to counter any fall in blood pressure. They are useful in combination with ACE inhibitors or angiotensin 2 receptor blockers. Potassium-sparing diuretics are the least effective diuretics but their use is not associated with potassium loss, which occurs with both thiazide and loop diuretics. In refractory oedema these agents may be useful, but rarely necessary, in combination with the loop diuretics when hypokalaemia is problem. The antihypertensive effect of thiazide diuretics manifests at relatively low dosages and there is no additional benefit from higher doses in terms of blood pressure reduction. In contrast, it is possible to increase the diuretic response with higher dosages but this also leads to greater potassium loss and other metabolic changes. There is an increasing use of spironolactone which acts by blocking the aldosterone receptor in resistant hypertension.

Clinical pharmacology

Thiazides are well absorbed orally, widely distributed and subject to a variable amount of hepatic metabolism. The effects on the kidney depend upon excretion of drug into the renal tubule, and thiazide diuretics become less effective with increasing renal impairment, while loop diuretics retain some efficacy. With thiazides, the onset of the diuretic effect is usually observed within 1 hour and may last for about 12 hours, but with repeated dosing, the acute diuretic effect tends to diminish in the majority of hypertensive patients. The antihypertensive effect, however, is more gradual in onset and more long-lasting so that, at steady state, the antihypertensive effect persists for more than 24 hours and once-daily dosing is therefore appropriate for most agents.

Pharmacologically predictable adverse effects

Hypokalaemia
Severe hypokalaemia may precipitate cardiac arrhythmias (especially in patients also receiving digoxin). It may be necessary to provide potas-

sium supplements or to use a combination diuretic treatment with both a thiazide diuretic and a potassium-sparing diuretic. Persistent hypokalaemia with low-dose thiazide treatment should raise the suspicion of an underlying abnormality of potassium homeostasis such as mineralocorticoid excess (Conn's syndrome).

Hyperuricaemia
Thiazide diuretics interfere with the excretion of uric acid, and may result in an increased blood level of uric acid and, rarely, the provocation of acute gout.

Hyperglycaemia
Long-term diuretic therapy is associated with an impairment of glucose tolerance and an increased incidence of non-insulin-dependent diabetes mellitus, particularly if used in combination with beta-blockers. The mechanism appears to be mainly related to interference with the action of insulin in peripheral tissues (so-called 'insulin resistance'). This adverse effect is dose dependent and new onset diabetes is rare with current low doses of thiazides.

Hypercalcaemia
This is a rare adverse effect of thiazide diuretics resulting from reduced renal excretion of calcium.

Other adverse effects

Hyperlipidaemia
By mechanisms that are not entirely clear, long-term use of thiazide diuretics is associated with modest changes in the plasma lipid profile with increases in total and low-density lipoprotein (LDL) cholesterol, increases in triglycerides and a reduction in high-density lipoprotein (HDL) cholesterol.

Impotence
This is a well-recognised but occasional problem with long-term diuretic treatment especially at higher doses. The mechanism is not known and the problem is usually reversible on treatment withdrawal. However this is also a problem seen with other anti-hypertensives.

Others
Thrombocytopenia and skin rash occur rarely.

Clinical comment

Thiazide diuretics (for example, bendroflumethiazide 2.5 mg daily; hydrochlorothiazide 12.5 or 25 mg daily; chlortalidone (chlorthalidone) 12.5 or 25 mg daily) are widely used and are effective antihypertensive drugs in mild, moderate and severe hypertension. Where the hypertension is complicated by chronic renal failure (serum creatinine >150 mmol), or is proving refractory to treatment, it may be necessary to use a loop diuretic. If hypokalaemia is a problem a combination of diuretic with an ACE inhibitor or an angiotensin receptor antagonist is a very effective well-tolerated regimen. Serum potassium can rise in renal failure, when a potassium-sparing diuretic should be avoided. Potassium-sparing diuretics should be avoided or used with caution in combination with ACE inhibitors or angiotensin receptor antagonists.

Calcium antagonists

Mechanism of action
Increased peripheral vascular resistance depends upon increased constrictor 'tone' in peripheral blood vessels, which, in turn, reflects increased contractility of vascular smooth muscle. This process is calcium-dependent, and calcium antagonists (calcium entry blockers) are able to promote vasodilator activity by reducing calcium influx into the cell by interfering with the voltage-operated calcium channels (and to a lesser extent the receptor-operated channels) in the cell membrane of vascular smooth muscle.

Interference with intracellular calcium influx is also important in cardiac muscle, cardiac conducting tissue and the smooth muscle of the GI tract. Thus, the potential cardiac effects of calcium antagonism are negative inotropic, chronotropic and dromotropic activities and the GI effects lead to constipation. These effects vary with different agents according to the ability to penetrate cardiac and other tissues and, in particular, because the receptor or recognition site close to the calcium channel is slightly different for each drug class.

Thus, although they are often considered as a single class, there are structural and functional distinctions to be made between the three principal types of calcium antagonist drug:

1 Dihydropyridine derivatives: nifedipine, amlodipine
2 Phenylalkalamines: verapamil
3 Benzothiazipine derivatives: diltiazem

The dihydropyridine derivatives have pronounced peripheral vasodilator properties, whereas verapamil and diltiazem also have cardiac effects and reduce heart rate.

Clinical pharmacology
Most of these agents have low and variable oral bioavailability because all are subject to extensive first-pass metabolism. The exception is amlodipine which, although it is extensively metabolised, has a substantially longer half-life (more than 40 hours compared to less than 10 hours) (see Table 5.3).

Table 5.3 Clinical classification of calcium antagonist drugs.

Drugs		Half-life (h)	Dosing frequency
Dihydropyridines			
Short-acting	Nifedipine	4–6	Multiple*
	Nicardipine	4–6	
Intermediate	Isradipine	8–12	Once or twice daily
Long-acting	Amlodipine	>40	Once
	Nifedipine	(Special formulation)	Once
Verapamil		8–12	Multiple*
Diltiazem		6–10	Multiple*

*Unless special formulation.

Both diltiazem and verapamil have short half-lives because of extensive first-pass metabolism. During chronic treatment they have a tendency to inhibit hepatic drug metabolism and therefore their own half-lives during steady-state treatment are slightly longer than those following the first dose. This enzyme inhibitory effect is a potential source for drug interactions, e.g. with ciclosporin.

Pharmacologically predictable adverse effects

1 *Dihydropyridines*: These, particularly with rapid onset and short-acting agents, have a well-recognised pattern of vasodilator side effects with headache and facial flushing and an associated reflex activation of the sympathetic nervous system which provokes cardioacceleration and palpitations. These symptoms usually decline with time. Longer acting agents and the longer acting formulations are less likely to promote these acute vasodilator effects. Swelling of the ankles and occasionally of the hands is a long-term effect of the dihydropyridine derivatives, including the long-acting agents. This does not appear to be attributable to a generalised fluid retention and instead reflects a drug-related disturbance of the haemodynamics of the microcirculation in the periphery, plus the effect of gravity.

2 *Verapamil*: The early onset vasodilator effects are less common with verapamil but the cardiac effects may manifest as bradycardia or atrioventricular (AV) conduction delay. Constipation is a well-recognised symptomatic complaint.

3 *Diltiazem*: The early vasodilator effects are again less apparent but bradycardia and AV conduction effects are recognised. Skin rash occurs occasionally.

Clinical comment

All types of calcium-antagonist drugs are effective antihypertensive agents because of their peripheral vasodilator activity. The long-acting dihydropyridine drugs, such as amlodipine or others in long-acting once-daily formulations are generally preferred in the treatment of hypertension. The negative cardiac effects of diltiazem and vera-pamil lead to reduced myocardial oxygen demand such that these drugs tend to be the preferred types of calcium antagonist as monotherapy in angina (see Chapter 4). Dihydropyridine calcium antagonists may be useful in elderly patients with isolated systolic hypertension.

ACE inhibitors

Mechanism of action

ACE inhibitors inhibit competitively the activity of angiotensin-converting enzyme (which is also termed kininase II) to prevent the formation of the active octapeptide angiotensin II from its inactive precursor, angiotensin I. This occurs in blood and in tissues including the kidney, heart, blood vessels, adrenal gland and brain. Angiotensin II has a range of activities but most importantly it is a potent vasoconstrictor, it promotes aldosterone release and it facilitates sympathetic activity both centrally and peripherally. Whilst the reduction in blood pressure following ACE inhibition is greatest in patients with a stimulated renin–angiotensin system (such as in sodium depletion, or diuretic treatment, or renal artery stenosis or malignant phase hypertension), it is now recognised that ACE inhibitors also lower blood pressure in essential hypertensive patients with normal or low activity of the renin–angiotensin system.

The enzyme, kininase II, is also responsible for the breakdown of kinins that have vasodilator and other properties. Inhibition of ACE leads to an accumulation of kinins including bradykinin which promotes vasodilator activity and may make a contribution to the overall effectiveness of ACE inhibitor drugs.

Clinical pharmacology

All ACE inhibitor drugs are bound to tissues and plasma proteins and this gives rise to a characteristic concentration–time profile whereby free drug is relatively rapidly eliminated by the kidney, predominantly by glomerular filtration, such that there is little evidence of drug accumulation during chronic dosing. However, because of the binding to tissue sites the plasma drug

65

Table 5.4 Drugs acting on the renin–angiotensin system.

ACE inhibitors	Typical dose regimens
First generation	
Captopril	25 mg two or three times daily
Enalapril	5–20 mg once or twice daily
Lisinopril	5–20 mg once daily
Second generation	
Fosinopril	10–20 mg once daily
Perindopril	2–4 mg once daily
Quinapril	20–40 mg once or twice daily
Ramipril	2.5–5 mg daily
Trandolapril	1–2 mg daily

concentration–time profile shows a long-lasting terminal elimination phase of several days.

There are significant pharmacological differences between the ACE inhibitors. For example, the prototype drug captopril is absorbed rapidly but has a short duration of action and is usually administered twice or thrice daily. Enalapril, like many of the other later ACE inhibitors, is an inactive pro-drug that requires hydrolysis in vivo of the parent ester to its active acid form enalaprilat. Lisinopril is an analogue of enalapril and is itself active (see Table 5.4).

ACE inhibitors also vary in efficacy and duration of action with some but not others more suitable for once-daily dosing. The dose–response relationship for blood pressure reduction is linear initially, but a 'plateau' is quickly reached within the therapeutic dose range; further increases in dosage do not increase the intensity of effect, either on blood pressure reduction or on plasma ACE inhibition, but prolong the duration of action. The fall in blood pressure following ACE inhibition is not associated with a change in heart rate; in particular, there is no reflex tachycardia.

Pharmacologically predictable adverse effects

Hypotension may complicate the first dose of ACE inhibitor drugs especially in patients with sodium or volume depletion in whom the renin–angiotensin system is activated. This is less of a problem with newer longer acting ACE inhibitors. Hypotension occurs only rarely in uncomplicated essential hypertension but is more common in patients with cardiac failure.

Impairment of renal function is recognised particularly in patients with renovascular disease (bilateral renal artery stenosis). Reversible renal failure may be precipitated. However, ACE inhibitors can protect renal function in patients with chronic renal failure and hypertension.

Cough is the most frequent adverse effect and is probably attributable to the effect on the kinin system rather than upon ACE inhibition as it does not occur with angiotensin receptor antagonists (see later). A non-productive, irritant cough is widely reported in the treatment of hypertension in about 15% of patients. The reported incidence is considerably less in patients with cardiac failure, presumably as a reflection of their much higher background incidence of respiratory symptoms.

Other adverse effects

Angioneurotic oedema is a rare but well-recognised class effect that also has been attributed to the kinin potentiation. Increases in serum potassium and, occasionally, hyperkalaemia occur because ACE inhibitors have potassium-saving effects (mediated via the reduction in aldosterone). Taste disturbance and skin rash occur more frequently with captopril.

Clinical comment

Although many of these agents are recommended for once-daily dosing, for some such as enalapril or ramipril, a more consistent response is produced by twice-daily administration. In elderly patients, or in patients with compromised renal function, or in patients with cardiac failure, it is advisable to initiate treatment with lower than usual dosages. In general these drugs are well tolerated by patients. ACE inhibitor drugs combine well with thiazide diuretics, and with calcium antagonists, to produce overall antihypertensive effects that are additive. However, it is recommended that potassium supplements and potassium-sparing diuretics should not be used in combination because hyperkalaemia may result, especially if there is pre-existing renal impairment. Since the effectiveness of ACE inhibitors in both hypertension and cardiac failure may be compromised by non-steroidal anti-inflammatory drugs (NSAIDs), if possible, NSAIDs should be avoided in these patients. ACE inhibitors (and angiotensin receptor antagonists) are associated with a lower (25–30%) incidence of new onset diabetes compared to other classes.

Angiotensin (AT$_1$) receptor antagonists

Angiotensin II receptors are subclassified into two subtypes, AT$_1$ and AT$_2$. The AT$_1$-receptor mediates all of the classical pharmacological effects of angiotensin II, e.g. vasoconstriction and aldosterone release, whereas the functional role of the AT$_2$-receptor remains unclear. Because many tissues contain enzymatic pathways capable of converting angiotensin I to angiotensin II, independently of ACE, there are theoretical advantages in blocking the renin–angiotensin system via AT$_1$-receptor antagonism. Losartan was the first AT$_1$-receptor antagonist; irbesartan, valsartan, candesartan and others have followed (Table 5.5). All are well absorbed after oral administration but differ slightly in their pharmacokinetic and pharmacodynamic properties. Losartan is converted to an active metabolite, EXP 3174; candesartan is the active metabolite of the pro-drug candesartan cilexetil. Irbesartan, valsartan, candesartan and EXP 3174 bind to the AT$_1$-receptor in a manner which is competitive but only slowly surmountable, so the duration of blood pressure lowering effect is longer than the apparent half-life of the drug.

The angiotensin II antagonists produce reductions in blood pressure similar to ACE inhibitors and other antihypertensive classes, but they seem to be particularly well tolerated with very few side effects. Because AT$_1$-receptor antagonists do not influence kinin metabolism, these drugs are not associated with the dry cough seen with ACE inhibitors. Angiotensin II antagonists may also offer additional benefit to patients with type II diabetes complicated by hypertension and nephropathy and can be useful in congestive heart failure together with ACE inhibitors or in ACE I in tolerant patients. Like ACE inhibitor treatment, regimens based on AT$_1$-receptor antagonists reduce the risk of new onset diabetes. Since diabetes carries a huge risk of long-term cardiovascular complications, this is likely to represent a major advantage for drugs that block the renin–angiotensin system.

β-Adrenoceptor antagonists (beta-blockers)

Comment

Beta-blockers were, for many years, widely used as first or second line treatment of high blood pressure. There was evidence of improved outcome after long term treatment especially for cardiac complications. However more recent long term trials have found that treatment regimens based on beta-blockers were less successful than alternative approaches based on ACE inhibitors, angiotensin (AT1) antagonists or calcium antagonists. Beta-blocker regimens were also associated with an increase (25–30%) in new onset diabetes an additional potential risk factor. Beta-blockers are still used in hypertension but there use is targeted to patients with additional cardiac indications or those in whom the other first choice classes are ineffective or poorly tolerated.

Table 5.5 Angiotensin II (AT$_1$) receptor antagonists used in hypertension.

Drug	Pro-drug	Route of elimination	Half-life (h)
Losartan	Yes	Hepatic	6–9
Valsartan	No	Unchanged in urine	6
Irbesartan	No	Hepatic	15–17
Candesartan	Yes	Hepatic	6–12

Mechanism of action

Beta-blockers antagonise the effects of sympathetic nerve stimulation or circulating catecholamines. β-Adrenoceptors are widely distributed throughout the body systems and are subclassified as β_1- and β_2-receptors according to their location. β_1-Receptors are predominant in the heart and β_2-receptors are predominant in other organs such as the lung, peripheral blood vessels and skeletal muscle. This is a clinically useful subclassification but it is not absolutely accurate, for example, there are β_2-receptors in the heart and there are β_1-receptors in the kidney.

1 *Heart*: Stimulation of β_1-receptors in the sino-atrial node causes an increase in heart rate (a positive chronotropic effect) and stimulation of the β_1-receptors in the myocardium increases the force of cardiac contractility (a positive inotropic effect).

2 *Kidney*: Stimulation of β_1-receptors in the kidney promotes the release of renin from the juxtaglomerular cells and thereby increases the activity of the renin–angiotensin–aldosterone system.

3 *Central and peripheral nervous system*: Stimulation of β-receptors in the brainstem and stimulation of prejunctional β-receptors in the periphery promote the release of neurotransmitters and increased sympathetic nervous system activity.

β-Adrenoceptors are also found in the eye. β_2-Receptors control the formation of aqueous humour, and beta-blockers applied topically to the eye are used in the treatment of glaucoma. Beta-blockers may block both β_1-receptors (selective or cardioselective) and blockers.

Clinical pharmacology

Beta-blockers vary in the extent to which they are eliminated via the kidney or via the liver, usually with extensive first-pass metabolism (Table 5.6). The lipid-soluble beta-blockers, such as propranolol, typically depend upon hepatic metabolism for their clearance, whereas the relatively water-soluble beta-blockers, e.g. atenolol, are eliminated via the kidney. Propranolol is often quoted as a reference example of a drug that undergoes extensive first-pass hepatic metabolism: this is flow-limited because it is directly dependent upon hepatic blood flow (see Chapter 1). Thus, particularly for drugs eliminated by the liver, a wide range of doses will be required in clinical practice because of the wide inter-individual variability in bioavailability combined with the inter-individual variability in response. The half-life of most beta-blockers is relatively short: those which depend upon the liver usually require multiple daily dosing, whereas those eliminated via the kidney tend to have longer half-lives and may be suitable for once-daily administration, particularly at high doses.

Clinical class	Approved name	β_1– selectivity	Major route of elimination
Non-selective	Propranolol	–	Liver
Selective	Atenolol	++	Kidney
	Bisoprolol	++	Liver/kidney
	Metoprolol	++	Liver
Additional properties			
Intrinsic sympathomimetic activity (also, partial agonist activity)	Pindolol	–	Liver
Anti-arrhythmic properties	Sotalol	–	Liver
Dual antihypertensive mechanism	Labetalol	–	Liver

Table 5.6 Examples of the pharmacological properties and route of elimination of some beta-blockers in clinical use.

Pharmacologically predictable adverse effects of β-receptor blockade

Bradycardia and impairment of myocardial contractility

An excessive reduction in heart rate and bradycardia is relatively common but seldom symptomatic. Rarely, an excessive reduction in inotropic activity may precipitate or exacerbate cardiac failure in a susceptible individual. Whilst these depressant effects on cardiac function are occasionally deleterious, they also lead to a reduction in cardiac work and a reduction in myocardial oxygen demand which contributes to the anti-anginal efficacy of these agents (see Chapter 4). Although acutely beta-blockers can worsen left ventricular dysfunction, there is now good evidence that, under specialist supervision, β-adrenoceptor antagonists may improve symptoms and prolong survival in patients with congestive heart failure.

Peripheral vasoconstriction

The β2-receptors in the smooth muscle of peripheral blood vessels subserve a vasodilator role, especially in skeletal muscle beds, and blockade of these receptors leads to a relative vasoconstriction which typically gives rise to impairment of the peripheral circulation with cold hands and feet and, possibly, also the development of Raynaud's phenomenon or the worsening of peripheral vascular disease. This is usually a problem only in critical ischaemia. Because of unnecessary concerns, many patients have been denied the benefits of beta-blockers.

CNS effects

Blockade of CNS β-receptors is associated with reduced sympathetic outflow, which is the probable cause of a sense of malaise which may occur insidiously during long-term treatment. Additionally, vivid dreams, nightmares and, rarely, hallucinations may occur with highly lipid-soluble beta-blockers, and propranolol in particular, because of their greater penetration into the CNS.

Bronchospasm

β2-Receptors mediate dilatation of the bronchi, and blockade of these receptors may precipitate bronchospasm in susceptible individuals. Asthma is an absolute contraindication for all beta-blockers which should be used with caution in chronic obstructive pulmonary disease with significant reversibility. In patients with less severe chest disease, beta-blockers can be used without concern.

Tiredness and fatigue

Stimulation of β2-receptors in skeletal muscle is associated with increased muscle activity and blockade of these receptors leads to a sense of tiredness and ready fatigue during exercise.

Masking of hypoglycaemia

The awareness of hypoglycaemia in individuals with Type 1 Diabetes mellitus depends partly upon sympathetic nervous activation. This response will be blunted by beta-blockers. This effect is marginal with cardioselective beta-blockers.

Metabolic disturbances

Beta-blockers, especially non-selective agents, increase triglycerides and reduce HDL cholesterol. Beta-blockers in long-term use increase the frequency of diabetes mellitus, particularly in combination with thiazide diuretics.

Additional pharmacological characteristics

1 Partial agonist activity (sometimes known as intrinsic sympathomimetic activity) manifests as a beta-stimulant effect when background adrenergic activity is minimal (e.g. during sleep) but the drug's beta-blocker effect manifests when adrenergic activity is increased (e.g. during exercise).

2 Membrane-stabilising activity: This is a local anaesthetic and anti-arrhythmic effect.

3 Selectivity: The prototype beta-blocker, propranolol, is non-selective as it blocks the responses mediated via both β1- and β2-receptors. Because many of the potential adverse effects are mediated through β2-receptors and many of the desirable effects require blockade of β1-receptors in the heart, there has been the development of relatively β1-selective (or cardioselective) blockers. It is important to recognise, however, that this selectivity is not absolute. Selectivity is lost at high doses.

4 Additional pharmacological properties: It is possible to augment the beta-blocker molecule with an ability to also block effects mediated through peripheral α-adrenoceptors (e.g. labetalol and carvedilol) or to harness some β_2-agonist or direct vasodilator activity (e.g. celiprolol).

Clinical comment

All beta-blockers, irrespective of their additional characteristics, lower blood pressure to a similar extent. In hypertension those which are β_1-selective (cardioselective) and which can be administered once daily tend to be preferred, e.g. bisoprolol 10 mg daily, atenolol 25–100 mg daily. Irrespective of their apparent 'cardioselectivity', these drugs are contraindicated in people with asthma and should be introduced with caution in patients at risk of cardiac failure.

In addition to use in hypertension, beta-blockers are also used to treat the following conditions: cardiac failure, supraventricular cardiac arrhythmias, angina pectoris, anxiety neurosis, thyrotoxicosis, migraine and glaucoma. There is also some evidence that prophylactic treatment with propranolol reduces the risk of gastrointestinal (GI) bleeding among patients with chronic liver disease and proven oesophageal varices.

α_1-Antagonists

Prazosin and doxazosin act via selective blockade of peripheral α_1-adrenoceptors to produce their vasodilator effects but they are not widely used first-line agents. There is less clear evidence of reduction in cardiovascular risk when these agents are used. Instead they tend to be used as third-line agents or where other drugs are poorly tolerated.

Alpha-blockers may be associated with a 'first dose' hypotensive effect that constitutes a postural fall in blood pressure after the initial dosage, accompanied by reflex cardioacceleration and palpitations. In susceptible patients who cannot maintain a rapid heart rate there is the risk of a vago–vagal collapse leading to syncope. This first-dose effect was particularly associated with the short-acting prototype agent prazosin and is much

less of a problem with longer acting agents such as doxazosin.

Centrally acting agents

Agents acting on α_2-adrenoceptors, or related imidazoline receptors in the brainstem, reduce sympathetic outflow and lead to a reduction in blood pressure.

Clonidine is an α_2-adrenoceptor agonist that can cause sedation and drowsiness, dry mouth and interference with sexual function in men. In addition, this agent may give rise to a rebound hypertensive syndrome on abrupt cessation of treatment at high dose, presumably as a consequence of receptor up-regulation.

Methyldopa, which acts via its active metabolite α-methylnoradrenaline, has a profile similar to that of clonidine but in addition is known to give rise to immunological side effects, including pyrexia, hepatitis and, rarely, haemolytic anaemia.

These centrally acting agents are no longer used widely because of poor side effect profiles (particularly CNS depressant effects) and because of the development of newer, comparably effective but better-tolerated alternative agents. However, methyldopa is still used to treat hypertension in pregnancy, especially where hypertension precedes pregnancy or is identified in the first or middle trimester. This is justified by the long-term experience of maternal, fetal and later developmental safety. More recently centrally acting agents have been developed which preferentially bind to imidazoline binding sites in brain. Agents such as moxonidine are reported to have fewer adverse effects although dry mouth remains a problem; moxonidine is used mainly as third-line therapy. These drugs have not been studied in long-term outcome trials.

Hypertensive emergencies

There are no indications for the rapid (within seconds or minutes) reduction of blood pressure, even where there is severe hypertension and related complications. However, there are some indications for the controlled and progressive reduction of blood pressure (over a period of a few hours) when accelerated or malignant phase hypertension is complicated by hypertensive encephalopathy or acute left ventricular failure, or in other situations such as dissection of the aorta or in eclampsia of pregnancy.

In severe cases, with the above complications, there may be grounds for intravenous treatment that is titrated to produce a gradual and progressive reduction in blood pressure. The preferred agents are glyceryl trinitrate or sodium nitroprusside by infusion where the rate of the infusion can be controlled, minute by minute, according to the blood pressure response. The infusion of glyceryl trinitrate is not associated with significant adverse effects beyond those predicted by the blood pressure reduction, but with sodium nitroprusside there is the additional potential complication of thiocyanate accumulation and cyanide poisoning, especially in patients with impaired renal function. For this reason, and especially with sodium nitroprusside, these manoeuvres should only be undertaken in the setting of an intensive care unit with appropriate monitoring facilities.

Cholesterol and lipids

Aim

The overall aim of lipid-modifying treatment is to reduce the circulating levels of atherogenic lipids in order to slow, reverse or ideally prevent the development of atherosclerotic vascular lesions and thereby reduce the long-term risk of cardiovascular disease.

Relevant pathophysiology

Cholesterol is a major component of lipid-containing atherosclerotic plaques. Raised plasma levels of cholesterol – and related lipid disturbances – have been identified as a major risk factor (along with smoking and hypertension) for atherosclerotic cardiovascular disease and its consequences, particularly myocardial infarction. Cholesterol is derived both from the diet and by endogenous synthesis in the liver and it is a com-

ponent of all cell membranes, a precursor of steroid hormones and bile salts, and of glycoproteins and quinones.

The biochemistry and metabolism of cholesterol are complex. Cholesterol, and other lipid fractions, are transported in blood via lipoproteins of different densities. Increased total cholesterol and its major component fraction, LDL cholesterol, have been linked to accelerated atherosclerosis and increased coronary artery disease. LDL cholesterol is cleared from the circulation by specific receptors on the cell surface and the function of these receptors plays an important role in determining the plasma levels of LDL cholesterol. In contrast, HDL cholesterol appears to have a protective and anti-atherogenic effect because it is involved in the mobilisation of cholesterol from tissues and its transportation back to the liver.

Primary and secondary lipid disorders

Disorders of lipid metabolism occur as primary conditions that may be familial or polygenic in origin, or secondary to an underlying disease state or drug treatment.

Familial hypercholesterolaemia

Very high levels of LDL cholesterol occur in this rare genetic disease which involves the failure to express LDL receptors. It is inherited as an autosomal dominant condition such that homozygotes have no LDL receptors and heterozygotes have only 50% of the normal number of LDL receptors. In this condition LDL cholesterol (and therefore total cholesterol) is very high, and in the homozygotes there will be no response to drug treatments that exert their lipid-lowering effects via the up-regulation of LDL receptors. In such patients it may be necessary to remove cholesterol by physical techniques such as apheresis using LDL affinity columns.

Polygenic lipid disorders

This is by far the most common type of primary lipid disorder and reflects a variety of factors including a non-specific genetic predisposition, dietary factors such as high calorie and saturated fat intake and lifestyle influences including physical inactivity. In the most common pattern there are moderate increases in LDL and total cholesterol. This is the commonest lipid disorder found in westernised populations. In part, the disturbed lipid profile reflects down-regulation of LDL receptors.

Secondary lipid disorders

These manifest as mixed elevations of cholesterol and triglycerides in response to underlying diseases such as hypothyroidism, nephrotic syndrome and diabetes mellitus, as a manifestation of chronic alcohol abuse, or in response to drug treatments such as thiazide diuretics and beta-blockers.

Risks of hypercholesterolaemia

The central role of cholesterol in the development of atheroma and atherosclerotic cardiovascular disease is well established. The epidemiological evidence from population studies in different countries and from within the same country identify clear associations between both LDL and total cholesterol and the development of cardiovascular disease, particularly CHD. There are also weaker associations with elevated triglycerides and an inverse relationship with HDL cholesterol.

Benefits of lipid-lowering treatment

A number of large placebo-controlled randomised clinical trials have been performed to examine the effects of cholesterol-lowering therapy in the primary and secondary prevention of cardiovascular disease. Primary prevention refers to patients who might have one or more cardiovascular risk factors, but in whom overt atherosclerotic disease has not presented clinically. Secondary prevention refers to those patients who have, for example, suffered an acute myocardial infarction or who have angina or intermittent claudication. Clinical trials using statins to lower cholesterol have shown 30–40% reductions in coronary heart disease events in both primary and secondary prevention studies. Cholesterol-lowering therapy also reduces the risk of stroke. The absolute benefits of treatment are proportional to the magnitude of cholesterol reduction and the pre-treatment cardiovascular risk in an individual patient.

Principles of lipid-lowering treatment

1 Detection: Hypercholesterolaemia can be identified in patients at risk by the measurement of total cholesterol in a non-fasting blood sample. Although a more accurate assessment of the lipid profile can be obtained from a fasting blood sample that can be subfractionated to measure the triglyceride concentration and the HDL and LDL cholesterol fractions, random not fasting lipids are increasingly used to guide treatment in practice.

2 Patients should be counselled about hypercholesterolaemia, and its risk, and the relevance of other concomitant risk factors. The reason for long-term treatment should be carefully explained.

3 Hypercholesterolaemia should be treated as part of a management plan for reducing all identifiable cardiovascular risk factors in the 'at risk' patient and management decision based on overall cardiovascular risk assessment.

4 Secondary types of lipid disorder: These should be identified in order to undertake the specific treatment and management for the underlying condition. Thus, further investigations should be undertaken to exclude significant renal or hepatic disease, hypothyroidism, diabetes mellitus, or alcohol abuse or relevant drug treatments.

5 Non-pharmacological treatment should always be used initially and this centres around dietary modification.

Lipid-lowering treatment

Dietary and lifestyle advice

The principles of dietary advice revolve around the reduced intake of saturated animal fats and, in the obese patient, a reduced total calorie intake. In addition, it is desirable to increase the intake of unsaturated fats and, where possible, increase the level of physical activity. Ideally, dietary modification should be planned in discussion with the partner, or other members of the family, and it should take account of some of the social, cultural and economic circumstances of each patient. In a compliant and motivated patient total cholesterol may be reduced by about 10% within a few months of adherence to dietary modification, but in the long term, it is unusual for patients to be able to maintain or exceed this magnitude of change.

Lipid-lowering drugs

There are several different drugs available for cholesterol reduction and modification of the plasma lipid profile. The major classes in widespread use include 3-hydroxy-3-methoxyglutaryl coenzyme A (HMG CoA) reductase inhibitors ('statins'), fibrates, and bile acid sequestrant resins (see Table 5.7).

HMG CoA reductase inhibitors

Mechanism

HMG CoA reductase is the rate-limiting enzyme in the hepatic synthesis of cholesterol and inhibition leads to reduced cholesterol production and, as a consequence, an attempt by the liver to compensate by increasing its extraction of LDL cholesterol from plasma by up-regulating its LDL cholesterol receptors. The principal effect, therefore, is a re-

Table 5.7 Summary of the actions of lipid-lowering drugs.

Drug	LDL	HDL	Triglycerides
HMG CoA reductase inhibitors	↓↓	↑	→
Fibrates	↓	↑	↓
Resins	↓	→	→
Nicotinic acid	↓	↑	↓
Ezetemibe	↓	↑	→

LDL, low-density lipoprotein; HDL, high-density lipoprotein.

duction of LDL cholesterol (and, thereby, total cholesterol) by up to 40%, and there are only modest effects on the other lipid fractions. Some statin drugs also lower triglyceride levels by 15%. Because cholesterol is synthesised mainly during sleep, these drugs are usually administered at night. HMG CoA reductase inhibitors comprise the family of 'statins' – simvastatin, pravastatin, atorvastatin, fluvastatin and rosuvastatin. While the statins clearly have a major action via lowering LDL cholesterol, there are increasing indications that other mechanisms particularly anti-inflammatory effect may also be important in stabilising atheroma plaques and reducing cardiovascular events.

Side effects reported include headache, GI symptoms and non-cardiac chest pain. Raised liver enzymes can also occur. Rarely rash and hypersensitivity reactions have been reported. The most troublesome side effects are myalgia, muscle cramps and occasionally life-threatening rhabdomyolysis. These symptoms are more common at higher doses and when statin is combined with fibrates, nicotinic acid or immunosuppressants. In severe cases the creatinine kinase in blood is raised.

Clinical comment

The impressive clinical evidence from large randomised clinical trials that statin therapy reduces cardiovascular mortality and morbidity in both primary and secondary prevention has led to a dramatic increase in prescribing. From a public health and cost-effectiveness perspective, the challenge has been to target statin therapy at the higher risk patients, i.e. those who will benefit most from cholesterol reduction. Current guidelines in the United Kingdom advocate statin therapy regardless of total cholesterol levels following an acute myocardial infarction and for those patients with angina. There is also evidence for intensive lowering of cholesterol with high dose statin in particular patient groups, e.g. in acute coronary syndromes. For primary prevention the strategy has been to advocate statin therapy for patients who have an absolute risk of a cardiovascular event of 2% or more per year (20% 10-year risk). Various tables have been produced to allow clinicians to quickly risk-stratify an individual patient by entering basic clinical information, e.g. age, smoking status, cholesterol level and blood pressure. Thus, the decision to initiate statin therapy for primary prevention is not based solely on the level of cholesterol, but also on an overall clinical assessment of an individual patient's absolute cardiovascular risk. This approach is supported by the results of prospective studies like the Heart Protection Study which confirmed the benefit of a statin across a wide (including 'normal') range of cholesterol in high-risk patients.

Fibrates

These drugs lower LDL cholesterol by about 20% and they also cause a significant reduction in total triglycerides and an increase in HDL cholesterol. They have a number of effects on lipid metabolism including the activation of lipoprotein lipase to promote lipolysis of triglyceride-rich particles, which reduces the levels of triglyceride, and they may also inhibit HMG CoA reductase and promote a consequential up-regulation of LDL receptor activity. Bezafibrate and gemfibrozil are examples of fibrates in widespread use and there is evidence (with gemfibrozil) that CHD events can be reduced as part of a primary prevention strategy. As a group, these drugs are absorbed completely from the GI tract and are excreted largely unchanged via the kidney, but are liable to cause GI side effects and there is potential for drug interactions, most notably with oral anticoagulants.

The side effects most commonly associated with fibrates are GI upsets, headaches, fatigue and skin reactions. Less commonly, muscle cramps and loss of libido are reported. The fibrates as a class are thought to increase bile lithogenicity and, although this has not been conclusively demonstrated with the modern agents, these drugs should be regarded as relatively contraindicated in those patients with gall bladder disease or with a strong family history of gallstones.

Bile acid sequestrant resins

Resins such as colestyramine are not absorbed from the GI tract and as a consequence bind bile salts to prevent their normal enterohepatic recirculation. Hence, hepatic cholesterol synthesis increases and the receptor-mediated uptake of LDL cholesterol from plasma is also increased. The resins primarily lower LDL cholesterol and total cholesterol with associated small increases in HDL cholesterol but no effect on triglycerides. The adverse GI effects of the resins cause major symptomatic problems that few patients are able to tolerate when large doses are administered. For this reason, there is also a significant incidence of poor compliance or non-compliance. The taste and texture of the resins are unpleasant. Symptomatic adverse effects are confined to the GI tract with dyspepsia, flatulence and altered bowel habit. Use with statins may increase the risk of cramps and myositis.

Ezetimibe

This agent blocks intestinal absorption of cholesterol and can augment the effects of statin if given in combination. It may also be useful where statin is contraindicated or not tolerated in high doses. This agent appears to be better tolerated than bile acid sequestrants. Although this agent has been shown to lower cholesterol levels there has as yet been no evidence, unlike the statins, that they improve cardiovascular outcomes.

Other lipid-lowering drugs

Nicotinic acid and its derivatives are potent inhibitors of LDL and VLDL formation; probucol lowers LDL cholesterol but also inhibits the production of HDL cholesterol, although the significance of this latter effect remains to be established.

Fish oils, high in unsaturated fatty acids, are particularly useful for reducing excessively high triglyceride concentrations. Both omega-3 acid ethyl esters and marine triglycerides are available.

Antiplatelet drugs

Approach to the management of thrombosis

Both antiplatelet drugs and anticoagulants are effective in prevention of arterial, cardiac and venous thromboembolism. Antiplatelet drugs are preferred for routine cardiovascular prevention, because they are less likely to cause excessive bleeding. However, anticoagulants are more effective in treatment of venous thromboembolism and peripheral arterial embolism and are indicated in specific circumstances such as atrial fibrillation. Thrombolytic agents have a main role in the treatment of acute thrombotic arterial occlusion, especially coronary thrombosis. Anticoagulants, heparin products and thrombolytics are described in Chapter 18.

There are many potential targets for drug action in the biochemical pathways involved in platelet activation. Aspirin is cheap and effective and has been the drug of choice; clopidogrel and dipyridamole are other options.

Aspirin

Pharmacology

All of the pharmacological effects of aspirin (acetylsalicylic acid) are based upon inhibition of prostaglandin synthesis. Aspirin is used as an antiplatelet drug in doses lower than those employed for analgesia. Aspirin acetylates and inactivates cyclo-oxygenase, a key enzyme in the platelet biosynthetic pathway for the pro-aggregatory prostaglandin thromboxane A_2. The interaction of aspirin with cyclo-oxygenase is irreversible. As platelets are anucleate, recovery of thromboxane synthesis is dependent on the appearance of a new platelet population in the circulation. Recovery from the effects of aspirin therefore takes about 10 days. Aspirin also inhibits endothelial cyclo-oxygenase, in this case leading to a reduction in prostacyclin synthesis, an effect that would be theoretically undesirable. A predominant effect on thromboxane synthesis is

achieved because the endothelium can regenerate cyclo-oxygenase activity. Differential sensitivity of the platelet and endothelial enzymes, and pre-systemic hydrolysis of aspirin, limiting endothelial exposure to active drug, may also contribute to the achievement of some selectivity of action (see below). The lower the dose of aspirin, the greater the differential effect; but no dose at which useful inhibition of thromboxane synthesis is achieved is absolutely selective. In practice, aspirin doses of 75–300 mg/day appear as effective as higher doses in thrombosis prevention, and have fewer GI side effects.

Effects on haemostasis

Administration of aspirin results in prolongation of the skin bleeding time and a characteristic defect on testing platelet aggregation in the laboratory. As would be expected, coagulation tests are unaltered by aspirin. Very large doses of aspirin, e.g. in overdose, can, however, lead to a variable prolongation of the prothrombin time.

Pharmacokinetics

Aspirin, in standard formulation, is rapidly absorbed from the upper GI tract including both the stomach and duodenum. Slow-release formulations are available which have delayed and incomplete absorption characteristics. Aspirin undergoes extensive pre-systemic hydrolysis to salicylate. Platelet cyclo-oxygenase may therefore be irreversibly inhibited as platelets pass through the portal circulation, whilst the endothelium on the systemic side of the circulation is exposed to smaller concentrations of active aspirin.

Clinical use of aspirin

Low-dose aspirin has been shown to be clinically beneficial in acute myocardial infarction, unstable angina and acute ischaemic stroke; in the secondary prevention of arterial thrombosis; and in prevention of arterial, venous and cardiac thrombosis in persons at increased risk (see Table 5.8). There are several general points of importance.

Table 5.8 Clinical conditions in which low-dose aspirin is of proven benefit.

Myocardial infarction (acute and chronic)
Unstable angina
Ischaemic stroke (acute and chronic)
Transient cerebral ischaemia
Peripheral vascular arterial disease
Post-coronary artery bypass graft
Post-peripheral arterial surgery
Atrial fibrillation
Prophylaxis of venous thromboembolism
Primary prevention of cardiovascular disease in high-risk patients (e.g. risk $\geq$2% per year)

1 'Low-dose' aspirin refers to a range of doses from 75 to 300 mg daily. Doses less than 100 mg require several days to produce their full effects on thromboxane synthesis. Hence a loading dose of 150–300 mg/day is given in acute myocardial infarction, unstable angina and acute ischaemic stroke.

2 Presentation with one form of arterial disease is often associated with risk of another form of vascular disease on which aspirin may have an impact. For example, treatment of a patient with a transient ischaemic attack reduces not only the risk of ischaemic stroke, but also of myocardial infarction and death from other vascular causes.

3 In acute myocardial infarction, it has been shown that administration of aspirin has additive effects with streptokinase in reduction of mortality.

4 Cerebral haemorrhage should be excluded by brain scanning before administering (or continuing) aspirin to a patient presenting with a stroke.

5 In patients with acute ischaemic stroke who are unable to swallow, aspirin may be given per rectum.

Adverse effects of aspirin

1 Gastric erosions and GI bleeding. GI toxicity constitutes the main adverse effect of aspirin. This includes dyspepsia, ulceration and GI bleeding (one excess major bleed per 500 patient-years use). It is related to inhibition of prostaglandin synthe-sis in the GI tract as well as to the antiplatelet effects of aspirin. The GI effects are dose related, and incidence is reduced but not eliminated by the use of lower doses.

2 Hypersensitivity reactions.

3 Precipitation of asthma.

4 Precipitation of renal failure, especially in patients with renal artery stenosis and in patients taking ACE inhibitor drugs.

5 Intracranial haemorrhage (one per 2500 patient-years).

Contraindications

1 Peptic ulcer or GI haemorrhage

2 Underlying bleeding disorders, congenital or acquired (including anticoagulant therapy)

3 Severe renal or hepatic impairment

4 Known hypersensitivity to aspirin

5 Intracranial haemorrhage or aneurysm

6 Uncontrolled hypertension (risk of intracranial haemorrhage).

Clopidogrel

Clopidogrel is an antiplatelet drug that has a different mechanism of action on platelets to aspirin. It has an active metabolite that irreversibly modifies the platelet ADP receptor, reducing the aggregability of platelets for the remainder of their lifespan. A dose of 75 mg/day is used clinically, which reduces platelet aggregability and prolongs the skin bleeding time to a similar extent as low-dose aspirin (75–300 mg/day). A large study showed that clopidogrel was at least as effective as aspirin in reducing the risk of arterial thrombosis in patients with recent myocardial infarction, recent ischaemic stroke, or chronic peripheral arterial disease. Clopidogrel was also as safe as aspirin, with a lower risk of dyspepsia and GI bleeding, but a higher risk of diarrhoea and skin rash. As it is more expensive than aspirin, the main indication is secondary prevention of arterial thrombosis in patients who are intolerant of aspirin or in whom aspirin is contraindicated. The combination of clopidogrel and aspirin appears more effective than aspirin alone (or anticoagulants) in prevention of thrombosis following coronary angioplasty with stenting. There is a recognised and important drug interaction with reduced efficacy of clopidogrel when used in combination with the proton pump inhibitor omeprazole.

Dipyridamole

Dipyridamole is a vasodilator drug that provokes myocardial ischaemia and is used in cardiac stress testing: it is therefore contraindicated in patients with angina. It was observed to reduce platelet aggregation in whole blood but not in plasma: it may act by reducing red blood cell uptake of adenosine, a circulating endogenous platelet inhibitor. Dipyridamole (100 mg thrice daily, or 200 mg sustained release twice daily) appears similarly effective to aspirin in secondary prevention of stroke, but has been less extensively evaluated, is more expensive and has vasodilator side effects including headache. It may be used in secondary prevention

of stroke or transient cerebral ischaemia in patients who are intolerant of aspirin or in whom aspirin is contraindicated. Whether or not the combination of dipyridamole and aspirin is more effective than aspirin alone in secondary prevention of cardiovascular events after stroke or transient cerebral ischaemia is controversial.

Glycoprotein IIb/IIIa receptor antagonists

The final common pathway of platelet aggregation is the exposure in activated platelets of membrane glycoprotein IIb/IIIa receptors, which are linked by fibrinogen in platelet aggregation. Several antagonists of this receptor are currently under investigation as antithrombotic agents. Abciximab is a monoclonal antibody that blocks this receptor: it is used as a single intravenous injection in prevention of thrombosis following high-risk coronary angioplasty.

Chapter 6

Drugs used to treat respiratory disease

Introduction

The most frequently encountered respiratory diseases in a general medical setting are chronic obstructive pulmonary disease (COPD), asthma, respiratory tract infection, lung cancer, bronchiectasis, interstitial lung disease and pulmonary embolic disease. Respiratory tract infections including pneumonia are discussed in Chapter 9.

Asthma

The main features of asthma are:
- wheeze, variable breathlessness, cough; reversible airflow obstruction (>15% reversibility to inhaled bronchodilator or >15% variability in mean peak flow).

The disease is characterised by:
- respiratory tract inflammation with increased eosinophils and mast cells; damage to the airway epithelium; and in chronic disease, remodelling of the airway wall with increased smooth muscle mass and matrix deposition.

Therapy is aimed at minimising symptoms and inflammation when patients are stable and treating acute exacerbations.

Chronic obstructive pulmonary disease

The main features of COPD are:
- Exercise-related breathlessness with relatively little day-to-day variability.
- Fixed airflow obstruction with little or no reversibility to bronchodilator treatment.
- Cough with sputum production is a variable feature but prominent in some patients. Histologically there may be destruction of the lung parenchyma (emphysema) and/or structural changes to the airway wall resulting in airflow obstruction.

Therapy is aimed at maximising any bronchodilator response and treating acute exacerbations.

Greater than 90% of COPD in developed countries is related to smoking. Lung function decline on average occurs 2–3 times more rapidly in smokers than in non-smokers, and smoking cessation results in lung function decline reverting to the rate of non-smokers. Breathlessness is very variable and may not relate well to lung function with some patients having well-maintained exercise tolerance despite markedly reduced Forced Expiratory Volume in 1 second (FEV_1) values. In addition to the pharmacological interventions listed below, surgical intervention may improve symptoms in a small number of patients with severe air-flow obstruction who are suitable for lung volume reduction surgery or lung transplantation. Both asthma

Lecture Notes: Clinical Pharmacology and Therapeutics, 8th edition. By Gerard McKay, John Reid and Matthew Walters. Published 2010 by Blackwell Publishing Ltd.

and COPD are common conditions and may co-exist.

Management of asthma and COPD

National Guidelines exist in most countries on the management of asthma and COPD (e.g. see www.brit-thoracic.org.uk), and are sub-divided into the management of acute and chronic disease.

Many of the drugs used are common to both asthma and COPD, are delivered by several inhaler devices. There are two main ways of administering inhaled drugs:

1 as a suspension via a metered dose inhaler (MDI),

or

2 as a dry powder

Asthma and COPD are treated in a stepwise approach with several therapies. Below, the management of chronic (stable) asthma and COPD is approached first, and discussions regarding therapy are considered by drug class.

Treatment of chronic airways disease

Clinical scenario

A 70-year-old male presents with several years of worsening breathlessness, wheeze and non-productive cough. He had asthma as a child and suffers from hayfever. He has smoked 20 cigarettes a day for 50 years. Examination is unremarkable and spirometry shows moderate airflow obstruction. The differential lies between COPD and chronic asthma. What drugs can be used to treat this condition?

Bronchodilators

β_2-Adrenoceptor agonists

Mechanism of action

β_2-Adrenoceptor agonists act by stimulating the β_2-adrenoceptor present on airway smooth muscle and other structural cells in the airway. Stimulation of the β_2-adrenoceptor results in activation of

Table 6.1 β-Adrenoceptor agonists in asthma.

SABAs	LABAs
Salbutamol (Albuterol)	Salmeterol
Terbutaline	Formoterol
Fenoterol	

adenylyl cyclase and subsequent elevation of intracellular cyclic adenosine monophosphate (cAMP). This produces a range of downstream effects depending on the cell type, the most important of which is relaxation of airway smooth muscle which results in bronchodilation.

Pharmacokinetics

There are two main groups of β_2-adrenoceptor agonists, short-acting β_2-agonists (SABAs) and long-acting β_2-agonists (LABAs). A list of the most commonly prescribed drugs is given in Table 6.1.

These drugs are administered by the inhaled route and, in acute exacerbations of asthma or COPD), via nebuliser. Intravenous infusion of salbutamol is also used in acute asthma. Onset of bronchodilation with SABAs is within 1–2 minutes and sustained for 4–6 hours. LABAs produce sustained bronchodilation over a 12-hour period. Formoterol also has a rapid onset of action, whilst salmeterol, which is a partial agonist, has a slower onset of action of around 20 minutes.

Adverse effects

β_2-agonists produce hypokalaemia (via β_2-receptor-mediated effects on sodium-potassium exchange), tachycardia (via direct effects on the heart) and tremor. These effects are dose-related and are more severe with intravenous administration compared with inhaled administration.

There has been concern over possible links between monotherapy with β-agonists in asthma and increased exacerbations and (very rarely) death. SABAs should therefore be used on an as-required basis and LABAs should only be used in combination with an inhaled steroid in patients with asthma (see below).

Interactions

The only clinically important interaction occurs when these drugs are used in conjunction with theophylline which may worsen tachycardia and rarely produce supraventricular or ventricular arrhythmias.

Clinical use

β_2-Adrenoceptor agonists are the mainstay bronchodilators used for symptom control both in asthma and COPD. They are much more effective in asthma than in COPD because of the reversible nature of bronchoconstriction evident most asthmatics. SABAs should be used as required to relieve symptoms although they may be taken in advance of exercise in those asthmatics prone to exercise-induced bronchoconstriction. Further guidance on usage can be found in the guidelines shown in the text boxes 'Main groups of drugs used to treat airflow obstruction' and 'Drug treatment of asthma'. Asthmatics requiring SABAs more than once a day on an average should also be prescribed inhaled steroids (see step 2 in guidelines). As mentioned above LABAs should not be prescribed as monotherapy in asthmatics.

Key points – main groups of drugs used to treat airflow obstruction

- β-Adrenoceptor agonists, which increase cAMP in airway smooth muscle cells and mast cells
- Theophylline and related methylxanthines, which also increase intracellular cAMP by inhibiting phosphodiesterase, the enzyme that breaks down cAMP (whether this is their main mode of action is less certain)
- Antimuscarinic drugs, which inhibit cholinergic (vagal) bronchoconstriction
- 'Anti-allergy' drugs, which inhibit the production, release or effects of bronchoconstrictor or inflammatory mediators
- Corticosteroids, which reduce the inflammatory response in asthma in particular; the precise mechanism(s) underlying their action are unknown but reducing the release of inflammatory cytokines is probably important

---

Key points – escalation of drug treatment of stable/chronic asthma

Step 1	This is the use of an inhaled β_2-receptor agonist (one or two puffs a day) for patients with very mild or occasional asthma.
Step 2	For patients needing more than one or two doses of an inhaled β_2-agonist per day, the addition of inhaled prophylactic therapy is required, i.e. low dose of inhaled steroid, sodium cromoglicate or nedocromil sodium. Inhaled steroids are the most effective of these prophylactic agents.
Step 3	If symptoms persist substitute inhaled steroid for a combination steroid/LABA inhaler, or add leukotriene antagonist or increase dose of an inhaled steroid.
Step 4	If symptoms still persist, at least a 6 week therapeutic trail of a leukotriene antagonist (if not already given), an oral theophylline or oral β_2-agonist should be given.
Step 5	Despite the use of the above drugs, a small percentage of patients with severe chronic asthma will require in addition a daily maintenance dose of oral prednisolone.

Doses

Salbutamol 200 μg inhaled as required; Terbutaline 500 μg inhaled up to 4 times daily Salmeterol 50–100 μg inhaled twice daily; Formoterol 12/24 μg inhaled twice daily.

Anticholinergics

Mechanism of action

Anticholinergics act by preventing acetylcholine released upon vagal stimulation from contracting airway smooth muscle. The most frequently used drug is the non-selective anticholinergic ipratropium bromide. Recently, muscarinic M_3-receptor selective anticholinergics have been introduced into practice particularly for COPD (tiotropium).

Pharmacokinetics

Ipratropium bromide produces bronchodilation over 4–6 hours and is usually administered by inhalers or occasionally nebulisers. Tiotropium has a longer duration of action (18–24 hours) and is given once daily.

Adverse effects

Adverse effects with anticholinergic agents are rare although high doses of ipratropium may at least in theory worsen glaucoma or symptoms of bladder outflow obstruction.

Interactions

There are no major interactions with this class of drugs.

Clinical use

Ipratropium bromide and tiotropium are used as bronchodilators predominantly in the management of COPD although ipratropium bromide is also used in the management of acute asthma (see below).

Doses

Ipratropium bromide: inhaler 20–40 μg four times daily inhaled, nebulised 250–500 μg up to four times daily. Tiotropium: 10–18 μg inhaled once daily, depending on device.

Inhaled corticosteroids

Mechanism of action

Corticosteroids activate the intracellular glucocorticoid receptor to produce anti-inflammatory effects either by directly altering gene transcription or by transrepression (i.e. interacting with other important transcription factors for pro- and anti-inflammatory genes).

Pharmacokinetics

Corticosteroids should be administered wherever possible by the inhaled route and via a device that maximises lung distribution. The aim is to achieve the maximum anti-inflammatory effect in the lung whilst minimising systemic absorption and unwanted adrenal suppression. Twice-daily administration is usual. Nebulised steroids have been used in a small number of asthmatic patients although controlled trials are few. Oral steroid usage is discussed below.

Adverse effects

Side effects are usually due to local deposition with inhaled devices (hoarse voice, oral candidiasis). With high doses of inhaled corticosteroids/nebulised corticosteroids some adrenal suppression may occur: concerns of increased risk of osteoporosis or reduced growth rate in children have been raised particularly with high-dose inhaled/nebulised corticosteroids although these remain to be fully substantiated.

Interactions

There are no important interactions when corticosteroids are given through the inhaled route.

Clinical use

Inhaled corticosteroids remain the mainstay anti-inflammatory treatment for the management of asthma except for very mild patients (i.e. those at step 1 on the BTS [British Thoracic Society] guidelines). Clinical use should be tailored to give the minimum dose in the long term which controls disease: the dose–response relationship for corticosteroids is relatively flat and whilst some benefit may be obtained by doubling the dose of inhaled steroids in many patients, the benefit is relatively small. A dose of 400–800 μg of beclomethasone equivalent is usually adequate to control disease in most patients with asthma. Inhaled corticosteroids have not been shown to have clinically useful effects on lung function decline in patients with COPD but do reduce exacerbation rates and should be prescribed for patients experiencing more than one exacerbation per year.

There are a range of inhaled corticosteroids available including beclomethasone, budesonide, fluticasone and ciclesonide. Whilst there are theoretical differences between each steroid, both in pharmacokinetics and in the devices available for administering the drugs, in practice these differences are not large and the choice of drug is often determined by cost and patient preference.

Doses

Beclomethasone, budesonide: start at 200 µg twice daily, increase to a maximum of 800 µg twice daily if necessary. Fluticasone: fluticasone is roughly twice as potent as beclomethasone and is usually used at 100–250 µg twice daily, increasing depending on the severity of asthma. Chlorofluoro-carbons (CFC)-free inhaled steroids have different distribution characteristics and beclomethasone administered through a CFC-free inhaler can be given at half the dose to achieve the same lung deposition. In practice CFC-free preparations are packaged so that the same number of doses (1–2 puffs twice a day) can be administered as with CFC-containing inhalers.

Cys leukotriene receptor antagonists

Mechanism

Leukotriene D_4 (LTD$_4$) is the major bronchocon-strictor mediator in the leukotriene synthesis path-way and brings about airway smooth muscle con-traction via activation of the Cys leukotriene 1 receptor. A number of drugs have been devel-oped to interfere either with synthesis of LTD$_4$ or with its receptor. Whilst there have been clin-ical studies with 5-lipoxygenase inhibitors, the most frequently used leukotriene modifier drugs are antagonists of the Cys leukotriene 1 receptor. These drugs produce modest amounts of bron-chodilation and, in addition, have some anti-inflammatory properties.

Pharmacokinetics

All of the currently used Cys leukotriene receptor antagonists are administered by the oral route. There are differences in rates of absorption and metabolism between drugs in this class: mon-telukast is used once daily whereas zafirlukast is used twice daily.

Adverse effects

In general, Cys leukotriene receptor antagonists are well tolerated. Initial concerns regarding in-creased incidence of Churg Strauss syndrome have largely resolved.

Interactions

Zafirlukast has been reported to enhance the anti-coagulant effect of warfarin in some individuals.

Clinical use

Cys leukotriene receptor antagonists are generally used as add-on therapy at step 3 for manage-ment of asthma. Particularly in the United States, these agents are sometimes used as first-line anti-inflammatory therapy instead of inhaled steroids. Recent evidence have suggested that inhaled steroids are more effective at controlling mild-to-moderate asthma when compared to leukotriene antagonists, when used alone. Their use has also been suggested in individuals with mild to moder-ate asthma who are unable to take inhaled steroids for other reasons (e.g. severe oropharyngeal side effects or patients with poor manual dexterity). In addition, there is some evidence advocating the use of leukotriene antagonists in allergic rhinitis. The potential use of these agents in COPD remains to be evaluated.

Doses

Montelukast 10 mg once daily orally; Zafirlukast 20 mg twice daily orally.

Theophyllines

Mechanism

Although theophyllines were amongst the first drugs to be developed for the treatment of asthma and COPD, the precise mode of action remains contentious. The major possibilities include non-selective phosphodiesterase inhibition, antago-nism of effects of adenosine and possible effects on muscle fatigue. Theophylline is a methylxan-thine used orally, while aminophylline is the in-travenous equivalent. Because of the belief that theophylline may work by phosphodiesterase inhibition, there are a number of drugs in devel-opment which target specific phosphodiesterase isoforms (especially PDE$_4$).

Pharmacokinetics

Theophylline has a narrow therapeutic win-dow (therapeutic serum levels 10–20 mg/L).

Metabolism is via cytochrome P450 1A2 and 3A4 and hence can be influenced by other drugs metabolised via cytochrome P450 (important examples include macrolide antibiotics such as erythromycin, antifungals including fluconazole, the oral contraceptive pill, cimetidine and verapamil, all of which potentially can increase serum theophylline levels). Serum theophylline levels can also be increased by heart failure, by viral infections, in the elderly and in patients with cirrhosis. Serum theophylline levels may be reduced, as a consequence of enzyme induction, in individuals taking anticonvulsants, in those with a history of alcohol abuse and in smokers.

Adverse effects

The major limiting factor with theophylline is gastrointestinal side effects and especially nausea (around 10% of individuals). Toxicity may be associated with tachyarrhythmias and seizures: both are most frequently seen when aminophylline is used intravenously and because of this, general intravenous administration of aminophylline has been phased out in many centres. It is potentially dangerous to use intravenous aminophylline in a patient taking oral theophylline preparations unless a recent serum theophylline level is available.

Interactions

See 'Pharmacokinetics' above.

Clinical use

Oral theophylline is used as add on therapy at step 3 of the BTS guidelines in the management of asthma and is also effective in some patients with COPD. Intravenous aminophylline has been largely discontinued due to the lack of evidence of efficacy in acute asthma and/or COPD and the risk of tachyarrhythmias and/or seizures. It is still used in some patients with difficult asthma or severe COPD: its use should be limited to a high dependency unit or Intensive Care Unit (ICU) setting where appropriate monitoring is available. Intravenous aminophylline should be given by slow infusion and not by bolus injection.

Doses

Theophylline: various slow-release preparations are available and are the best way to administer the drug, the total dose administered usually being around 400 mg per day. For intravenous aminophylline the infusion rate is adjusted depending on the serum level (if known) and clinical setting: the usual dose is 0.5 mg per kg per hour. For patients not previously on oral theophyllines a loading dose of 5 mg per kg over 20 minutes may be given.

Mucolytics

Mucolytics are prescribed to aid the expectoration by reducing sputum viscosity. They are mainly used in patients with COPD and bronchiectasis. There are three main agents used: carbocisteine, erdosteine and mecysteine hydrochloride. In the management of stable patients, carbocisteine and erdosteine has been shown to reduce the exacerbation rates in patients with COPD. Erdosteine has been shown to reduce the time and symptoms associated with COPD exacerbations, when used in conjunction with antibiotics. The mechanism behind this is postulated as a consequence of the additional anti-inflammatory, anti-oxidant and anti-pertussive effect that erdosteine possesses. These drugs are generally well tolerated apart from gastrointestinal side effect. Caution should be used in patients with a history of peptic ulceration, as mucolytics might disrupt the gastric mucosal barrier.

Sodium cromoglicate

Cromoglicate derivatives were amongst the first anti-inflammatory drugs developed for the management of asthma and rhinitis. They have limited efficacy and their use has been largely superseded by inhaled steroids. The precise mode of action is unclear although it has long been hypothesised that stabilising effects on mast cell degranulation or effects on sensory nerve endings may be important.

Anti-IgE therapy

A humanised monoclonal antibody against IgE has recently been approved for the management of chronic persistent asthma. Administration is subcutaneously on a monthly basis. Use is limited by patient's weight (dose to be administered being calculated in part from body weight and in part by total IgE levels). Currently as of the time of writing, patients with very high IgE levels are not being considered for therapy partly because of the dose that would need to be administered and partly because of potential concerns over immune complex formation. The use of anti-IgE therapy should be limited to specialist centres. Anti-IgE therapy is much more expensive than other routinely used asthma medications, hence a cost-benefit analysis should be considered in each patient for whom therapy is suggested.

Prednisolone

Prednisolone remains the mainstay anti-inflammatory agent used for chronic asthma unresponsive to the BTS step 4 management and for symptomatic severe COPD patients who demonstrate evidence of steroid responsiveness. Short courses of high-dose prednisolone are also used in the management of acute exacerbations of asthma and of COPD.

Patients requiring long-term oral steroid usage should have bone density measurements (typically every 3 years) and be considered for bone protection (e.g. with a bisphosphonate and calcium supplements) if at high risk of osteoporosis.

Steroid-sparing agents in severe asthma

A small number of patients with chronic asthma require long-term treatment with prednisolone. As a consequence of adverse effects related to high-dose steroid therapy (osteoporosis, avascular necrosis, steroid-induced diabetes, weight gain, adrenal suppression), there have been a number of trials of steroid-sparing agents in this setting. Reasonable evidence exists for efficacy with low-dose methotrexate, cyclosporin and azathio-prine. These drugs should be used only in the setting of a specialist clinic with experience in this area.

Treatment of acute airways disease

Clinical scenario

A 20-year-old male presents with a several hours of worsening breathlessness, wheeze and non-productive cough. He has asthma and does not smoke. He has a respiratory rate of 30 breaths a minute, a moderate expiratory wheeze, a peak flow which is 30% predicted but normal arterial blood gases. A diagnosis of acute severe asthma is made. What drugs can be used to treat this condition?

The above has described drugs used in the treatment of chronic or stable airways disease. Many of these treatments are also in the management of patients with acute asthma or COPD. One additional therapy used in the acute setting is Magnesium Sulphate.

Magnesium sulphate

Magnesium sulphate ($MgSO_4$) is used intravenously (8 mmols over 20 minutes) in the management of life-threatening asthma, although this is an unlicensed indication). This produces some bronchodilation: the mechanism of action is unclear. The main side effects are gastrointestinal upset and hypotension.

Management of acute asthma

Acute asthma is a medical emergency that requires rapid assessment and treatment. Typically, patients present with worsening of symptoms, deterioration in peak flow, increased respiratory rate (>25 breaths/minute), an inability to complete sentences in one breath, and tachycardia (>110 beats per minute). Life-threatening features include a silent chest, cyanosis, confusion or coma, peak flow <33% predicted, oxygen saturations <92% predicted, hypoxia, acidosis or hypercapnoea on arterial blood gases.

Pharmacological management consists of:
- High flow rate oxygen (initially 40–60%)
- Nebulised salbutamol (5 mg in oxygen) repeated at 15- to 20-min intervals if necessary, also ipratropium 500 μg nebulised in oxygen 4-hourly if failure to respond to nebulised salbutamol
- Prednisolone 30–40 mg stat then continued for a minimum of 5 days: use i.v. hydrocortisone (100 mg q.d.s.) if life-threatening attack or if the patient is unable to take prednisolone orally (Note: it can take up to 6 hours for steroids to have their initial effect)
- MgSO$_4$ 8 mmol over 20 minutes by slow intravenous infusion if the attack is life-threatening.
- If patients fail to respond to the above i.v. salbutalmol, i.v. aminophylline (see notes above) and ICU referral should be considered.

Management of acute exacerbations of COPD

Clinical scenario

A 60-year-old male with COPD presents with a week's history of worsening breathlessness, wheeze and cough productive of green sputum. He has smoked 20 cigarettes a day for many years. On examination there was decreased air entry and a mild expiratory wheeze bilaterally. He is diagnosed as having an acute infective exacerbation of COPD. What drugs can be used to treat this condition?

Exacerbations of COPD usually present with worsening breathlessness, cough and sometimes sputum production. Treatment consists of the following:
- Oxygen: initially 28% (see section on 'Oxygen therapy' below)
- Nebulised salbutamol (5 mg) and ipratropium (500 μg) 4–6 times per day
- Prednisolone 30 mg daily for 7–10 days
- Antibiotics (e.g. amoycillin 500 mg three times a day or doxycycline 200 mg first day followed by 100 mg daily) if evidence of infection.

Patients failing to respond to the above measures sometimes respond to i.v. aminophylline. Non-invasive ventilation, usually Bi-level Positive Airway Pressure, benefits some patients and may avoid the need for intubation in patients for whom this is being considered.

Other therapy for airways diseases

Smoking cessation

In COPD patients, smoking cessation is currently the only effective measure that has a disease-modifying effects (see above).There is also an increased risk of exacerbation and a failure to respond to therapy in smoking asthmatics. Hence, smoking cessation remains an important part of the management of these and other conditions. Potential interventions that have been explored include non-pharmacological approaches (smoking support advice, acupuncture, etc.), nicotine replacement therapy and oral administration of bupropion or varinicline.

Nicotine replacement therapy

Nicotine replacement therapy is effective at aiding smokers to stop in addition to behavioural support. It is administered by transdermal patches, as chewing gum, or by nasal spray or inhalator. Side effects include gastrointestinal upset, headache and influenza-like illness. Caution is needed in patients with severe or unstable angina, arrythmias, recent stroke and diabetes.

Bupropion

Bupropion was originally developed as an antidepressant but has been shown to increase rates of smoking cessation in motivated individuals. The exact mode of action of the drug is uncertain although bupropion is a noradrenaline reuptake inhibitor with some additional effects on dopamine reuptake. Side effects may be related to antimuscarinic activity (dry mouth, AV block, tachycardia and gastrointestinal side effects), and there is also a potential to increase seizure frequency. Insomnia may also be a problem. There are many important potential interactions because of inhibition of cytochrome P450 activity. The recommended dose is

150 mg daily for 6 days followed by 150 mg twice daily for a maximum of up to 9 weeks.

Varenicline

Varnicline is a selective nicotine receptor partial agonist and has been shown to improve abstinence from cigarette smoking in the longer term. Side effects are again related to antimuscarinic activity (see above),and there are also reports of increased suicidal behaviour in susceptible individuals. Varenicline is commenced at 500 μg daily and gradually increased to 1 milligram twice daily over a week if tolerated for 11 weeks.

Oxygen

Acute oxygen therapy

Use of oxygen in hospitals is often poorly supervised. The new BTS guidelines indicate oxygen concentrations, mode of delivery (e.g. face mask or nasal cannulae), and target saturations should be prescribed in order to ensure that patients receive appropriate therapy. This is particularly important in patients dependent upon hypoxic drive to maintain ventilation (especially patients with severe COPD and type II respiratory failure). In such patients the concentration should not initially exceed 28% via a Venturi mask with target oxygen saturations of between 88 and 92% Patients may require higher oxygen concentrations but repeated monitoring of arterial blood gases is required to ensure the hypoxic drive is not lost. In contrast, in acute asthma high flow rates of oxygen are safe and appropriate.

Chronic oxygen therapy

Domicillary oxygen should be considered in patients who do not smoke and are hypoxaemic. Oxygen treatment can be divided into short burst or long-term oxygen therapy (LTOT).

Short-burst oxygen therapy

This can be prescribed for intermittent use for episodes of breathlessness not relieved by other measures. In general this is for patients who desaturate markedly on exercise despite having resting PaO_2 values above the recommended threshold for consideration for LTOT. It is important to advise patients not to over rely on short burst oxygen treatment instead of seeking medical help if appropriate. Short-burst oxygen therapy can be administered using bottled or liquid oxygen.

Long-term oxygen therapy

Patients with chronic respiratory disease who are hypoxic at rest often benefit symptomatically from long-term oxygen therapy (LTOT). Some studies have shown a survival advantage for patients with a PaO_2 <7.3 kPa and who use O_2 >15 hours per day. Patients with secondary polycythaemia, nocturnal hypoxaemia, peripheral oedema or evidence of pulmonary hypertension are eligible for LTOT if their PaO_2 <7.3 kPa. Long-term oxygen therapy should only be recommended for individuals with resting hypoxia, which improves on LTOT (initially 24% O_2 via a concentrator) without a concomitant rise in $PaCO_2$ (in general $PaCO_2$ must rise by <1 kPa to allow LTOT). Formal assessment is required before LTOT therapy can be recommended and because of the obvious risk of explosion, patients should not still be smoking. Installation of tubing within the patient's accommodation allows movement between rooms for patients who are still ambulant.

Notes on other respiratory diseases

Bronchiectasis

Clinical scenario

A 40-year-old male presents with a several year history of cough productive of purulent sputum. He had pertussis as a child and has never smoked 20. Examination reveals finger clubbing and bilateral basal crackles. Imaging confirms bronchiectasis. What drugs can be used to treat this condition?

Bronchiectasis is a chronic inflammatory condition where there is saccular dilatation of the terminal airways and/or thickening of the segmental bronchi. Patients usually present with productive cough with or without haemoptysis and may have variable amounts of airflow obstruction. There are a number of causes including previous pneumonia (including tuberculosis), cystic fibrosis (see below), obstructed major airway (e.g. inhaled foreign body), fibrotic lung disease (traction bronchiectasis), immunodeficiency and ciliary dysfunction syndromes. Management is aimed at treating infection and reversing airflow obstruction if possible. Patients with immunodeficiency syndromes (e.g. common variable hypogammaglobulanaemia) may also benefit from immunoglobulin replacement therapy although this will not reverse structural damage that has already occurred. Colonisation with pseudomonas is a particular problem that may require specialist microbiological input to determine the most appropriate antibiotic regimen. Treatment options for patients with stable bronchiectasis includes education airway clearance techniques, inhaled combination steroid/LABA therapy, mucolytics, long term macrolide therapy (such as Azithromycin) and surgical intervention. Acute exacerbations are managed by targeted antimicrobial therapy and treating any associated airflow obstruction.

Cystic fibrosis

Clinical scenario

A baby is diagnosed as having cystic fibrosis after a positive Guthrie (antenatal genetic) testing. What drugs may be required for potential respiratory complications of this condition?

Cystic fibrosis presents with early onset bronchiectasis. Advances in specialist care with early treatment of infection, avoidance of colonisation, regular postural drainage and treatment of pancreatic insufficiency have meant that the prognosis has improved markedly over the last 20 years such that patients frequently survive into their early forties. Treatment should be in a specialist centre and as with bronchiectasis is aimed at treating infection and airflow obstruction. In addition, particular attention should be made in improving nutritional status of patients (which may include pancreatic supplementation), reduce airway colonization with bacteria (such as *Staph. aureus*), additional aids to expectoration (e.g. recombinant human DNAse), and consideration for lung transplantation if indicated.

Interstitial lung disease

Clinical scenario

A 70-year-old male presents with a several year history of worsening breathlessness and non-productive cough. He has never smoked. Examination shows finger clubbing and bilateral basal crackles. Physiology and radiology is highly suggestive of idiopathic interstitial pneumonia. What drugs can be used to treat this condition?

A wide range of systemic inflammatory conditions can cause interstitial lung disease (e.g. sarcoidosis, vasculitis) and treatment is aimed at controlling the underlying disease process usually with high-dose immunosuppression. There is also a group of specific inflammatory conditions affecting predominantly or exclusively the lung, including hypersensitivity pneumonitis, idiopathic interstitial pneumonia (now subdivided into a range of conditions), and a number of rarer conditions. Treatment is with high-dose immunosuppression, initially using high-dose oral prednisolone and then introducing steroid-sparing agents (e.g. azathioprine). There is also evidence that N-acetylcysteine slows the progression of fibrosis when used in conjunction with other immunomodulatory agents. The prognosis depends upon the underlying disease process which may be good if the disease process is characterised by an acute inflammatory response. In patients with long-standing fibrotic changes or with usual interstitial pneumonia (UIP), response to treatment is often limited at best. Lung transplantation remains an option for selected patients.

Pulmonary hypertension

Clinical scenario

A 30-year-old female presents with a several month history of worsening breathlessness and marked peripheral oedema. She has systemic lupus erythematosus and has never smoked. Examination reveals an elevated jugular venous pressure, ankle oedema, a loud second heart and a pan systolic murmur heard best over the left lower sternal edge. Investigations reveal pulmonary hypertension felt secondary to her connective tissue disorder. What drugs can be used to treat this condition?

Pulmonary hypertension may be primary or secondary, the latter usually due to chronic respiratory disease, connective tissue disorders, cardiac disease or thromboembolic disease. Secondary pulmonary hypertension may respond in part to reversing underlying causes (e.g. right to left shunts in the heart) although by the time of presentation often little improvement is possible. LTOT is the most useful treatment in this situation, together with treating any underlying element of heart failure.

Primary pulmonary hypertension is a rare condition that most frequently affects middle-aged females. In addition to LTOT, pulmonary artery pressure can potentially be reduced by the use of prostacylin analogues (iloprost, epoprostenol), voltage-dependent calcium channel antagonists and the endothelin 1 receptor antagonist bosentan. Treatment should be in a specialist centre with experience of the use of these agents.

Chapter 7

Drugs used to treat neurological disease

Introduction

This chapter will provide an overview of drugs used in neurological practice. A broad range of conditions is encountered by neurologists and this diversity is reflected in the range of pharmacological strategies described. The emergence of immunotherapy in the management of certain neurological disorders has brought a new dimension to the management of many chronic, disabling conditions; recent developments in this field will be discussed. Drugs may also play a role in the development of neurological symptoms, and this causal relationship is considered.

Epilepsy

Clinical scenario

A 22-year-old woman is referred to hospital following a witnessed collapse with generalised seizure activity. She had swiftly regained consciousness but remained confused for a few minutes thereafter. On questioning, she gives a history of several previous episodes of collapse with loss of consciousness, after which she had awoken feeling confused, with stiff, sore muscles and bleeding from a bitten tongue. Following neurological evaluation and discussion a decision to commence antiepileptic medication is made. What factors may affect the choice of treatment strategy?

Lecture Notes: Clinical Pharmacology and Therapeutics, 8th edition. By Gerard McKay, John Reid and Matthew Walters. Published 2010 by Blackwell Publishing Ltd.

Pathophysiology

A seizure is a paroxysmal event resulting from abnormal, hypersynchronous discharges of cortical neurons which will cause symptoms or signs. These are not rare, and around 5% of the population will experience a seizure at some time in their life. Epilepsy is a disease causing a tendency to recurrent unprovoked seizures and will affect around 0.5% of the population at any time.

For the clinician, epilepsy can be categorised as either 'partial' (also known as localisation-related) where discharges arise from an area of abnormality in an otherwise normal brain (perhaps as a result of infection, trauma, or vascular disease) or 'generalised' where a presumably genetic abnormality causes a widespread lowering of seizure threshold. This categorisation is useful as the two epilepsies may cause differing seizure types and respond to different therapies. Clinical assessment may highlight focal changes which will help localise the site of origin.

Both types of epilepsy may cause one of the most commonly observed seizures, the generalised tonic-clonic seizures, but symptoms and signs of focal onset focal onset of symptoms will only occur in a secondary generalised seizure.

If seizure discharges remain restricted to a particular area, this causes a partial seizure. A simple partial seizure causes neurological symptoms with full awareness throughout. A complex partial seizure, however, will cause awareness to be impaired, often with staring and automatisms. If seizure activity spreads through the brain, the commonly observed phases of tonic then clonic activity will cause a generalised tonic-clonic seizure (previously known by the obsolete term 'grand mal' seizures).

In generalised epilepsies, seizure types do not conform to such anatomical limitations; while seizures may be manifest as a primary generalised tonic clonic convulsion, this type of epilepsy can also cause seizures that are myoclonic, atonic, clonic, or childhood absences.

Other terms describing epilepsy take into account aetiology. Epilepsies occurring as a consequence of identifiable brain pathology (trauma, tumour or infarction) are symptomatic. Those arising from a presumed but so far unidentified focus are known as cryptogenic. Those thought to arise from a genetic disorder (including most generalised epilepsies) are termed idiopathic. The risk of mortality ensures that special mention should be made of *generalised status epilepticus* where epileptic activity persists for 30 minutes or more. Treatment protocols for status epilepticus are well defined in national and local guidelines.

Aim and principles of therapy

Achieving seizure freedom will be possible in 70–80% of those with epilepsy. A wide range of treatments are available, and the choice of drug will depend on a number of factors, including epilepsy classification, fertility, concomitant drug therapy, and presence of other medical conditions.

The largest studies have confirmed sodium valproate as the first choice for generalised epilepsies such as juvenile myoclonic epilepsy (JME), but where future pregnancy is a possibility (taking into account recommendations in 2003 from the Committee on Safety of Medicines in the UK), lamotrigine is an alternative. Levetiracetam is increasingly used in such patients without the same level of evidence of safety in pregnancy. Topiramate has been found to be useful but again should be avoided in pregnancy. Ethosuximide is the only available alternative to valproate for absence seizures (previously known as 'petit mal');

phenytoin or carbamazepine are ineffective. Clonazepam and clobazam can be used as an adjunct for treating myoclonic seizures for seizures occurring in clusters (e.g. during menstrual periods).

For partial epilepsies, studies suggest that lamotrigine is first choice (better tolerability) while carbamazepine, oxcarbazepine, topiramate, and levetiracetam have been shown to be useful as monotherapy. Phenytoin continues to be used in generalised status epilepticus, but long-term side effects and pharmacokinetic unpredictability mean that it is not used as a first line treatment in other settings. Barbiturates such as phenobarbital and primidone are cheap and effective treatments for generalised seizures but poor tolerability, tolerance, and the risk of withdrawal seizures limit their widespread use.

The therapeutic goal in epilepsy treatment is complete remission of seizures without side effects, using a single drug (monotherapy). Table 7.1 is a list of anti-epileptic drugs (AEDs) with their doses, common side effects and interactions. It is fair to say that the newer drugs represent an advance in tolerability but not necessarily efficacy. Many anticonvulsants have important interactions with other drugs, including other anticonvulsants and oral contraceptives that are highly protein bound or are metabolised by the liver. Interactions between the older AEDs are complex and may enhance toxicity without a corresponding increase in the anti-epileptic effect. There is good correlation between therapeutic effect and drug level with phenytoin and to lesser degree with phenobarbital and carbamazepine; valproate and newer AEDs do not require monitoring of plasma levels. If ineffective, medications should be increased to the maximum tolerated dose on clinical grounds rather than serum levels. Approximately one-third of patients will require polytherapy with two or more drugs.

Newer anti-epileptic drugs

It says much about the conservative nature of neurology that drugs licensed in the early 1990s are considered 'new' antiepileptic drugs. Those that are still under patent are relatively expensive.

Table 7.1 Anti-epileptic drugs.

Generic name	Principal uses	Typical dosage and dosing intervals	Half-life	Therapeutic range	Adverse effects			Drug interactions
					Neurologic	Systemic		
Carbamazepine	Partial Epilepsy – all seizure types including partial and secondary generalised seizures	600–1800 mg/day (15–35 mg/kg, child) b.i.d.–q.i.d.	12–17 h	4–12 mg/L (17–42 μmol/L)	Ataxia, dizziness, diplopia, vertigo, worsening of idiopathic generalised epilepsies (e.g. provoking myoclonic jerks)	Aplastic anaemia, leukopenia, gastrointestinal irritation, hepatotoxicity		Level decreased by erythromycin, propoxyphene isoniazid, cimetidine
Clonazepam	Absence, atypical absence, myoclonic	1–12 mg/day (0.1–0.2 mg/kg) q.i.d.–t.i.d.	18–48 h	10–70 pg/L	Ataxia, sedation, lethargy	Anorexia		Increased sedation with hypnotics
Ethosuximide	Absence (petit mal)	750–1250 mg/day (20–40 mg/kg) q.d.–b.i.d.	60 h, adult; 30 h, child	40–100 mg/L (283–708 μmol/L)	Ataxia, lethargy, headache	Gastrointestinal irritation, skin rash, bone marrow suppression		No known significant interactions
Gabapentin	Focal-onset	900–2400 mg/day t.i.d.–q.i.d.	5–9 h	Not established	Sedation, dizziness, ataxia, fatigue	Gastrointestinal irritation		No known significant interactions
Lamotrigine	Partial and generalised epilepsies, Lennox–Gastaut syndrome	150–500 mg/day b.i.d.	15–25 h (with enzyme-inducers); 5–9 h (with valproic acid)	Not established	Dizziness, diplopia, sedation, ataxia, headache	Skin rash, Stevens–Johnson syndrome		Level decreased by carbamazepine, phenobarbital, phenytoin; level increased by valproic acid

(Continued)

have shown it to have best efficacy in patients with generalised epilepsy. It is effective against most seizure types as well as migraine prophylaxis, neuralgia, and bipolar disorder. It is well absorbed, extensively protein bound and metabolised in the liver, and thus contraindicated in active liver disease and porphyria. Rarely, fatal hepatic failure has occurred in children under 3 years of age and those with metabolic or degenerative disorders. Common adverse effects include weight gain, gastric irritation, ataxia, tremors, polycystic ovary-like symptoms in women. Other rarer serious complications include pancreatitis, leukopenia and bone marrow depression. Some patients may notice loss of hair followed by regrowth of curly hair. Use in pregnancy should be avoided if possible; the risk of spina bifida in babies exposed in utero is 2–3%. Parenteral preparations are available for continuation or initiation of valproate treatment when oral therapy is not possible. There is evidence for use of intravenous valproate in *status epilepticus*.

Phenytoin

Phenytoin acts by neuronal membrane stabilisation and blockade of sodium channels. Despite efficacy in tonic–clonic and partial seizures, phenytoin is no longer a first-line therapy because of its narrow therapeutic window and long-term side effects. The relationship between dose and plasma concentration is non-linear; small dosage increases in some patients may produce large rises in plasma concentration at saturation (zero-order) kinetics. Monitoring of plasma concentration is extremely useful with phenytoin. It is also an enzyme inducer and is commonly implicated in drug interaction. Phenytoin is also effective in neuralgia and myotonia. Cosmetic side effects (coarse facies, acne, hirsutism and gingival hyperplasia) make it less useful in long-term. It is to be avoided in porphyria and in second degree or complete heart block. Phenytoin is the cause of a common drug-induced systemic lupus erythematosus (SLE). Concentration-dependent side effects include anorexia, insomnia, nausea, cerebellar symptoms (nystagmus and ataxia), peripheral neuropathy, chorea, obtundation and seizures. Long-term use

can cause osteomalacia (vitamin D malabsorption), megaloblastic anaemia (folate malabsorption), Dupuytren's contracture and generalised lymphadenopathy that may appear indistinguishable from Hodgkin's lymphoma on histology. Rarely, blood dyscrasias (agranulocytosis), hepatitis, skin rash and erythema multiforme are reported.

The parenteral preparation of phenytoin is the first-line therapy in patients with status epilepticus. The injection must only be given intravenously. The injection solution is strongly alkaline and if extravasated, it can cause intense irritation of tissues and in the hands, swelling and discoloration ('purple glove' syndrome). Because of its alkaline pH, phenytoin should not be mixed with solutions with acidic pH, e.g. 5% dextrose in water, which will precipitate the salt (dihydantoin sodium). Rapid intravenous injections may also cause cardiovascular and central nervous system (CNS) depression, heart block, hypotension and respiratory arrest; patients over the age of 50 years are more susceptible. The rate of infusion should not exceed 50 mg/min; resuscitation facilities and a cardiac rhythm monitor must be available.

Fosphenytoin

Fosphenytoin is a water-soluble prodrug of phenytoin that is suitable for intramuscular or intravenous injections. Once administered, the compound is de-esterified to produce serum phenytoin. It is more neutral in solution and is better tolerated at infusion sites. Doses of fosphenytoin are expressed as phenytoin equivalents (PE), which may lead to confusion on the ward. While fosphenytoin can be administered more rapidly than phenytoin, the serum levels of phenytoin rise at an equivalent rate, lessening the advantage. Although cardiovascular complications are less likely, cardiac monitoring is still recommended during intravenous infusion.

Lamotrigine

It acts by blocking the neuronal sodium and calcium channels and is effective as monotherapy in partial and generalised seizures. It is well absorbed, fully bioavailable and is metabolised largely as a glucuronide conjugate in the liver. We know that there is a risk of enzyme induction leading to interactions with oestrogen containing contraceptives. While licensed for used in both partial and generalised epilepsies, lamotrigine is usually used more in the former. It is contraindicated in hepatic impairment. Elimination half-life of lamotrigine is reduced to around 15 hours by the enzyme-inducing AEDs (carbamazepine and phenytoin), whereas sodium valproate inhibits its metabolism and doubles the half-life to nearly 60 hours. It must be given at a very low dose (12.5 mg daily or 25 mg every alternate day) with slow weekly dose increment in patients on concomitant valproate therapy. A pharmacodynamic interaction is common when used alongside carbamazepine and the symptoms of neurotoxicity (headache, nausea, dizziness, diplopia and ataxia) can be avoided or ameliorated by reducing the carbamazepine dose. The commonest side effect of lamotrigine is skin rash (3–5%) and there is good evidence that lower starting doses reduce this risk. Other side effects that are concentration dependent include dizziness, nausea, diplopia and ataxia.

Topiramate

Topiramate has a number of actions on neuronal function including blockade of sodium and calcium channels, mild carbonic anhydrase activity, and increasing effect of GABA. It has effect both alone and in combination in partial and generalised epilepsies. Metabolism is largely hepatic and excretion is in urine and faeces after glucuronidation. There is increasing use of this drug in migraine prophylaxis, and in treatment of headaches, bipolar disorder, and neuralgia. Common side effects include sedation, drowsiness, and distal tingling; these are most common at early stages and during titration. Renal stones occur more commonly, especially where fluid intake is low or where there is a family history of nephrolithiasis.

Levetiracetam

One of the more recently introduced drugs, levetiracetam has good efficacy in both generalised and partial epilepsies. It has stable and linear pharmacokinetics and has no known pharmacokinetic drug interactions. It can be titrated rapidly, quickly achieving therapeutic doses. Serious adverse effects are rare. In some patients, the drug can cause some anxiety and behavioural difficulties.

Anti-epileptic drug therapy in pregnancy

Ongoing surveillance studies confirm the risk of teratogenicity with AED use. Sodium Valproate is most culpable, especially at higher doses, while carbamazepine and lamotrigine have the most favourable profile. Evidence is increasing that levetiracetam may be safely used in pregnancy. Polypharmacy with AEDs causes a further increase in risk. In view of the increased risk of neural tube and other defects all women taking AEDs who may become pregnant should be informed of the risks and must be screened antenatally (α-fetoprotein measurement and a second trimester ultrasound scan) if they become pregnant. High dose folic acid (5 mg/day) is recommended both before and during pregnancy for women receiving established AEDs.

As well as structural effects on fetal development, there is an emerging body of evidence that valproate may reduce IQ in babies exposed prenatally. This risk needs to be quantified, and comparison needs to be made with other AEDs.

In view of the increased bleeding associated with carbamazepine, phenobarbital and phenytoin, prophylactic Vitamin K_1 should be given to the mother on any of these drugs before delivery. Breast feeding is acceptable with most AEDs.

Status epilepticus

The treatment protocol for convulsive (tonic–clonic) status epilepticus is outlined in Table 7.2.

Key points – epilepsy

- Approximately 80% of patients with epilepsy achieve seizure freedom with treatment
- A wide range of drugs to treat seizures are available, they differ in mechanism of action, side effect profile and relative efficacy in particular types of seizure disorder
- Choice of optimal strategy can be complex and is driven by the characteristics and preferences of the patient and the type of seizure disorder

Headache

Headache is the most common neurological symptom. Primary headache disorders (e.g. migraine, tension-type headache, cluster headache) are not associated with an underlying pathology whereas secondary headache disorders result from an underlying pathological condition (infectious, vascular or neoplastic). Secondary causes of headache should be considered if there is a new-onset or change in headache for patients over 50 years, if the headache has a sudden onset (i.e. the headache reaches its maximum intensity within 5 minutes), if neurological examination is abnormal, if the

Table 7.2 Therapy for convulsive status epilepticus.

Time frame (min)	Intervention
(continuing seizures) 0–5 minutes	Monitor vital signs, administer O_2, establish i.v. access, collect blood for biochemistry, blood gases and toxic screen; drug levels (phenytoin, carbamazepine) if on treatment.
	Consider investigation for previous infection (e.g. chest X ray, MSU, LP)
	If compliance in doubt, replace usual doses of antiepileptic medication
	Put patient in recovery position. 50 mL of 50% dextrose i.v. (+100 mg thiamine i.m./i.v. if possible alcoholic)
	If seizures have been continuing for longer than 5 minutes
	Lorazepam 0.1 mg/kg i.v. at 2 mg/min (maximum dose: children 2 mg and adults 8 mg)
	Do not repeat dose more than once – further treatment required, use phenytoin
	If seizures continue
	Phenytoin 15–20 mg/kg i.v. at 50 mg/min (typically 1 g in an adult)
25–30 minutes	*If seizures continue*
	Patient must be admitted to an ICU
	EEG monitoring if possible
>30 minutes	General Anaesthesia with
	Thiopental (thiopentone) (2.5% solution), given i.v. 100–150 mg in adults over 10–15 s (2–7 mg/kg in children), then maintained at 0.5–1 mg/kg/h
	If EEG facilities are available, dose may be adjusted on the basis of EEG monitoring, maintaining burst-suppression pattern in the EEG with intervals of <1 s between bursts
	Additional treatment possible with:
	Midazolam (loading dose 0.1–0.2 mg/kg slow i.v., then maintained at a dose of 0.75–10 µg/kg/min)
	Clomethiazole (chlormethiazole) as an 0.8% solution intravenously 40–120 mg/min up to a maximum of 800 mg (80 µg/kg in children), then maintained at a rate of 4–8 mg/min
	Propofol (loading dose 1–2 mg/kg i.v., followed by 2–10 mg/kg/h)
	Phenobarbital 5–10 mg/kg (not exceeding a cumulative total dose of 20 mg/kg or 1 g)
	Alternatively
	Paraldehyde by deep intramuscular injections (5 mL in each buttock, maximum 10 mL using all glass equipment with a steel needle)

patient is awakened from sleep by the headache or if the headache is worsened by change in posture.

Migraine

Migraine is a common episodic disorder characterised by spontaneous or triggered attacks of moderate-to-severe headache typically lasting 4–72 hours. The headache is often unilateral and pulsating. It builds up over minutes to hours and is associated with nausea and/or vomiting, photo- and phonophobia (sensitivity to light and sound). It often limits the patient's ability or work or study and is aggravated by routine physical activity. It is more common in females and often there is a positive family history.

Up to one-third of patients experience migraine with aura. The aura refers to focal neurological symptoms (visual, sensory, motor or language dysfunction) which accompany or precede the headache. It is also possible to experience aura without developing headache.

Aim and principles of treatment

Management of migraine consists of: (i) avoidance of specific precipitants or triggers (patients often discover these themselves); (ii) pharmacological treatment of acute attacks and (iii) prophylaxis.

Treatment of acute attack

This should begin at the onset of headache when symptoms are mild. Non-steroidal anti-inflammatory drugs (NSAID) such as aspirin or ibuprofen, often combined with an anti-emetic (metoclopramide, domperidone or phenothiazine), is the first choice. Paracetamol is also effective. Opiate analgesia should be avoided in patients due to the risk of developing medication overuse headache.

As serotonin (5-hydroxy tryptamine or 5-HT) plays a key role in the neurovascular inflammation seen in migraine 5-HT$_1$ agonists (known as 'triptans') are used in the treatment of an acute attack in those patients who do not respond to simple analgesics. There are multiple preparations of trip-

tans available and patients should not be considered as non-responders to triptans unless they have tried every triptan. Triptans do not improve nausea or vomiting and often an additional anti-emetic is required. With severe nausea or vomiting nasal sprays and injectable preparations of triptans may be useful. If response is suboptimal, triptans can be used in combinations with NSAIDs. Triptans should be avoided in the aura phase of the attack and are contraindicated in hemiplegic migraine, ischaemic heart disease, previous stroke or uncontrolled hypertension. Prolonged use of triptans can also give rise to 'rebound headache'.

Ergotamine has largely been replaced by NSAIDs and triptans in the treatment of acute migraine. Side effects include nausea, vomiting and abdominal cramps. It should be avoided in patients with cardiovascular or cerbrovascular disease. However, unremitting severe migraine lasting for days ('status migrainosus') may require the parenteral therapy with anti-emetics and ergotamine-based drugs.

Migraine prophylaxis

Migraine prophylaxis should be considered in patients when migraine is frequent (>1 attack per week), interferes with activities of daily living or when it is severe and does not respond to acute treatments. The aim of prophylaxis is to reduce the frequency and severity of migraine. The most commonly used drugs are propanolol (80–240 mg/day) and amitriptyline (25–150 mg/day). There is also evidence for the use of sodium valproate (800–1500 mg/day), topiramate (50–200 mg/day), gabapentin (1200–2400 mg/day), venlafaxine (75–150 mg/day), pizotifen (0.5–3 mg/day) and methysergide (2–6 mg/day). Each drug should be commenced at low dose and gradually increased over time. It may take up to 6 months for the drug to reach full efficacy.

Antimigraine drugs in common use

Sumatriptan

A 5-HT$_{1D}$ agonist, sumatriptan is used for acute attacks of migraine (oral preparation, intranasal

spray or subcutaneous injections) and cluster headache (subcutaneous injections only). It
should not be taken until 24 hours after stopping
any preparation containing ergotamine. It has
poor bioavailability and less than half of the orally
administered dose is absorbed. Further reduction
may occur in patients with migraine-induced gas-
troparesis and vomiting. The dose by mouth is
50 mg (some patients may require 100 mg) and
patients not responding should not take a second dose for the same attack. In responders, the
dose may be repeated if migraine recurs (maximum 300 mg in 24 hours). It is available as an
intranasal spray and subcutaneous injection for
prompt relief. The dose by subcutaneous injection
using an auto-injector is 6 mg (maximum 24 mg
in 24 hours) and 1 spray (20 mg) intranasally
(maximum 40 mg in 24 hours). Sumatriptan is
also effective in cluster headache. None of the
5-HT agonists should be used for prophylaxis
and all are contraindicated in ischaemic heart
disease, previous myocardial infarction, coronary
vasospasm, uncontrolled hypertension and in attacks of migraine with brain stem dysfunction
('basilar migraine'). Side effects of triptans include
sensations of tingling, heat, heaviness, pressure or
tightness in the chest, flushing, dizziness, weakness, vomiting and fatigue.

Beta-blockers

Propranolol, a non-selective beta-blocker, is effective in reducing the frequency of migraine attacks
in daily doses of 40–120 mg (this may be increased
up to 480 mg according to effectiveness) given
orally. Other cardioselective beta-blockers (bisoprolol or atenolol) are better tolerated and probably equally effective. Their mechanism of action
in migraine prophylaxis is unknown.

Amitriptyline

The anti-migraine effect of amitriptyline (and
other TCAs) is not a result of its antidepressant property and small doses are often effective
(20–50 mg/day). Sedation and dry mouth are two
common side effects. The detailed pharmacology
of amitriptyline is given elsewhere in this book.

Pizotifen

It is an antihistamine and serotonin antagonist
structurally related to the tricyclic antidepressants.
It affords good prophylaxis for migraine but may
cause weight gain and drowsiness. The treatment
may be started at 500 μg at night; maximum dose
is 3 mg/day.

Methysergide

A $5-HT_2$ antagonist, methysergide is a very effective drug for prophylaxis of migraine and cluster
headache but carries serious long-term side effects
(retroperitoneal, pleural and cardiac valvular fibrosis, arterial and coronary vasospasm) that widely
limit its use now. These risks can be minimised
by taking periodic 'drug holidays' (5 months on
the drug and 1 month off in a 6-month cycle). The
usual dose is 1–2 mg 2–3 times daily. Methysergide
is also used in 'serotonin syndrome' and to treat
diarrhoea caused by carcinoid tumour in higher
doses.

Key points – headache

- Headache is the most common neurological symptom
- Simple analgesia is sufficient in the management of
the vast majority of cases
- Triptans are effective in the relief of migraine when
simple analgesia fails
- Prophylactic therapy to reduce frequency of migraine
should be considered in the context of frequent, severe
attacks

Cerebrovascular disease

Pathophysiology

A stroke is the sudden onset of neurological deficit
from a vascular mechanism. Eighty per cent of
strokes are a consequence of ischaemia; a transient
ischaemic attack (TIA) is an ischaemic neurodeficit
that rapidly resolves. The accepted boundary between a TIA and a completed stroke is 24 hours.

The remaining 20% of strokes are primary haemorrhages, including subarachnoid, lobar and hypertensive deep cerebral haemorrhages. Multiple factors, both non-modifiable (age and sex) and modifiable (e.g. hypertension and diabetes), influence the risk of cerebrovascular disease. Prolonged hypertension and diabetes are specific risk factors for small vessel cerebral stroke (lacunar infarcts); smoking is a risk factor for all vascular mechanisms causing stroke. Cerebral venous thrombosis may be spontaneous (as seen during pregnancy) or may be secondary to a hypercoagulable state, focal intracranial or ear infections.

Aim and principles of treatment

Intracranial haemorrhage

The specific treatment is often surgical and pharmacological interventions are directed to the reduction of raised intracranial pressure (ICP). Nimodipine, a calcium channel blocker that crosses the blood–brain barrier, may be effective in minimising symptomatic vasospasm following subarachnoid haemorrhage if begun early (by day 4). Cerebral vasospasm after aneurysm surgery is best treated by improving cerebral perfusion with vasopressor agents.

Acute treatment of ischaemic stroke

Patients with TIA or an established ischaemic stroke should receive aspirin (75–300 mg/day) as soon as the diagnosis is confirmed. If fever and/or hyperglycemia are present, these should be treated promptly. Anticoagulation is strictly reserved for patients with high risk of venous thromboembolism, cerebral venous thrombosis without major haemorrhage, recurrent thromboembolic arterial stroke from a known source (e.g. cardiogenic emboli with atrial fibrillation) and progressive stroke in the basilar artery territory. Systemic or selective intra-arterial thrombolytic therapy with recombinant tissue plasminogen activator (rtPA) may be offered in patients seen within the first 4.5 hours of the ischaemic event in the absence of any major infarction or haemorrhage on brain imaging

with computed tomography (CT). Despite a higher risk of cerebral haemorrhage as a consequence of thrombolytic therapy in ischaemic stroke, both short-term outcome and long-term disabilities significantly improve in thrombolysed patients.

Secondary prevention of stroke

Lifestyle and risk factor modifications will remain the cornerstone of secondary stroke prevention. All patients with ischaemic stroke or TIA should receive life-long aspirin (75–300 mg daily), ideally incombination with sustained-release dipyridamole (200 mg twice daily). Higher doses of aspirin have little advantage and only worsen gastrotoxicity. Clopidogrel (75 mg/day) is an alternative for patients intolerant of aspirin or dipyridamole. Warfarin is indicated for patients with atrial fibrillation or cardioembolic stroke. Dual treatment with aspirin plus clopidogrel, or aspirin plus warfarin, carries a high risk of bleeding complications. These combinations are not routinely used in the secondary prevention of stroke.

Blood pressure reduction should be considered in all patients with cerebrovascular disease. Existing data favours the use of a diuretic/ACE inhibitor combination, introduced a few weeks after the onset of the symptoms. Strategies to lower blood pressure may need to be modified in the context of significant carotid stenosis: aggressive blood pressure reduction in such patients may theoretically aggravate cerebral ischaemia. A more detailed account of blood pressure lowering agents can be found in Chapter 5.

Statin therapy modestly reduces risk of further vascular events in patients with ischaemic stroke, and statins are indicated in such patients.

Key points – cerebrovascular disease

- In highly-selected patients, acute treatment of ischaemic stroke with thrombolytic therapy reduces disability and improves outcome
- Blood pressure reduction is effective in the secondary prevention of ischaemic and haemorrhagic stroke
- Antiplatelet treatment and statin therapy prevents further vascular events in patients with ischaemic stroke

Infections of the nervous system

Treatment for suspected acute bacterial meningitis and herpes simplex encephalitis (HSE) must begin as soon as possible (before the lumbar puncture). The most common causes of bacterial meningitis are *Streptococcus pneumonia*, *Neisseria meningitides* and *Haemophilus influenzae*. Current guidelines for community acquired bacterial meningitis recommend intravenous ceftriaxone (2 g BD) and intravenous dexamethasone (10 mg QDS). If listeria meningitis is suspected (age >55 years or immunosuppression or pregnant) add intravenous amoxicillin (2 g QDS). If pneumococcal meningitis is suspected add vanocomycin +/− rifampicin. Immunocompromised patients (e.g. AIDS, immunosuppressive chemotherapy, transplantation) may be at risk of fungal (Cryptococcus, Candida, Aspergillus), CMV or tuberculous meningitis. Brain abscesses and subdural empyemas are focal suppurative infections of the brain and require surgical drainage in addition to antibiotics.

HSE presents clinically with headache, confusion, seizures and focal neurological signs. If suspected, intravenous acyclovir should be commenced (10 mg/kg TDS).

The tick-borne Lyme disease (*Borrelia burgdorferi*) can present with meningism, cranial neuropathies and painful radiculopathies. Treatment is with intravenous benzylpenicillin (2.4 g QDS), ceftriaxone (2 g OD) or oral doxycycline (100–200 mg BD).

In tropical countries, cerebral malaria (caused by choloroquine-resistant forms of *Plasmodium falciparum*) and tuberculous meningitis are important causes of mortality and morbidity. AIDS patients are at risk of toxoplasmosis and progressive multifocal leucoencephalopathy (PML).

Leprosy is the commonest infection of the peripheral nerves in the world. Please see Chapter 9 for discussion of the pharmacology of antimicrobial chemotherapy.

Drug-induced neurological disorders

See Table 7.3.

Table 7.3 Drug-induced common neurological disorders.

Exacerbation of myasthenia
  Aminoglycosides
  Erythromycin
  Phenytoin
  Polymyxin
Extrapyramidal effects
  Butyrophenones, e.g. haloperidol
  Methyldopa
  Metoclopramide
  Phenothiazines
Myopathy
  Colchicine
  Corticosteroids
  Penicillamine
  Quinine
Headache
  Drugs causing benign intracranial hypertension (hypervitaminosis A, corticosteroids, tetracycline)
  Ergotamine (withdrawal)
  Nitrites
  Vasodilators (e.g. hydralazine)
Seizures
  Amfetamines (amphetamines)
  Ciclosporin (cyclosporin)
  Isoniazid
  Lidocaine
  Lithium
Peripheral neuropathy
  Amiodarone
  Chlorpropamide
  Clofibrate
  Didanosine
  Ethambutol
  Ethionamide
  Isoniazid
  Metronidazole
  Nalidixic acid
  Nitrofurantoin
  Vincristine
Optic neuritis
  Aminoquinolenes
  Ethambutol
  Isoniazid
  Phenothiazines
Sleep disturbances
  Dopamine agonists/levodopa
  MAO inhibitors
Stroke
  Oral contraceptives

Table 7.4 Neurological disorders with a proven or presumed immunological mechanism.

Central nervous system (CNS)	
Acute	Disseminated encephalomyelitis
	Haemorrhagic leukoencephalitis
	Demyelinating optic neuritis
	Transverse myelitis
	CNS vasculitis (isolated angiitis of CNS)
Subacute	Neuro-systemic lupus erythematosus (SLE)
	Subacute cerebellar degeneration and limbic encephalitis (usually paraneoplastic)
Chronic	Multiple sclerosis (MS)
	Stiff-person syndrome
Peripheral nervous system	
Acute	Acute inflammatory demyelinating polyneuropathy (AIDP) (Guillain–Barré syndrome)
	Vasculitis of peripheral nerves
Chronic	Chronic inflammatory demyelinating polyneuropathy (CIDP), MMN (multi-focal motor neuropathy)
	Acquired neuromyotonia
Neuromuscular junction	
	Myasthenia gravis
	Lambert Eaton Myasthenic Syndrome (LEMS)
Skeletal muscles	
	Polymyositis and dermatomyositis

Neuroimmunology

Pathophysiology

Immunological mechanisms are recognised to play an important role in the pathogenesis of a number of neurological diseases (Table 7.4). Treatment of an acute attack following neuroimmunological injury can utilise one of three main methods: (i) high doses of corticosteroids (e.g. intravenous methylprednisolone); (ii) intravenous human immunoglobulin (IVIg) or (iii) plasma exchange. Established autoimmune mechanisms require long-term immunosuppression: most commonly this is with oral corticosteroids but azathioprine, cyclophosphamide, ciclosporin, methotrexate and mycophenalate mofetil may avoid many steroid-related long term problems if aggressive immunosuppression is necessary.

Methylprednisolone

Intravenous methylprednisolone is usually used for rapid suppression of inflammatory disorders

and has equivalent side effect profile and mechanism of action as prednisolone. Patients often experience a metallic taste at the time of infusion, and psychosis and restlessness are reported occasionally. It is usually given in short courses (1 g daily for 3 days or 500 mg daily for 5 days). When steroids are used for long-term immunosuppression, care must be taken to avoid long-term complications like osteopenia. To counter this, prophylactic use of bisphosphonates may be desirable in high-risk cases (e.g. post-menopausal women). For the pharmacokinetics and adverse effects of corticosteroids and immunosuppressive drugs, please refer to the relevant sections in this book.

Intravenous human immunoglobulin (IVIg)

IVIg is derived from pooled immunoglobulin. It is screened for viruses (e.g. hepatitis, human immunodeficiency virus). The mechanism of action of IVIg in acute and chronic neuroimmunological disorders is unclear, but it is thought that exogenous anti-idiotype antibodies in IVIg may neutralise putative autoantibodies. It is possible that administered IVIg increases the catabolism of endogenous IVIg including the circulating autoantibody fraction. The usual dose is 2 g/kg given over 3–5 days. Prior to administration of IVIg serum Immunoglobulin A (IgA) levels should be checked as IgA-deficient patients may develop anaphylaxis. Other common side effects include headache, fever, urticaria, hypotension and increased blood viscosity. Rarer side effects include renal failure, venous thrombosis and aseptic meningitis. Advantages of IVIg over plasma exchange are that it can be given promptly and without central venous cannulation.

Multiple sclerosis

In the UK approximately 1 in 800 people are affected by multiple sclerosis (MS). In MS there is destruction of myelin within the central white matter. An acute attack causes demyelination, which results in focal neurological symptoms. Recurrent attacks may cause destruction of axons leading to permanent loss of function and disability. Relapsing-remitting MS is the commonest clinical form, and steroids can be used to reduce duration and severity of relapses. Disease-modifying treatments aim to reduce the number and extent of clinical relapses, so reducing disease load and functional loss. Once permanent damage has occurred, drug treatment aims to improve symptoms (pain, sensory symptoms, trigeminal neuralgia, fatigue, depression, sphincter and sexual dysfunction, and spasticity).

Relapses are treated with short courses of high dose intravenous methylprednisolone (1 g/day for 3 days or 0.5 g/day for 5 days) or oral methylprednisolone (500 mg/day for 5 days) which speed up natural recovery. With short-term administration, there is no need to taper the steroids. Worsening of MS symptoms may result from infection and it is always worth ruling out a urinary tract infection prior to treating a 'relapse' with steroids. When relapses are severe or unresponsive to steroids intravenous immunoglobulin or plasma exchange can be helpful.

Disease modifying therapies in MS aim to reduce the frequency of relapses and disability accrued over time. Their use and availability has been controversial due to their high costs. Interferon beta (IF-β) and glatiramer acetate reduce annual relapse rates by about 30%. Current UK treatment guidelines advise that patients should have experienced at least 2 clinically significant relapses in the previous 2 years, be able to walk, and usually be over 18 years of age. There are several commercially available interferons administered by either subcutaneous or intra-muscular injection (usually self-administered). Side effects include flu-like symptoms, headache, injection site reactions, mood disturbance, bone marrow suppression, deranged liver function and the development of neutralising antibodies. Regular monitoring of blood count and liver function is required. Glatiramer acetate (Copaxone) is given as a daily subcutaneous injection and is generally better tolerated. These drugs are effective in relapsing forms of MS only.

Mitoxantrone is a cytotoxic agent (an anthracenedione derivative) that has been shown to reduce relapses in relapsing-remitting and secondary-progressive MS. It is given via monthly intravenous infusion. Side effects include nausea and vomiting, bone marrow suppression, amenorrhea, irreversible cardiotoxicity and leukaemia. It is reserved for those patients with aggressive disease, or who have failed previously on disease modifying drugs.

Natulizamab (Tysabri®) is a monoclonal antibody which binds α4-integrins on leukocytes, inhibiting cell adhesion and reducing leukocyte transmigration across the blood–brain barrier into the CNS. It reduces relapse rate by nearly 70% and reduces disability accrual over 2 years by 50%. It is administered by monthly intravenous infusion and side effects include anaphylaxis, infection, depression and menstrual irregularities. In addition, it is rarely associated with the development of progressive multifocal leukoencephalopathy which can be fatal.

Newer, more effective therapies are in development, including orally active agents (e.g. cladribine and fingolimid). Other immunosuppressive

Table 7.5 Symptomatic treatment of chronic neurological disability.

Nature of symptoms	Drugs available
Spasticity	Oral and intrathecal baclofen (GABA agonist) Diazepam (GABA agonist) Dantrolene (direct effect on skeletal muscles) Tizanidine (α2-adrenoreceptor agonist) Botulinum toxin (local injections to spastic muscles)
Muscle spasms	Clonazepam Baclofen
Bladder symptoms	Antimuscarinics: flavoxate and oxybutinin for increased frequency; tolterodine, propiverine may also be effective in urge incontinence: *all may cause retention and precipitate angle-closure glaucoma*; cholinergics (carbachol, bethanecol) for retention *in the absence of urinary obstruction*; adrenergic blockers (prazosin, doxazosin) improve urinary flow by reducing the tone of external uretheral sphincter
Nocturnal enuresis	Adults: desmopressin or propantheline Children: tricyclics (imipramine, amitriptyline)
Dysesthesia	Carbamazepine, lamotrigine
Pain	Tricyclics (amitriptyline, imipramine) Anti-epileptics (carbamazepine, gabapentin)
Fatigue	Amantadine or modafinil
Depression	SSRI (sertraline, citalopram)
Impotence	Sildenafil

therapies are sometimes used – e.g. azathioprine, methotrexate, cyclosphosphamide.

Symptomatic therapies are helpful, and Table 7.5 lists some of the drugs available for patients with chronic neurological disability as seen in MS. These treatments can be delivered in any chronic neurological disorder where similar symptoms emerge.

Movement disorders

Clinical scenario

An 81-year-old man is referred to the geriatric assessment unit with a 2-year history of worsening mobility and frequent falls. On examination he is found to have an expressionless face, reduced arm swinging on walking and increased tone in his limbs. A provisional diagnosis of parkinsonism is made and a trial of drug treatment is discussed. What options are available when considering a treatment plan?

Pathophysiology

Movement disorders are either hypokinetic (where there is too little movement – bradykinesia, rigidity) or hyperkinetic (where there is too much movement – tremor, chorea, dystonia, myoclonus). The most common hypokinetic movement disorder is parkinsonism. The cardinal features of parkinsonism are bradykinesia (slowness in the initiation of voluntary movements with progressive reduction in speed and amplitude of repetitive movements), resting tremor, muscular rigidity and postural instability. The most common cause of parkinsonism is Parkinson's disease (PD), although cerebrovasular disease and long-term administration of dopamine depleting drugs are also causes.

Parkinson's disease

In addition to the motor features, PD also causes a variety of non-motor symptoms (e.g. dementia, depression, apathy, anxiety, constipation, erectile dysfunction, REM sleep behaviour disorder, anosmia, pain and fatigue) that are increasingly recognised. PD results from degeneration of dopaminergic cells within the substantia nigra pars compacta of the midbrain, resulting in reduced dopamine concentration within the nigrostriatal (and other dopaminergic) pathways. The cause of neuronal cell death in is unknown in idiopathic PD but 8 genes have recently been implicated in the development of familial PD.

The mainstay of drug therapy in PD is levodopa, the amino acid precursor of dopamine. It gets converted to dopamine within the presynaptic cells in the striatum. Patients with Parkinson plus disorders (e.g. multiple system atrophy or progressive supranuclear palsy) or vascular parkinsonism are less dopa-responsive.

Aim and principles of therapy

The goal of treatment in early PD is to improve motor and non-motor symptoms and to slow the neurodegenerative process (neuroprotection). There is much debate about the correct time to start antiparkinson medication, but it is common practice to initiate medication when the patient becomes functionally disabled by their symptoms. In more advanced disease, drug treatment may focus on managing motor complications. Typically patients are commenced on one antiparkinson drug (often a dopamine agonist in younger patients and levodopa in older patients), the dose titrated according to clinical effect, and further drugs added as necessary.

Drugs used for parkinsonism

See Table 7.6.

Levodopa

Levodopa remains the most efficacious treatment available for PD and most patients will eventually be commenced on it. Common side-effects of levodopa include nausea, hypotension and confusion. Long-term use of levodopa will invariably result in development of motor complications ('wearing off', 'on-off' fluctuations and dyskinesias). Approximately 50% of patients experience motor complications after 5 years of levodopa therapy.

Levodopa is always given in combination with a peripheral dopa-decarboxylase inhibitor (carbidopa or benserazide) which prevents peripheral degradation of levodopa to dopamine reducing cardiovascular side-effects (hypotension and arrhythmias). The preparations available are: co-careldopa or Sinemet (levodopa + carbidopa) and Madopar (levodopa + benserazide). Levodopa is initiated at low doses (typically 50 mg BD) and can be gradually increased until the patient is on 300–400 mg/day. Further increases can be made according to response (maximum dose is around 1.5 g/day). Heavy protein meals should be avoided when taking levodopa as dietary amino acids compete with levodopa for absorption. The dopamine antagonist domperidone (10–20 mg TDS) is useful in improving nausea and postural hypotension since, unlike prochlorperazine and metoclopramide, it does not cross the blood–brain barrier and therefore does not worsen motor symptoms.

Patients should be warned not to discontinue levodopa suddenly as this can result in the parkinsonism-hyperpyrexia syndrome which is clinically similar to neuroleptic malignant syndrome. A small proportion of those prescribed antiparkinson medication develop a characteristic pattern of behaviour known as dopamine dysregulation syndrome. These patients obsessively over-medicate with their antiparkinson drugs and may be become very dyskinetic.

The half life of levodopa is 90 minutes and its pulsatile administration is implicated in the development of motor complications. Modified release preparations of Madopar and Sinemet prolong the half-life of levodopa through continuous

Table 7.6 Commonly used anti-parkinsonian drug therapy.

Drug	Dose	Side effects
Levodopa		
Levodopa/carbidopa, regular dose	100/10 to 250/25, increase slowly to t.i.d. or q.i.d.	Orthostatic hypotension, gastrointestinal complaints, hallucinations, confusion, chorea, dyskinesias
Slow-release dose	100/25 to 200/50 b.i.d. or t.i.d.	
Dopamine agonists		
Bromocriptine	7.5–30 mg daily in divided doses	Postural hypotension, nausea, vomiting, hallucinations, psychosis, dyskinesias
Pergolide	0.05–3 mg daily in divided doses	Nausea, dizziness, hallucinations, confusion, constipation, postural hypotension, dyskinesias
Ropinirole	0.5–9 mg daily in divided doses	Nausea, somnolence, leg oedema, abdominal pain, vomiting, syncope, dyskinesia, hallucinations
Pramipexole	264 mcg – 3.3 mg (base)	Nausea, somnolence, drowsiness, confusion, insomnia, hallucinations, leg oedema
Amantadine (acts by NMDA-receptor blockade)	100–200 mg	Livido reticularis, diarrhoea, depression
Apomorphine (subcutaneous injections)	3–30 mg daily in divided doses	Nausea, vomiting, confusion, hallucination, postural hypotension, dyskinesias, local reaction to injections (nodule and ulcers)
Enzyme inhibitors		
Selegeline (inhibits MAO-B)	5 mg b.i.d.	Nausea, dizziness, insomnia, hallucination
Entacapone (inhibits COMT)	200 mg with each dose of levodopa; maximum 2 g	Nausea, vomiting, abdominal pain, dizziness
Antimuscarinics		
Trihexiphenidyl	2–5 mg t.i.d.	Dry mouth, blurred vision, confusion
Benzatropine (benztropine)	0.5–2 mg t.i.d.	Dry mouth, confusion

absorption, but this is at the expense of reduced bioavailability. There are also dispersible preparations of Madopar which have a faster onset of effect, which can be useful if a rapid response is necessary or if the patient has difficulty swallowing tablets. An intrajejunal preparation of levodopa+carbidopa (Duodopa) has recently been licensed for patients with advanced PD and motor complications. It is administered via a gastrostomy tube and is able to achieve more stable plasma levels of levodopa. Its use is limited by its considerable expense.

COMT inhibitors

Catechol-O-methyltransferase (COMT) inhibitors prevent the breakdown of levodopa and are prescribed as an adjunct in patients who have developed motor complications. Entacapone is a COMT inhibitor that prevents conversion of levodopa to 3-O-methyldopa within peripheral tissues such as the liver and erythrocytes. Tolcapone is another COMT inhibitor which acts centrally as well as peripherally. Entacapone is available either alone as Comtess (200 mg tablets, taken 15 minutes before levodopa dose) or in combination with levodopa and carbidopa as Stalevo.

Dopamine agonists

Dopamine agonist (DA) drugs stimulate the striatal postsynaptic dopamine receptor and have longer plasma half-lives than levodopa. They are useful as monotherapy in early PD and in combination with levodopa and/or monoamine-oxidase B inhibitors with more advanced disease.

DA monotherapy in early PD, when compared with levodopa monotherapy, has been shown to delay development of motor complications. More common side-effects of agonists include nausea and vomiting, daytime somnolence (with occasional sudden onset of sleep), ankle swelling and confusion. DA therapy is often poorly tolerated in the elderly and therefore levodopa may be chosen as monotherapy in early PD in this group. Pathological gambling (and other impulse control disorders) and hypersexuality are

also recognised with DA therapy. The older DA's are ergot-derived (bromocriptine, cabergoline, pergolide and lisuride) and have been available for many years but their use has been limited recently by the association of lung, cardiac valve and retroperitoneal fibrosis with long-term usage.

Newer non-ergot agonists (pramipexole, ropinirole, apomorphine and rotigotine) are not associated with fibrotic reactions. Pramipexole has additional antidepressant effects (due to stimulation of the D3 receptor). Rotigotine is administered via a transdermal patch and apomorphine is administered subcutaneously either via a single injections or a continuous pump infusion. Adherence in PD can be problematic and both ropinirole and pramipexole have recently become available in once daily oral preparations.

Monoamine–oxidase B inhibitors

Monoamine-oxidase B (MAO-B) inhibitors (selegiline and rasagiline) prevent the breakdown of levodopa within the synapse and are used as either early monotherapy or as add-on therapy in later disease. Selegiline is available in 5 mg or 10 mg tablets (Eldepryl) or as a dissolvable buccal preparation (Zelepar, 1.25 mg). MAO-Bs may precipitate a hypertensive crisis if used in combination with tyramine-containing foods (e.g. some cheeses, avocados, processed foods). Selective serotonin reuptake inhibitors (SSRIs) should not be prescribed alongside an MAO-B due to the (small) risk of developing serotonin syndrome.

Amantadine

Amantadine (originally developed for its antiviral activity) has modest anti-parkinsonian effects resulting from dopamine and noradrenaline reuptake blockade and antagonism of N-methyl-D-aspartic acid (NMDA). It is used for its antidyskinetic effect. Starting dose is 100 mg and this can be increased to TDS.

Anticholinergics

Anticholinergic drugs (e.g. trihexphenidyl, orphenadrine, benzatropine and procyclidine) may be useful in treating tremor in PD. However, their use is limited by confusion and they should be avoided in the elderly. They are believed to exert their anti-tremor effect by correcting the relative cholinergic excess that occurs in the striatum as a result of dopamine deficiency. Anticholinergics are also useful in reducing drooling. Anticholinergics are contraindicated in patients with closed-angle glaucoma or prostatism. Common side effects also include dry mouth, nausea and urinary retention.

Key points – Parkinson's disease

- Parkinson's disease is caused by a failure of dopamine transmission due to degeneration of dopaminergic cells
- Choice of treatment strategy is determined by the characteristics of the patient and the nature of the symptoms
- Levodopa-based treatment is highly effective but associated with side effects in the longer term
- Dopamine agonists are of particular use in early disease as they alleviate symptoms and delay motor complications
- Anticholinergic therapy should be considered in cases where tremor is problematic

Chapter 8

Treatment of psychiatric disorders

Introduction

The last 50 years have seen major changes in psychiatric practice, with the advent of effective psychotropic drugs and the trend away from custodial to community care. The introduction of the phenothiazines in the 1950s transformed the lives of many patients with schizophrenia by abolishing troublesome symptoms and permitting a return to more normal behaviour. Next came the antidepressants, a welcome alternative to the effective but to some, controversial, electroconvulsive therapy. Since the 1960s lithium has been used effectively in acute mania, as prophylaxis in bipolar affective illness and more recently as adjunctive therapy for refractory depression. The 1960s also saw the introduction of chlordiazepoxide, the first clinical use of benzodiazepines. These sedative and anxiolytic agents were a welcome improvement upon the more dangerous barbiturates they replaced but their widespread use has led to concerns over dependency. A relatively quiescent couple of decades then gave way to an explosion of new pharmacotherapies. Antidepressant treatments expanded, first with the introduction of selective serotonin reuptake inhibitors (SSRIs) followed by a range of other novel agents. Lithium now shares a stage with several anticonvulsant drugs shown to be effective as mood stabilisers. The management of schizophrenia and related psychoses has benefited from a new generation of antipsychotics with improved side effect profile and, particularly in the case of clozapine, evidence of improved efficacy. Most recently, pharmacotherapy for substance use disorders and dementia has also been the focus of renewed interest.

The classification of psychiatric disorders remains heavily dependent upon the identification of clusters of symptoms, and as a result diagnostic categories have a disconcerting tendency to merge. In general, where a particular illness does not fall clearly into a diagnostic category, treatment is best directed at relief of the predominating symptoms. A working outline of the major categories in which drug treatment is likely to be required is given below.

Elucidation of the cause of psychiatric symptoms is frequently difficult. It is important to try to characterise the principal underlying abnormality, as specific drug treatment is available for most of these categories. Misdiagnosis may exacerbate psychiatric symptoms; for example, sedative benzodiazepines given to a depressed patient may lead to further impairment of function and even increased risk of suicide. Tricyclic antidepressants may precipitate or aggravate psychotic symptoms in a patient with schizophrenia.

Lecture Notes: Clinical Pharmacology and Therapeutics,
8th edition. By Gerard McKay, John Reid and Matthew Walters. Published 2010 by Blackwell Publishing Ltd.

Clinical scenario

A 22-year-old man with a history of heavy consumption of cigarettes and alcohol is brought to hospital by the police having been found exhibiting odd behaviour in the street. On examination he was withdrawn and made little eye contact. Careful psychiatric assessment revealed a number of recurring paranoid delusions with complete lack of insight. His family revealed recent homicidal ideation towards his brother. He was transferred to a psychiatric unit for further evaluation and treatment. What strategies can be considered?

Antipsychotic drugs

Aims

The main aims are to inhibit the most florid subjective and behavioural disturbances of psychosis, and to restore the patient to as near normal a life in society as possible. Some atypical antipsychotics also aim to diminish 'negative symptoms' of schizophrenia such as amotivation, flattened affect and social withdrawal.

Adverse effects of conventional antipsychotics

Dose-related adverse reactions from known pharmacological properties

1 Extrapyramidal side effects, caused by dopamine receptor blockade, including: (i) acute dystonia; (ii) parkinsonism; (iii) akathisia; and (iv) tardive dyskinesia – involuntary choreoathetoid movements which, unlike other EPS, may persist even after withdrawal of the antipsychotic drug. Tardive dyskinesia may be aggravated by anticholinergic drugs and treatment is generally unsatisfactory. Benzodiazepines, diazepam and clonazepam may be helpful
2 Increased prolactin (also resulting from dopaminergic blockade), e.g. galactorrhoea, infertility and impotence
3 Anticholinergic effects, e.g. blurred vision, constipation, urinary hesitancy, dry mouth, tachycardia or arrhythmias
4 α_1-Adrenoceptor blockade, e.g. postural hypotension
5 Histamine$_1$-receptor blockade, e.g. sedation
6 Antipsychotic malignant syndrome (potentially fatal hyperthermia, muscle rigidity and autonomic dysfunction)

7 Hypothermia in the elderly
8 Other adverse effects such as confusion, nightmares and insomnia and weight gain
Hypersensitivity reactions not related to dose
1 Cholestatic jaundice with portal infiltration occurs in 2–4% of patients, usually early in treatment. It presents the biochemical features of cholestasis and resolves slowly on drug withdrawal
2 Agranulocytosis (rare)
3 Skin rashes, including photosensitivity dermatitis and urticaria may occur

---

Relevant pathophysiology

The antipsychotics are used in acute schizophrenia to diminish disturbance as a consequence of delusional thinking, hallucinations, inappropriate behaviour and anxiety. In chronic schizophrenia maintenance antipsychotic therapy reduces risk of relapse. Atypical agents may also reduce negative symptoms more resistant to conventional antipsychotics. In affective disorders antipsychotics are used to control manic symptoms, and in depression where delusions, or anxiety and agitation are prominent. They are also used to treat drug-related psychoses and in organic syndrome like delirium they can be helpful given their rapid onset of tranquilisation and ability to be given by an intramuscular route.

The pathophysiology of the psychoses is still unclear and the mechanisms by which drugs exert their effect are still largely hypothetical. The 'dopamine hypothesis', which proposes an over-activity of the brain dopamine system in schizophrenia, is the most favoured explanation for the antipsychotic effects of these drugs. The finding of increased dopamine concentrations in the brains of both treated and untreated patients with schizophrenia, together with the dopamine receptor antagonistic effects of antipsychotics, is in keeping with this hypothesis. On the other hand, 'atypical' antipsychotics such as clozapine, which have additional pharmacological properties, may be effective where typical antipsychotics have failed. Furthermore, traditional antipsychotic agents have little effect upon the 'negative' symptoms of schizophrenia. Thus it is important to recognise that although the 'dopamine hypothesis' might help to explain some of the therapeutic effects of antipsychotics, it does not in itself explain the pathophysiology of schizophrenia.

Conventional antipsychotics

Mechanism

Conventional antipsychotics act as competitive antagonists of dopamine (particularly D_2) receptors in the central nervous system and compete for dopamine binding sites *in vitro*. Although all have similar efficacy, they show a range of other pharmacological properties that might contribute to their therapeutic effects and which are also of importance in determining the profile of adverse effects for any individual drug.

1 Muscarinic blockade causing anticholinergic activity is considerable with thioridazine and much less with fluphenazine and haloperidol.

2 α_1-Adrenoceptor blockade is prominent with chlorpromazine and thioridazine and less so with fluphenazine.

3 Histaminergic (H_1) blockade results in sedation most commonly with chlorpromazine and thioridazine.

4 Dopaminergic blockade is greater with 'high-potency' drugs such as haloperidol. This is also closely linked to propensity for adverse extrapyramidal (Parkinsonian) side effects (EPS).

EPS may need to be controlled by reduction in the dose of antipsychotic or temporary co-administration of anticholinergic drugs such as procylidine, trihexyphenidyl (benzhexol), orphenadrine or benzatropine (benztropine) (see 'Movement disorders', Chapter 7).

Pharmacokinetics

Chlorpromazine, the prototype antipsychotic, is absorbed orally and metabolised by the liver to many active and inactive metabolites. It has a plasma half-life of over 16 hours that, together with the long-lived active metabolites, makes once-daily dosing practical although rarely used. No clear-cut therapeutic range can be defined because of the presence of unmeasured active metabolites and a wide range of individual responses in patients. Plasma or urine drug levels are only of help in assessing compliance. First-pass metabolism is immense, of the order of 80%, making intramuscular administration considerably more potent than the oral alternative.

Adverse reactions

Dose-related adverse reactions from known pharmacological properties include those listed below.

Clinical use and dose

Chlorpromazine: orally 75–300 mg daily, increasing up to 1 g gradually if required. Chlorpromazine: intramuscular injection, 25–50 mg 6- to 8-hourly as required to control acute symptoms. Haloperidol: orally 1.5–3 mg, 2–3 times daily with doses of up to 30 mg daily in treatment resistant cases.

Antipsychotics administered in lower doses are used in nausea and vomiting (see 'Nausea and vomiting', Chapter 3), hiccough, vertigo and labyrinthine disturbances, and during drug withdrawal reactions. They are also widely used as premedication in anaesthesia (see 'General anaesthesia', Chapter 20). Other psychiatric indications are mentioned above.

Atypical antipsychotics

These include aripiprazole, clozapine, risperidone, olanzapine, quetiapine, zotepine and amisulpride. They differ from conventional antipsychotics (and from each other) in their pattern of receptor binding, e.g. clozapine has affinity for 5-hydroxytryptamine (5-HT) and D_4 receptors in addition to the more conventional sites listed above. All atypicals share a reduced propensity to cause EPS (most importantly tardive dyskinesia). Claims have been made for their effectiveness in treating negative symptoms but only clozapine has been demonstrated clearly to be superior to conventional antipsychotics in treatment-resistant patients.

Other adverse effects of atypicals include weight gain (most commonly with clozapine, olanzapine and quetiapine) and sedation. Clozapine may cause agranulocytosis and prescription is restricted initially to hospital patients who can be provided with weekly blood monitoring.

Depot antipsychotics

Long-acting depot antipsychotic preparations play an important part in the community maintenance of more disabled and therefore poorly compliant psychiatric patients. A number of different antipsychotics are used in this way. Commonly used examples are fluphenazine and flupentixol (flupentixol). Fluphenazine is a phenothiazine derivative. As the decanoate or enanthate ester it can be given as a depot by intramuscular injection at intervals of 14–40 days. Adverse effects of fluphenazine are similar to those of chlorpromazine but sedation and anticholinergic adverse effects are less common. EPS are correspondingly more common, particularly dystonia and akathisia or restlessness. Liver and bone marrow toxicity and skin rashes have been reported, as with most other phenothiazines. Flupentixol is a thioxanthine, and as such is somewhat less sedating than other classes of antipsychotic. It is more likely to cause EPS.

Dose

Fluphenazine decanoate: 25–100 mg by injection into the gluteal muscles every 15–40 days, determined by response and side effects. A test dose (12.5 mg) should be given when treatment is begun, to assess possible extrapyramidal reactions.

Flupentixol decanoate: 40–400 mg (test dose 20mg) similarly administered.

Comment. Antipsychotic drugs play a central role in the initial treatment and long-term management of psychoses. The dose should be determined individually from response and adverse effects. Novel drugs (with the exception of clozapine) are increasingly prescribed now as first-choice interventions. Ineffectiveness after a minimum of 6 weeks treatment on any one drug should result in a trial of a second drug of a different class. Clozapine should be considered if there is lack of response to two antipsychotics. Depot intramuscular preparations are useful for long-term outpatient management. Adverse effects are common and may be disabling or even dangerous. Patients on long-term antipsychotic medication should remain under close medical supervision.

Antipsychotics should not be used in the management of simple anxiety as an alternative to anxiolytics, minor tranquillisers or other forms of treatment.

Clinical scenario

A 47-year-old man presents to his general practitioner with fatigue, loss of appetite, headache and diffuse lumbar and thoracic back pain. These symptoms have been present for several months and are associated with a subjective reduction in the quality of his sleep. His family report irritability and an increase in alcohol consumption over this period. The general practitioner makes a diagnosis of depression and decides upon pharmacological treatment as a first line strategy. What options can be considered and what factors may inform the choice of drug?

Antidepressants

Aims

The main aims are to relieve symptoms of depression, restore normal social behaviour and prevent further episodes.

Relevant pathophysiology

Depression is common in all populations. Its prevalence is increasing worldwide and it is anticipated to become the second commonest cause of global morbidity (after ischaemic heart disease) by 2020. Pathological feelings of sadness and despair may be associated with physical and emotional withdrawal. Depressive illnesses are a common factor in suicide.

Major depression is characterised by low mood and anhedonia (loss of pleasure). Other key symptoms include psychomotor changes, cognitive impairment and changes in sleep, appetite and weight. Psychotic symptoms, such as delusions of unworthiness, may also occur. Episodes may be recurrent (unipolar depression) or alternate with mania (bipolar affective disorder).

A range of drugs, including sedatives, steroids, opiates and the antihypertensive methyldopa may cause depressive symptoms. The causative drug should be withdrawn if possible.

The neurobiological basis of depression is thought to involve underactivity of central neuronal pathways where noradrenaline or serotonin act as transmitters. This amine hypothesis is supported by biochemical measurement of these transmitters and their metabolites *in vivo* in cerebrospinal fluid and in brain tissue at post-mortem, and from neuroendocrine evidence of abnormal aminergic neurotransmission in depressed patients. There is further support from the therapeutic actions of drugs that modify amine turnover. It is currently thought that mona-aminergic change is the beginning of a molecular cascade in depression. Most modern antidepressants are concerned with aminergic reuptake inhibition. As a result of this there is associated pre-synaptic autoregulatory desensitisation, up- and down-regulation of post-synaptic receptor sites, receptor-mediated second messenger and neurotrophic intracellular signalling effects.

Monoamine oxidase inhibitors (MAOIs) block the intrasynaptic breakdown of noradrenaline and serotonin and thus increase transmitter activity.

Tricyclic antidepressants block neuronal reuptake (uptake 1) of noradrenaline and/or serotonin into noradrenergic/serotonergic neurones, altering transmitter levels in the synaptic cleft.

The SSRIs selectively inhibit the reuptake of serotonin.

Other 'atypical' antidepressants influence noradrenergic and/or serotonergic neurotransmission in a variety of other ways.

Comment. The diagnosis of depression is complicated by frequent non-specific somatic symptoms of anorexia, malaise, weight loss and constipation. Conversely, the symptoms of depression often accompany non-psychiatric physical illness

and understandably depressing adjustments such as bereavement. Nevertheless, pathological depression is common, responsive to drug treatment and therefore important to identify and treat appropriately. Suicide is a serious and well-recognised complication of depression.

Tricyclic antidepressants

Mechanism

This group of drugs includes the closely related agents amitriptyline, nortriptyline, imipramine and clomipramine. They competitively block neuronal uptake of noradrenaline and serotonin into nerve endings and in the short term increase transmitter levels in the synaptic cleft. In the long term these agents lead to down-regulation of pre- and post-synaptic adrenoceptors and serotonin receptors in the brain.

All tricyclics have a range of other pharmacological properties that may contribute to their therapeutic actions and adverse effects:

1 α-Adrenoceptor blockade
2 Anticholinergic effects
3 Antihistaminergic effects
4 Other non-specific sedative actions.

The therapeutic response to tricyclics develops over 3–4 weeks. Suicide by overdose of antidepressant is a risk during this lag period during treatment. There is some evidence that long-term tricyclic treatment is superior to placebo in reducing the frequency of recurrent depressive symptoms. Amitriptyline, which has more sedative properties, may be useful in agitated depression or where insomnia is troublesome. Imipramine, with less sedative properties, is indicated in those who have marked motor retardation.

Pharmacokinetics

Tricyclics are extensively metabolised by the liver. The half-life of amitriptyline is >24 hours and the formation of metabolites with antidepressant activity further extends the duration of drug activity. Once-daily dosing, ideally at night, is indicated for most tricyclics.

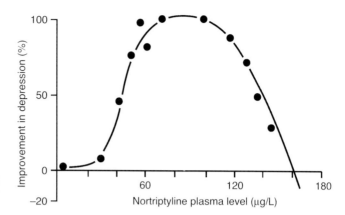

Figure 8.1 Relationship between drug plasma level and effect with nortriptyline.

Hepatic metabolism of tricyclics is determined by genetic and environmental factors. There are wide differences in plasma level when the same dose is given to a group of individuals. Thus the dose of tricyclic should be titrated individually, with therapeutic response or adverse effects as end points.

Studies with nortriptyline have shown an unusual relationship between drug plasma level and effect (Fig. 8.1). At low drug levels and also at high drug levels there is little effect, while optimal effect is seen within a very narrow concentration range (50–150 µg/L) or therapeutic window. This has led some to propose drug level monitoring as a guide to antidepressant therapy, but this is not routine clinical practice.

Adverse effects of tricyclics

1 Sedation and confusional states, especially with amitriptyline
2 Anticholinergic effects, e.g. dry mouth, constipation, urinary symptoms, sexual dysfunction and precipitation of glaucoma
3 Postural hypotension, especially in the very young and old
4 Cardiac tachyarrhythmias (seen in overdose) and conduction defects that are quinidine/procainamide-like. May occur more frequently in patients treated with long-term tricyclics
5 Self-poisoning by tricyclic overdose is common and its management is discussed further in Chapter 26
6 Fits may occur on withdrawal of tricyclics

Adverse effects

Clinical use and dose
As the many side effects can limit adherence, it is often prudent to begin with a relatively low dose and titrate upwards to a therapeutic dose over a period of 1–2 weeks: 25–75 mg orally, titrated to 100–200 mg daily. Imipramine may also be useful in nocturnal enuresis and hyperactivity syndrome in childhood. Amitriptyline is also used in some forms of neurogenic pain.

Other related antidepressants
Monocyclic, bicyclic and tetracyclic drugs have been developed with similar therapeutic properties to the tricyclics

Selective Serotonin Re-uptake Inhibitors (SSRIs)

Drugs in this group include fluoxetine, fluvoxamine, paroxetine, sertraline and citalopram

Mechanism
These drugs inhibit the reuptake of serotinin 5-HT into neurones in the central nervous system.

Pharmacokinetics
SSRIs have good oral bioavailability and are eliminated by liver metabolism. They have long half-lives (e.g. fluoxetine 2 days) and can be given once daily.

Adverse effects

SSRIs have the same *incidence* of adverse effects as the tricyclics but the nature of these effects is different: nausea, diarrhoea, headache, insomnia and agitation are the main problems. They are less sedative than tricyclics and safer in overdose. Those with shorter half-lives should be withdrawn slowly – a discontinuance syndrome is recognised. SSRIs increase the levels of carbamazepine, phenytoin, MAOIs (2 weeks should elapse between treatments and 5 weeks in the case of fluoxetine), benzodiazepines, lithium and possibly warfarin.

Comment. Tricyclic antidepressants and SSRIs have similar efficacy but a different range of side effects. The main significance of SSRIs is that they have much reduced toxicity in overdose.

Monoamine oxidase inhibitors

Mechanism

Phenelzine, tranylcypromine and iproniazid are non-competitive irreversible antagonists of monoamine oxidase (MAO). They block MAO type A, in contrast to selegiline, which is described in Chapter 7. The enzyme is blocked not only in brain monoamine neurones but also in peripheral neurones, enterocytes in the gut wall and platelets. Inhibition of MAO leads to increases in serotonin, noradrenaline and dopamine in the brain.

The problems with MAOIs result from widespread enzyme inhibition, and as a result other drug treatments for depression have been favoured. There are now reversible MAOIs, such as moclobemide, which promise a safer alternative. Apart from therapeutic failure with other antidepressants, indication for the use of MAOIs include phobic states and 'agitated' depression.

When used, the response may be delayed for 2–3 weeks. After the use of irreversible MAOIs the enzyme recovers slowly (2–3 weeks) after the drug is stopped, as it requires re-synthesis. This problem does not accompany the use of reversible MAOIs.

Adverse effects

1 Postural hypotension
2 Headache

3 Anticholinergic side effects
4 Drug-induced liver damage (phenelzine and iso-carboxazid)
5 Hypertensive crisis.

The most important adverse effect is hypertensive crisis following amine-containing foods, beverages or drugs. Inhibition of MAO in the gut wall allows absorption of tyramine and other sympathomimetic substances in food or drink. MAO usually metabolises these to inactive products during absorption. The amines are taken up from the circulation by peripheral sympathetic nerve endings. They displace endogenous noradrenaline from storage sites (indirect sympathomimetic action) leading to hypertension, tachycardia and headache.

Severe paroxysmal hypertension may cause a cerebrovascular accident. Foods rich in tyramine, particularly cheese, meat, yeast extract and red wine, should be avoided.

Comment. The dangers of hypertension, the limitations on food intake and the availability of alternatives have greatly reduced the role of MAOIs in depression. They are rarely used as first-line agents.

Other antidepressants

Mianserin

A tetracyclic compound with sedative properties and low cardiotoxicity. Blood dyscrasias can occur in patients (particularly the elderly) treated with this drug. A 30–60 mg daily dose is given at bedtime, increasing if necessary and if tolerated to 200 mg daily.

Nefazodone

Causes 5-HT reuptake inhibition and $5-HT_2$ blockade. The commonest side effects of nausea and restlessness can be minimised by building up the dose gradually to an optimal range of 300–600 mg daily. There is a beneficial effect on sleep.

Venlafaxine

A combined serotonin and noradrenaline reuptake inhibitor (SNRI) but without the anticholinergic and sedative effects commonly seen with the tricyclics. Dosage should be 75 mg daily or greater and a once-daily slow-release form is available. The most frequent side effect is nausea, usually resolving after a week, but blood-pressure elevation may occur at higher doses.

Mirtazepine

Termed a 'noradrenergic and specific serotonergic antidepressant' this drug has a novel action in enhancing noradrenaline and (indirectly) serotonin transmission by blocking pre-synaptic α_2-adrenergic receptors. It also causes 5-HT$_2$- and 5-HT$_3$-receptor blockade, minimising serotonergic side effects. Dose range is 15–45 mg, with sedation more prominent at lower doses.

Reboxetine

Specifically causing noradrenaline reuptake inhibition, reboxetine is administered in a dose range of 4–12 mg daily. Claims have been made for its greater effect on social functioning. Dry mouth is the commonest side effect.

Mood stabilising agents

Relevant pathophysiology

Mania and hypomania are characterised by a pathologically elevated mood and disinhibited behaviour. They usually occur as part of a bipolar affective (manic depressive) disorder. Mania is characterised by elated mood and irritability with motor over-activity, non-stop talk, flight of ideas, grandiosity and a progressive lack of contact with reality.

Treatment of an acute manic episode includes sedation with haloperidol or other major tranquillisers, together with general supportive measures. Specific therapy with lithium salts is used both in the acute attack (the main disadvantage to its use as sole agent being its delayed onset of effect) and for prophylaxis between attacks. Lithium is also now recognised to have a place in the prophylaxis against recurring depressive disorder and as adjunctive therapy in antidepressant-resistant depression. The anticonvulsants carbamazepine and sodium valproate are also used as prophylactic agents in bipolar disorder.

Lithium carbonate

Mechanism

The monovalent lithium cation, given as the carbonate salt, modifies the effect in mania. The mechanism of action of lithium is not clear. It appears to substitute for sodium and potassium cations in cellular transport processes. It has effects on the release of monoamine neurotransmitters and alters intracellular and extracellular ion concentrations, fluxes across excitable membranes and the concentrations of 'second messengers' such as inositol phosphate. Lithium may take several days to achieve its effect.

Pharmacokinetics

Lithium is rapidly and completely absorbed after oral dosing. It is not metabolised and is excreted unchanged by the kidney with a half-life of 12 hours. Lithium is distributed in total body water, and it slowly enters cells and reaches steady-state levels after dosing for 5 days. There is a narrow therapeutic range for lithium (0.5–1.0 mmol/L, with higher levels sometimes used in acute mania), with severe adverse effects occurring at higher levels. Monitoring of drug levels in plasma is essential for optimal control of therapy. Change in renal function is the most important factor modifying elimination and thus plasma levels. Lithium clearance is 0.2 times the creatinine clearance, and the dose must be modified in the presence of renal impairment and in the elderly. The sodium and potassium status of the patient also influences lithium levels and response. Thus dehydration, salt depletion or diuretic therapy all tend to increase the plasma drug concentration.

Adverse effects (see above)

These are more common and severe when the plasma lithium level exceeds 1.2 mmol/L or in the presence of salt depletion or diuretic therapy.

Drug interactions

Lithium levels rise following the introduction of diuretics. Other drugs altering sodium balance (e.g. steroids, ACE inhibitors and non-steroidal anti-inflammatory drugs) may have the same effect. Lithium potentiates the neurotoxicity of haloperidol and flupentixol. Owing to the wide range of further possible interactions, always check carefully before administering another drug with lithium.

Adverse effects of lithium carbonate

1 Nausea and vomiting
2 Drowsiness, confusion and fits
3 Ataxia, nystagmus and dysarthria
4 Hypothyroidism by interference with iodination; rarely hyperthyroidism
5 Oedema and weight gain
6 Nephrogenic diabetes insipidus

Dose

Lithium carbonate: 0.4–2.0 g daily in divided doses, depending on renal function and drug plasma levels achieved.

Other mood stabilisers

Carbamazepine

This commonly used anticonvulsant is an effective treatment both for acute mania and as prophylaxis in bipolar disorder. Trials suggest that its prophylactic effect is less marked than lithium and so should be reserved for those where lithium is contraindicated or has proven ineffective. There is an uncertain relationship between blood levels and treatment response. A dose of 600–800 mg should be aimed for, depending on response and side effects.

Sodium valproate

While there is not as much evidence available for valproate, what there is suggests effectiveness in treatment of acute mania and prophylaxis of

bipolar disorder. Blood levels above 45 mg/L are associated with response but side effects are prominent at levels above 100 mg/L.

Antipsychotic drugs

Haloperidol and other antipsychotic major tranquillisers have long been used in the management of acute mania. Symptoms are controlled, but it is not clear whether the duration of the manic episode is reduced. These drugs are useful in the treatment of acute attacks.

Haloperidol or chlorpromazine have been used successfully and may be used either alone or in combination with lithium carbonate so long as the dose of haloperidol does not exceed 15 mg/day and the plasma lithium concentration does not exceed 0.8 mmol/L. For adverse effects, see drug induced neurological disorders in Chapter 7.

Comment. Lithium carbonate is used for long-term prophylaxis in bipolar affective disorder and recurring depressive illness, and it is used together with phenothiazines for control of symptoms in acute attacks. The daily dose of lithium depends on renal function and should be determined individually. Monitoring of lithium plasma levels is essential for optimal treatment without unacceptable adverse effects.

Carbamazepine and valproate may be more effective in lithium-resistant cases (e.g. rapid-cycling affective disorder, mania with depressive symptoms) and combinations of any two of the three mood stabilisers may be more effective than monotherapy.

Anxiolytics

Aim

The aim is to control symptoms of anxiety without interfering with normal physical or mental function.

Relevant pathophysiology

The experience of anxiety, with physical and psychological symptoms, is a universal phenomenon.

Furthermore, better defined and clearly morbid anxiety disorders such as agoraphobia are amongst mankind's commonest seriously disabling conditions. As a result there has always been widespread and excessive use of whatever anxiolytic agents are available. Since the introduction of chlordiazepoxide in 1960, the anxiolytic benzodiazepines have become the most widely prescribed group of drugs in the United Kingdom and in the United States (15–20% of the population at any one time). Medical practitioners, conditioned to 'treat', often find it extremely difficult to resist demands for a pill to relieve anxiety even though such problems invariably require other forms of intervention.

The principal groups of drugs used in the management of anxiety are the benzodiazepines, the β-receptor blockers and recently developed agents affecting 5-HT systems. There is also growing interest in the use of imipramine and SSRIs in the treatment of patients with panic attacks, the use of serotonergic agents in the treatment of patients with obsessional or compulsive disorders and the use of MAOIs in the treatment of certain phobic conditions.

Comment. Anxiety in appropriate circumstances is a normal response. If anxiety symptoms are frequent or persist in a severe form, they may interfere with normal function. Such pathological anxiety is an indication for assessment and appropriate treatment, which might include a pharmacological agent.

Benzodiazepines

Mechanism

Benzodiazepines have a relatively selective action on the limbic system, cerebral cortex and the ascending amine systems that govern arousal. They potentiate gamma-aminobutyric acid (GABA) transmission. The identification of specific binding sites for benzodiazepines has led to speculation that these 'receptors' are normally present to be activated by an, as yet, unidentified 'endogenous benzodiazepine', deficient in anxiety states. Clear proof of this has yet to emerge.

The amnesic action of benzodiazepines is useful in addition to sedation for use as pre-medication for minor investigative procedures like gastroscopy and bronchoscopy.

The benzodiazepines currently available range from very short-acting drugs such as flurazepam or temazepam, which are used as hypnotics, to longer-acting agents such as diazepam, chlordiazepoxide and oxazepam, which are most useful as anxiolytics. Variations in pharmacokinetics and metabolism are responsible for these differences.

Pharmacokinetics

Diazepam is rapidly absorbed from the gastrointestinal tract and extensively metabolised by oxidation in the liver. It forms several active metabolites, including oxazepam, which is used therapeutically in its own right. The plasma half-life is long (24 hours) and its duration of effect even longer, as the active metabolites have half-lives of several days. The half-life may be increased in the elderly, who may also be more sensitive to the drug.

Oxazepam is an active metabolite of diazepam. It is cleared by conjugation in the liver and has a half-life of 10–20 hours.

Chlordiazepoxide was one of the earlier benzodiazepines. It is still used as an anxiolytic, and is the drug of choice in serious alcohol withdrawal states.

Adverse effects

Benzodiazepines are drugs of dependence. The risk of physical dependence is apparently greater with short-acting agents. Prescriptions should be limited to short-term use (no longer than 6 weeks) and in the case of anxiety only if the condition is severely disabling.

Other adverse effects are listed below.

Drug interactions

Benzodiazepines, have, additive, or, synergistic, effects with other centrally acting drugs – antihistamines, alcohol, barbiturates. This may increase the impairment of motor or intellectual function or worsen respiratory depression.

Adverse effects of benzodiazepines

1 Drowsiness, agitation, ataxia and lightheadedness, especially in the elderly
2 Incontinence, nightmares and confusion
3 Excessive salivation
4 Changes in libido
5 Respiratory depression, hypotension
6 Impaired alertness with motor and intellectual dysfunction, e.g. driving, operating machinery
7 Paradoxical stimulant effects in some violent patients
8 Disinhibition can lead to suicidal behaviour
9 Withdrawal can be associated with rebound increased agitation, hallucinations and epileptic seizures
10 Thrombophlebitis may follow intravenous diazepam
11 Psychological adjustment to bereavement may be inhibited by benzodiazepines

Diazepam and chlordiazepoxide do not interfere with the metabolism of other drugs and do not interact with warfarin.

Clinical use and dose

Benzodiazepines are appropriate in the short-term management (2–4 weeks) of severe disabling anxiety. Chlordiazepoxide is the treatment of choice in severe alcohol withdrawal states including delirium tremens.

Diazepam: orally, 4–30 mg daily in divided doses titrated to control symptoms and continued only as long as is necessary; intramuscularly or slow intravenous injection, 10 mg repeated after 4–6 hours if required. Diazepam is used as a sedative in acutely agitated hospitalised patients or as premedication before minor procedures.

Comparable doses of the benzodiazepines are shown in Table 8.1.

Comment. Use the lowest possible dose.

The use of benzodiazepines to treat mild anxiety is unjustifiable. Long-term use is to be avoided. If a patient has taken a benzodiazepine for a long time, the drug should be withdrawn slowly, at a rate determined by the severity of the withdrawal syndrome.

Other drug treatment of anxiety

β-Receptor blockers

β-Receptor blockers reduce cardiovascular and other β-receptor mediated effects of increased sympathetic activity. Most experience has been acquired with propranolol, a non-selective beta-blocker. Their value in the treatment of morbid anxiety is limited but occasional use in patients disabled by performance anxiety can be of value. The clinical pharmacology and adverse effects of beta-blockers are discussed in Chapter 4. Beta-blockers should be used with caution in patients with a past history of asthma, peripheral vascular disease, cardiac failure or bradyarrhythmias.

Dose

Propranolol: 40 mg before a predictably anxiety-provoking situation.

Serotonergic agents

Buspirone is a 5-HT$_{1a}$ receptor agonist for which reasonable evidence of clinical efficacy exists. It does not appear to interact with the same receptors as the benzodiazepines, but early claims of

Table 8.1 Anxiolytic drugs and dose range used.

Drug	Group	Dose (mg)
Chlordiazepoxide	Benzodiazepines	75–100
Diazepam		4–30
Lorazepam		1–10
Medazepam		10–30
Oxazepam		30–120
Propranolol	Beta-blocker	40 (when need anticipated)
Buspirone	5-HT$_{1a}$-receptor agonist	15–30

freedom from physical dependence should be treated with caution.

Clomethiazole

Clomethiazole has few advantages over benzodiazepines, and prolonged use may lead to dependence and severe respiratory depression can occur.

Tricyclic antidepressants, SSRIs and MAOIs

Imipramine and SSRIs have a part to play in the treatment of patients disabled by recurrent panic attacks. SSRIs and clomipramine are used in the treatment of obsessive-compulsive disorder, and MAOIs used in the treatment of certain phobic disorders. Their effects are probably a result of long-term changes in central noradrenergic and/or serotonergic activity. Optimal treatment of such patients also involves an appropriate psychological intervention. Use of these agents depends upon careful assessment of the clinical problem and requires specialised advice.

Comment. Anxiety symptoms should only be treated with drugs if they are severe and interfere with the patient's lifestyle or if alternative social or psychotherapy is not possible or appropriate. Treatment should be regularly revised and stopped as soon as possible. Benzodiazepines are effective but beta-blockers may be an alternative, with fewer dependence problems and less abuse potential. The treatment of more severely disabled patients with anxiety disorder may benefit from one of the various noradrenergic or serotonergic agents traditionally used in the treatment of depression, but such use should be restricted to specialised services.

Hypnotic drugs and the treatment of insomnia

Aim

By short-term use the aim is to restore normal restful sleep without a residual hangover the next day and to aid a return to normal sleep without drugs.

Relevant pathophysiology

Insomnia is an interference with the quality or quantity of sleep and is a very common complaint. Insomnia is a subjective symptom and reflects what the patient considers to be the 'normal' length and quality of sleep. Individuals vary in their expectation of sleep. Requirements for sleep may vary and diminish with advancing age. A reduced duration of total sleep is common in the elderly and may not be pathological.

The treatment of sleep disorders requires:

1 Assessment of the type of sleep disorder
2 Assessment of accompanying symptoms of anxiety or depression and their treatment
3 Diagnosis and treatment of other physical symptoms interfering with sleep, e.g. pain, nocturnal dyspnoea or urinary frequency
4 Consideration of non-pharmacological strategies, including changes in lifestyle. Simple measures like bathing, exercising or enriched milk drinks at bedtime may help.

Drug treatment should be offered only when the alternatives given above have been excluded, and where there is evidence of frequent and marked sleep impairment. Hypnotics should ideally be used for short periods of days or weeks when required, and not given for regular long-term use.

Comment. A successful hypnotic should act rapidly, allow the subject to wake if necessary without severe sedation and be free from residual hangover effects in the morning. Unfortunately, few of the available agents meet these criteria.

Benzodiazepines

Mechanism

Benzodiazepines exert hypnotic effects by similar mechanisms to their anxiolytic actions but at higher doses. At the peak of drug action, in addition to the anxiolytic effect, the drugs affect brain arousal systems by potentiating the inhibitory effects of GABA.

Nitrazepam, flurazepam and temazepam are widely used (Table 8.2). They induce sleep within 20–40 minutes of dosing and produce sleep with a

Table 8.2 Benzodiazepine hypnotic drugs.

Drug	Plasma half-life (hour)	Active metabolite
Nitrazepam	20+	None
Flurazepam	2–4	Yes, with long half-life
Temazepam	5–6	None

reduction in deep sleep (stage 4) and a reduction in rapid eye movement (REM) sleep.

Residual hangover effects with cumulative adverse reactions in chronic dosing may occur with nitrazepam and flurazepam, which have a long half-life and an active metabolite, respectively.

Temazepam appears to have the advantage of a short half-life and no active metabolites. Residual impairment is less with temazepam than with other benzodiazepines.

Adverse effects

Benzodiazepines are drugs of dependence. Particular problems relevant to their use as hypnotics include oversedation (especially in the elderly), 'hangover' effect, paradoxical agitation, and withdrawal phenomena including rebound insomnia, vivid dreams and fits.

Clinical use and dose

Benzodiazepines are indicated in the short-term management of severe, disabling insomnia. Normal doses before going to bed are;
Temazepam: 10–30 mg
Nitrazepam: 5–10 mg
Flurazepam: 15–30 mg

Comment. Hypnotic drugs should only be used for short periods of time. They should certainly not be prescribed without very careful thought. Other physical, psychiatric and social factors may well require attention.

Zopiclone, zolpidem and zaleplon

These are non-benzodiazepine hypnotic agents which act through a similar mechanism. They have a short duration of action and are commonly-used in the management of short term sleep disturbance. Long-term use is not encouraged as dependence may occur.

Drug-induced psychiatric disorder

Central nervous system adverse effects of drugs are common, especially in the case of lipid-soluble drugs with specific effects on:
1 Receptors
2 Transmitter synthesis
3 Degradation of transmitters
4 Electrophysiological effects on excitable membranes.
A careful history of recent drug ingestion is an essential feature of the evaluation of a patient with psychiatric illness and, where possible, the first step in the management of drug-induced psychiatric symptoms should be withdrawal of the offending drug.

There are many well-documented examples of drugs causing behavioural adverse effects, and these are summarised in Table 8.3.

Abuse of psychoactive drugs

Abuse of drugs and related agents is a major social problem amongst young people, especially in urban communities. Therapeutic drug use may also lead to dependence, e.g. benzodiazepines used for anxiety or insomnia, or opiate analgesic abuse in patients first treated for chronic severe pain. However, the concept of drug misuse or abuse must be judged in a cultural and historical context. Attitudes to the non-therapeutic use of cannabis and even opiates differ greatly throughout the world.

The problems of drug abuse are:
1 The direct specific toxic effects, e.g. respiratory depression with opiates
2 Generalised actions on mood, disinhibition of social behaviour and impaired level of consciousness
3 Short-term consequences of drug withdrawal, e.g. psychological and physical symptoms of dependence

Table 8.3 Drug-induced psychiatric disorder.

Depression

Antihypertensives
  Methyldopa
  Clonidine
  Reserpine
  Propranolol
  Guanethidine
  Non-steroidal anti-inflammatory drugs

Sedatives
  Benzodiazepines
  Alcohol
  Barbiturates

Steroids
  Corticosteroids
  Oral contraceptive pill

Analgesics
  Opiates

Others
  Levodopa   Cimetidine
  Tetrabenazine   Triamcinolone
  Methysergide   Mefloquine

Antipsychotics
  Phenothiazines and other antipsychotics

Psychotic states
  Sympathomimetics (amfetamine (amphetamine)) and the amfetamine-derived 'designer' drug Ecstasy
  Anticholinergic drugs (atropine, trihexyphenidyl (benzhexol))
  Levodopa and dopamine agonists (bromocriptine, apomorphine)
  Steroids (prednisolone, dexamethasone)
  Phencyclidine (PCP: 'angel dust')
  Cannabis

Anxiety and anxiety symptoms
  Sympathomimetics (amfetamine, ephedrine, phenylpropanolamine, etc.)
  β_2-Adrenoceptor agonists (isoprenaline, salbutamol, terbutaline)

Drug-withdrawal states
  Benzodiazepines, clonidine, barbiturates, opiates and alcohol

4 Long-term medical complications of the contemporary drug 'subculture', e.g. hepatitis, septicaemia, acquired immunodeficiency syndrome (AIDS) and bacterial endocarditis.

Psychoactive drugs, like analgesics or sedatives, have a high potential for abuse because of:

1 *Central effects.* They modify mood or behaviour, leading to either pleasurable experiences, depersonalisation or intoxication and amnesia.

2 *Tolerance.* If there is tolerance to the effect with regular use, and thus a need to increase the dose to get the same effect, then not only is the drug-taking habit reinforced but there is a greater risk of chemical toxicity or adverse effects at the higher doses.

3 *Withdrawal symptoms.* Symptoms on withdrawal of the abused drug further reinforce the need for continued drug use (or abuse). While these withdrawal symptoms may often be psychological, in the case of benzodiazepines, opiates and barbiturates, physical symptoms on withdrawal create further dependence or 'addiction'.

Drugs with a high abuse potential can be divided into:

1 Therapeutic agents:
  • Benzodiazepines
  • Barbiturates
  • Other hypnotics and sedatives
  • Opiate analgesics and analogues, including dextropropoxyphene.

2 Non-therapeutic agents ('street' drugs):
  • Cannabis
  • Cocaine
  • Opiates

- Amfetamines (amphetamines); their therapeutic use now is very limited
- LSD, psylocybin, phencyclidine and other hallucinogens
- Solvents
- Alcohol.

The following agents are used in the management of psychoactive substance misuse.

Benzodiazepines

Their primary use is in the management of severe alcohol withdrawal states, which may present with autonomic overarousal and fits, and delirium tremens. Long-acting compounds such as chlordiazepoxide are preferred and prescribed on a reducing dose regime over 5–7 days. Initial doses are judged on symptom severity and may range from 60 to 160 mg/day. Vitamin supplementation B_1 ought to also be given to minimise risk of amnesic (Wernicke–Korsakoff) syndrome. Vitamin deficiency and malabsorption require high doses to be used.

Disulfiram

The metabolism of ethanol is blocked by disulfiram, which causes inhibition of aldehyde dehydrogenase (ALDH) leading to accumulation of acetaldehyde. Symptoms of the alcohol–disulfiram reaction include flushing, tachycardia, headache, nausea, vomiting and hypotension. Rarely, significant medical complications can arise. The practice of patients receiving a test challenge has now been abandoned and disulfiram therefore acts as a deterrent to drinking in patients who are motivated toward abstinence. Enzyme inhibition (and thus potential for reaction) lasts up to 7 days and patients must be warned of potential interactions with alcohol in foods and over-the-counter medications.

Acamprosate

Acamprosate enhances GABA inhibitory neurotransmission and antagonises glutamate excitation. This is thought to be the mechanism by which it reduces craving for alcohol. It is pre-scribed in a usual dose of 666 mg three times daily. It should be commenced while abstinent but can be maintained during brief relapses.

Opiate dependence

May be treated by use of substitute prescribing (methadone) or by drugs that abolish the euphoric effects of opiates (naltrexone). Drugs such as lofexidine are used to minimise symptoms of opiate withdrawal.

Comment. The management of drug abuse is not easy and involves:

1 Management of acute pharmacological toxicity
2 Treatment of any acute medical complications, e.g. septicaemia, endocarditis
3 Psychiatric assessment and treatment of any underlying psychopathology, e.g. depression
4 Controlled planned withdrawal of the drug, if necessary, with temporary substitution, e.g. methadone for heroin
5 Long-term measures such as family or community support (Alcoholics Anonymous), psychotherapy or drug therapy (disulfiram for alcoholics).

Treatment of dementia

Aim

Traditionally, drugs have been used to minimise behavioural disturbance in dementia. New agents, such as donepezil, stabilise or reverse cognitive decline, albeit temporarily.

Relevant pathophysiology

Dementia is a chronic, progressive organic brain disorder resulting in memory decline and eventual loss of all aspects of cognitive functioning. A small number of cases are reversible where certain specific aetiologies can be found (e.g. vitamin B_{12} deficiency, normal pressure hydrocephalus, hypothyroidism). The majority, however, are irreversible, the commonest being Alzheimer's disease (and its variant, Lewy Body dementia) and multi-infarct dementia.

Alzheimer's disease is characterised by post-mortem findings of senile plaques, neurofibrillary tangles and reduced neurotransmitter levels, particularly of acetylcholine, the severity of which correlates with neuronal loss. Acetylcholinesterase inhibitors have recently been introduced in the management of mild to moderate Alzheimer's disease. Compounds currently available include donepezil and rivastigmine. They may slow the rate of cognitive and non-cognitive decline in 40% of patients.

Donepezil

This is prescribed in an initial dose of 5 mg daily, rising to 10 mg/day after 1 month. Side effects, which include nausea, vomiting and diarrhoea, are minimised by careful dose titration.

Rivastigmine

Similar side effects to donepezil are seen. Rivastigmine is prescribed twice daily in doses of 6–12 mg/day, titrated weekly to maximum tolerated dose.

Comment. While drugs may slow cognitive decline, they do not alter ultimate disease progres-sion and, on withdrawal, rapid deterioration may occur, even when no clear response has been seen. This should be explained to patients and their relatives. Baseline assessment of cognitive functioning should precede treatment and patients should be reassessed again at 3 months. If no clear improvement has occurred the drug should be stopped. Other drugs, including antidepressants and antipsychotics are often used to control behavioural disturbance. However, antipsychotics should be avoided if at all possible in patients with Lewy Body dementia, where they may cause severe EPS.

Key points – psychiatric disorders in which drug treatments are commonly used

- Acute and chronic organic brain syndromes (including delirium, dementia and drug-related psychoses)
- Bipolar affective (manic-depressive) disorder
- Unipolar depression (psychotic and non-psychotic)
- Schizophrenia and delusional disorders (paranoid psychoses)
- Generalised anxiety and panic disorders
- Phobias
- Obsessive compulsive disorder
- Complications of drug dependence, alcohol misuse and personality disorder may require drug treatment

Chapter 9

Antimicrobial therapy

Aim

The aim is to cure or control infection without harm to the patient and with minimal ecological impact.

Clinical scenario

A 56-year-old man is admitted to hospital with fever and breathlessness. A diagnosis of lower respiratory tract infection is made and empirical treatment with broad spectrum antibiotic therapy is initiated. After 5 days of treatment he remains pyrexial and unwell. Cultures of blood and sputum are negative and his antibiotic therapy is augmented with the addition of a second broad spectrum agent. His symptoms begin to improve; however, after a further 6 days of dual antibiotic therapy he complains of abdominal pain and develops profuse foul-smelling diarrhoea. Stool analysis is positive for the presence of Clostridium difficile toxin and his antibiotic treatment is stopped. What factors guide selection of appropriate antimicrobial drugs, and how may complications such as C. difficile diarrhoea be avoided?

Principles of drug treatment

One of the greatest of all therapeutic advances was the introduction of drugs to treat bacterial infec-

Lecture Notes: Clinical Pharmacology and Therapeutics, 8th edition. By Gerard McKay, John Reid and Matthew Walters. Published 2010 by Blackwell Publishing Ltd.

tions in man. Whilst the introduction of immunisation markedly reduced the prevalence of serious infection, the introduction of sulphonamides in 1936 and penicillin in 1941 was associated with marked reductions in infection-related mortality. Since the 1940s there has been a vast increase in the number of antimicrobial agents available for clinical use. The ready availability of new agents has enhanced the likelihood that a suitable agent can be found for a particular infection, but it has also resulted in a confusing range of choice and a readiness to prescribe antimicrobial agents even when the presence of bacterial infection is poorly documented. Moreover, poor regulation of antibacterial use has been associated with increasing rates of resistance and potential life-threatening complications including *C. difficile*-associated diarrhea and intravenous line related infection. Newer antibiotics are usually expensive, not necessarily better than established agents and are increasingly broad in spectrum. When prescribing an antimicrobial agent, careful consideration should be given to patient factors, the suspected (or proven) organism's biological characteristics and the chemical and biological properties of the antimicrobial agent. The interaction of the three is essential in understanding antimicrobial therapeutics. The goal is to utilise an antimicrobial agent which will reach and concentrate at the site of infection with an optimal therapeutic response without deleterious consequences for the patient or the environment. In practice this requires the selection of an agent with the narrowest spectrum of activity (for the suspected or proven microorganism), delivered at the optimum dose and duration via the most appropriate route of administration.

The patient

Recognition and documentation of infection and its severity

It is good clinical practice to document clinical signs of infection including evidence of a systemic inflammatory response and other severity markers. Site and severity of an infection will directly influence choice (spectrum of activity), route (parenteral or oral) and duration of therapy. Systemic inflammatory response may be blunted or masked in the elderly and in those receiving anti-inflammatory drugs, immunomodulatory agents or beta-blockers. The clinical suspicion of infection should be supported by laboratory investigation but these should not delay life-saving therapy. Appropriate specimens, e.g. sputum, urine, pus, blood, etc., should be obtained before treatment is commenced whenever practical. In hospitalised patients with sepsis syndrome, blood cultures are mandatory. Failure to isolate a micro-organism does not however exclude infection. Presence of an organism from non-sterile sites may imply colonisation rather than infection and should be interpreted with caution.

Age

Drug kinetics are influenced by age-dependent changes in pathways of elimination (Chapter 23). Clinically important examples involving antimicrobial agents include:

1 Relative deficiency of hepatic glucuronyl transferase in neonates, leading to an accumulation of chloramphenicol with an increased likelihood of cardiovascular collapse at excess serum concentrations.

2 Physiological decrease in renal function with age, leading to potential accumulation of amino-glycosides in the elderly with a risk of toxicity: dose modification per creatinine clearance is necessary.

3 Other antimicrobials contraindicated in specific age groups are:

- Sulphonamides in the neonate (displacement of bilirubin, leading to kernicterus)
- Tetracyclines in growing children (tooth discoloration)

Renal and hepatic function

Many commonly used antimicrobials are eliminated by the kidney (e.g. penicillins, quinolones, aminoglycosides) while a few undergo hepatic metabolism. Dose modification is likely to be necessary if renal function is moderately or severely impaired (see 'Influence of impaired renal function', Chapter 22) (Table 9.1). Drug level monitoring is mandatory for antimicrobials with concentration-related toxicity (e.g. aminoglycosides and glycopeptides).

Drug sensitivity

Always ask about previous exposure to drugs and clarify possible reactions. Penicillins and cephalosporins are the antimicrobials most frequently associated with sensitivity reactions and there is a 5–10% cross-sensitivity between these two drug groups because they both contain the β-lactam ring. Minor sensitivity reactions to penicillins, such as rash, should not prevent prescription of a cephalosporin, but a life-threatening allergic reaction to penicillin is an absolute contraindication to the use of cephalosporins and carbapenems.

Increased susceptibility to infection

Patients with malignant disease or who receive cytotoxic or immunosuppressant drugs are susceptible to infections with commensal bacteria as well as less common organisms, e.g. some viruses, yeasts, fungi and protozoa. In particular, neutropaenia (less than 500×10^6/L) is accompanied by a high risk of bacteraemia with both Gram-negative and -positive organisms. Fever in such

Table 9.1 Examples of antimicrobials for which dose modification or caution is required in the presence of renal impairment or liver disease.

Renal impairment				Liver disease
Dose adjustment required (or avoid) based on creatinine clearance (mls/minute)				Close monitoring of liver function required (or avoid)
Any creatinine clearance	<50–60	<30	<10	
Aminoglycosides, Vancomycin	Aciclovir Nitrofurantoin	Trimethoprim	Flucloxacillin,	Anti-tuberculous therapy, Anti-Antiretroviral therapy
Amphotericin B	Meropenem Fluconazole Itraconazole Lamivudine Quinine	Oseltamivir Amoxicillin Co-amoxiclav Ciprofloxacin Cotrimoxazole	Ceftriaxone Doxycycline	Fluconazole and itraconazole Ceftriaxone, Co-amoxiclav, Flucloxacillin Sodium fucidate, Moxifloxacin

patients must be assumed to have an infective aetiology and should be treated aggressively before a definitive bacteriological diagnosis is available. HIV infection, as immunocompromise progresses, will put patients at risk of a range of opportunistic infections with viral, bacterial, fungal and parasitic microbes. Diabetes predisposes to an increased risk of bacterial infection through a number of different mechanisms including poor vascularity, neuropathy and impaired host defenses. Hospitalised patients in general are more susceptible to bacterial infection as a consequence of medical interventions including surgery, prosthetic material and use of intravascular and urethral catheters which become conduits for potentially pathogenic bacteria.

Comment. The patient's age, gender, general state of health, comorbidity site and severity of infection must be considered when choosing both the drug and its dose.

The organism

Antimicrobial agents exert their effect on their target organism by either direct killing of the organism ('cidal' effect) or by disabling or inhibiting cell function ('static' effect), enabling host defences to complete killing. Resistance to antimicrobial agents is a phenomena common to all classes of agents. It is an evolutionary response of the target organism to the agent and is a consequence of frequency of use, dosing and duration, mode of action and pharmacokinetics of the agent. There can be local, regional, national and international differences in susceptibility and these data should inform rational empirical therapy and treatment guidelines.

Bacteria

Bactericidal drugs kill the organisms against which they are effective. Bacteriostatic drugs do not kill the organism but inhibit its ability to replicate usually through inhibition of protein synthesis. Testing in vitro is available for most antibacterial drugs. Susceptibility testing is based upon the concentration of antibiotic required to inhibit growth. This is determined by a standardised, laboratory devised measurement, the mean inhibitory concentration (MIC; mg/L). The MIC divides bacteria into 3 susceptibility categories, resistant, sensitive or indeterminant. Generally the 'break point' is an MIC measurement used to determine if an agent will be effective or not against a particular organism. Application of such in vitro findings to the patient assumes that adequate drug concentrations are achieved at the site of infection. The relationship between antibiotic concentration and the MIC is important in determining drug dosage and frequency. Some agents display concentration dependent killing, with optimum activity associated with peak concentrations (e.g. aminoglycosides). Others display time-dependent killing with optimum activity associated with time of drug concentration above the MIC (e.g. beta-lactams).

Resistance

Some bacteria have always been resistant to the effects of certain drugs, while others have developed resistance in the course of repeated exposure to antimicrobials. The two major mechanisms by which resistance is produced are gene mutation and DNA exchange between bacteria. Resistance may take three main forms:

1 An alteration in the bacterial component on which the drug acts, e.g. changes in the 30S ribosomal subunit in organisms developing resistance to aminoglycosides.

2 The drug might be destroyed by the organisms, as in the case of penicillins that are inactivated by β-lactamases produced by resistant bacteria. Bacteria have evolved a complex armamentarium of β-lactamases, such as extended spectrum β-lactamases that are able to degrade recently developed drugs such as third-generation cephalosporins (e.g. cefotaxime).

3 Cell membrane permeability to drugs is reduced, as in resistance to tetracyclines.

The development of resistance may be reduced if antimicrobials are not given indiscriminately, are adequately dosed and in certain circumstances 'cycled', avoiding constant use of a particular class of agent. Drug combinations also limit the appearance of resistant organisms in conditions such as tuberculosis (TB) where prolonged treatment against slow growing intracellular organisms is necessary.

Viruses

Many viral infections are self-limiting and entirely controlled by the host immune response. In chronic viral infections, antiviral agents seldom eradicate infection but reduce viral load and rely on a functioning or recovering immune system for longer term control. In the context of HIV antiretroviral therapy, *genotypic* resistance pertains to specific viral gene mutations associated epidemiologically with treatment failure, and *phenotypic* resistance which describes in vitro resistance akin to bacterial resistance. The former is used more frequently in clinical practice and is also applicable to hepatitis B infection. Resistance in other viral infections is not routinely reported but may be important clinically in some infections (e.g. influenza). Combination antiviral therapy (using at least three agents from at least two classes) has proven long term benefit in control of HIV and substantially reduces the risk of resistance, an inevitable consequence of single or dual agent therapy. Combination therapy is also emerging in the management of viral hepatitis.

Fungi and protozoa

Resistance is not formally assessed in many fungal or protozoal infections but is implied by treatment failure when other causes can be eliminated. Epidemiological data are key in assessing the likely success of a particular agent in a specific scenario, e.g. community-acquired candidiasis is more likely to respond to standard therapy (fluconazole) than candidiasis acquired in the intensive care unit. Likewise *P. falciparum* malaria is more likely to be resistant to mefloquine in South-East Asia, where there has been unregulated use, than in West Africa.

Comment. Antimicrobial treatment must take appropriate account of the organism's anticipated susceptibility (based on local epidemiology), should adjust in the context of laboratory proven susceptibility and be appropriate for the patient's intrinsic ability to combat infection.

The drug

Absorption

Certain antimicrobials, e.g. the aminoglycosides, can only be given parenterally because absorption from the gastrointestinal tract is negligible. Where a choice exists between oral and parenteral

CSF	Bile	Urine	Lung
Chloramphenicol	Penicillins	Penicillins	Penicillins
Penicillins	Cephalosporins	Cephalosporins	Cephalosporins
Pyrazinamide		Aminoglycosides	Doxycycline
Isoniazid		Sulphonamides	Levofloxacin
Rifampicin		Nitrofurantoin	Linezolid
Linezolid		Trimethoprim	
Fluconazole		Ciprofloxacin	

Table 9.2 Examples of antimicrobials for which therapeutic concentrations in specific tissues are achieved.

drug formulations, the decision must rest on the severity of the illness, the site of the infection, the need to achieve high tissue concentration and the likelihood of absorption. In severely ill patients, those vomiting or with diarrhea, absorption of drugs from the gut may be unreliable necessitating use of intravenous preparations. However, when gut function recovers or the clinical condition improves, a switch to an oral preparation reduces the risk of catheter-associated infection and is generally cheaper.

Tissue distribution

The principles determining drug distribution are described in Chapter 1. In addition to these general considerations of blood concentration, protein binding, lipid solubility, etc., a further factor influencing antimicrobial distribution is the presence of inflammation, which tends to improve tissue penetration (e.g. vancomycin cerebrospinal fluid (CSF) penetration improves in the presence of meningitis). However, it must not be assumed that the presence of inflammation greatly transforms the penetration of drugs. For example, gentamicin crosses poorly into the CSF even in the presence of meningitis. Table 9.2 indicates those agents with high penetration to CSF, bile, urine and lung.

Route of elimination

This is usually renal or hepatic metabolism or in some case biliary excretion; see Chapter 1 and the section above on renal and hepatic function.

Adverse effects

These are of three general types:

1 Hypersensitivity reactions that are either immediate or delayed. The former produce anaphylaxis while the latter manifest themselves in various ways, the most common being rashes. Hypersensitivity reactions usually occur with no prior warning and are most commonly seen with penicillins, cephalosporins and sulphonamides.

2 The other type of adverse reaction is usually predictable in being concentration related; aminoglycoside renal toxicity is an example. Aminoglycosides may also accumulate within the inner ear following prolonged therapy and this may, despite adequately monitored and dose adjusted therapy, result in oto-vestibular toxicity. Fortunately, the toxic concentrations of most antimicrobials in common use greatly exceed the required therapeutic concentrations. Where this is not the case, e.g. gentamicin, therapeutic drug monitoring (TDM) is mandatory (see Chapter 21). Adverse reactions to antimicrobials are summarised in Table 9.3 and discussed in more detail under specific agents.

3 Antimicrobials are unique amongst therapeutic agents in that they also exert an ecological effect on other commensal organisms (in the gut, mucus membranes and skin) not deliberately targeted by the prescriber. In the individual patient certain broad spectrum agents will increase the risk of C. difficile associated diarrhoea, meticillin- resistant Staphylococcus aureus (MRSA) and extended-spectrum beta-lactamase producing coliforms.

Table 9.3 Major adverse reactions of antimicrobial drugs.

Organ system	Drug	Comment
Kidney	Aminoglycosides	Concentration-related
	Glycopeptides	Concentration-related
	Amphotericin B	
Bone marrow suppression	Linezolid	
	Glycopeptides	Concentration-dependent
	Amphotericin B	
	Flucytosine	
	Chloramphenicol	
	Sulphonamides	Rare
Haemolytic anaemia	Sulphonamides	Two distinct mechanisms: immune and glucose-6-phosphate deficiency
	Nitrofurantoin	
	Quinolones	Rare
	Penicillins	Rare
	Cephalosporins	Rare
Thrombocytopenia	Sulphonamides	Rare
	Linezolid	
	Cephalosporins	Rare
	Glycopeptides	Rare
	Rifampicin	Intermittent therapy
Neutropenia	Penicillins	Rare: mainly ampicillin, carbenicillin
	Cephalosporins	Rare
	Sulphonamides	Rare
	Chloramphenicol	
Neurological eighth nerve	Aminoglycosides	Concentration-related
	Vancomycin	Rare
Optic nerve	Ethambutol	
	Linezolid	Rare
Peripheral neuropathy	Isoniazid	Prevented by pyridoxine
	Metronidazole	Prolonged treatment
	Linezolid	
	Nitrofurantoin	
Convulsions	Penicillins	Large intrathecal or massive intravenous doses
	Imipenem with cilastin	
	Quinolones	Large doses
Benign intracranial hypertension	Tetracyclines	
	Penicillins	
	Nalidixic acid	
Neuromuscular blockade	Aminoglycosides	
Gastrointestinal system		
Liver	Pyrazinamide	Commonest agent implicated in TB therapy
	Isoniazid	More often slow acetylators

(Continued)

Table 9.3 (*Continued*)

Organ system	Drug	Comment
	Rifampicin	Usually mild – worse in alcoholics/preceding damage
	Tetracyclines	Massive doses
	Erythromycin estolate	Cholestasis
	Sodium fucidate	Cholestasis
	Flucloxacillin	Cholestasis
	Co-amoxiclav	Cholestasis
	Cephalosporins	Cholestasis
Clostridium difficile-associated diarrhoea	Cephalosporins Quinolones Clindamycin Broad spectrum penicillins (co-amoxiclav, piperacillin-tazobactam)	
Other adverse reactions		
Hypersensitivity	Penicillins Sulphonamides	10% cross-sensitivity with cephalosporins
Stevens–Johnson syndrome	Sulphonamides Penicillins	
Bone development/tooth staining	Tetracyclines	Contraindicated in childhood and pregnancy
Pulmonary fibrosis	Nitrofurantoin	Associated with prolonged use
Rashes	Commonly penicillins and sulphonamides but virtually any drug can cause rashes	

Drug interactions

These can be either kinetic, e.g. enzyme induction or inhibition, or dynamic, e.g. two drugs adversely affecting the same organ. Examples include the following:

1 Aminoglycosides and frusemide have an additive nephrotoxic effect.

2 Rifampicin induces the same enzymes that metabolise the contraceptive pill and can cause failure of contraception.

3 Sulphonamides inhibit the enzymes that metabolise phenytoin and can cause phenytoin toxicity.

4 Tetracyclines form insoluble complexes in the gut lumen with both antacids and iron, leading to treatment failure.

5 Quinolones may trigger side effects of theophylline as a result of its decreased elimination.

6 Amphotericin B and aminoglycosides or vancomycin display increased nephrotoxicity and ototoxicity.

Antimicrobial prophylaxis

Antimicrobial agents are sometimes given to people who do not have an infection but who are considered to be at risk from a specific organism.

Examples include the use of rifampicin or ciprofloxacin in close contacts of patients with meningococcal meningitis, and the long-term use of trimethoprim in children with repeated urinary tract infections and evidence of vesicoureteric reflux. Perioperative prophylaxis in certain types of surgery where the risk of infection is high (e.g. colorectal with gentamicin and metronidazole) or the consequences of infection are life-threatening (e.g. open heart with gentamicin and flucloxacillin) is now standard practice. As with antibiotics for treatment, peri-operative prophylaxis may have adverse consequences. Good practice is to limit antibiotics to a single (intravenous) dose administered at the time of anaesthesia or just prior to the procedure.

Comment. An antimicrobial agent might be quite ineffective, or even dangerous, unless its clinical pharmacology is viewed in relation to the whole clinical situation. The drug chosen must reach the site of infection, in an effective concentration, without producing toxicity or adversely influencing any concurrent therapy. In most circumstances antibiotics are chosen before results of culture are available. Some guidelines for empirical therapy of a variety of infections are shown in the Table 9.4.

Antibacterial drugs

Penicillins

Mechanism

Penicillins have a bactericidal action. They inhibit cell wall synthesis by preventing the formation of peptidoglycan cross-bridges in actively multiplying bacteria.

Pharmacokinetics

Oral absorption

Not absorbed: Piperacillin

Moderately absorbed: Phenoxypenicillin (penicillin V),

Well absorbed: amoxicillin, flucloxacillin, co-amoxiclav

Even relatively well-absorbed penicillins are destroyed to some extent by gastric acid and should therefore be given at least 30 minutes before meals.

Distribution

The penicillins have good penetration to most tissues but poor entry to CSF. However, meningeal inflammation increases CSF penetration allowing the use of these agents in the treatment of

Table 9.4 Examples of empirical antibiotic therapy for adults.

Source of infection	Antibiotic
Lower urinary tract infection	Trimethoprim or nitrofurantoin
Upper urinary tract infection	Co-trimoxazole or ciprofloxacin or gentamicin
Cellulitis (mild)	Flucloxacillin or erythromycin or doxycycline
Cellulitis (severe)	(flucloxacillin *or* vancomycin) + clindamycin
Community-acquired pneumonia	
Mild	Amoxicillin or clarithromycin or doxycycline
Severe	Amoxicillin + clarithromycin
Suspected staphylococcal pneumonia	Add flucloxacillin *or* vancomycin to above regimen
Exacerbation of COPD	Amoxicillin or doxycycline
Pharyngitis	Usually viral. If group A Streptococcus suspected use Penicillin or erythromycin
Gastroenteritis	No antibiotic usually required. If invasive Salmonellosis suspected, ciprofloxacin
Peritonitis	Gentamicin + metronidazole + Amoxicillin
Bacterial meningitis	Ceftriaxone (and amoxicillin if age >55 years or immunocompromised)
Severe sepsis – uncertain origin	Benzyl penicillin + flucloxacillin + gentamicin
	or vancomycin + gentamicin (if penicillin allergy or health care associated)

Table 9.5 Examples of doses of penicillins.

1	Benzylpenicillin: intramuscular 300–600 mg two to four times daily (children 10–20 mg/kg daily); intravenous up to 14.4 g daily; intrathecal 6–12 mg daily
2	Phenoxymethylpenicillin (penicillin V): oral dose 500 mg 1g 6-hourly (children, 125–250 mg 6-hourly)
3	Ampicillin: oral dose 250–1000 mg 6-hourly; intravenous or intramuscular 500–1000 mg 6-hourly (children, half doses)
4	Amoxicillin: oral 250–500 mg 8-hourly (children, half dose)
5	Carbenicillin: intravenous (rapid infusion) 5 g 4- to 6-hourly (children, 250–400 mg/kg daily divided doses); intramuscular 2 g 6-hourly (children, 50–100 mg/kg divided doses)
6	Ticarcillin: intravenous infusion (rapid) or intramuscular 15–20 g daily divided doses
7	Azlocillin: 2 g 8-hourly by intravenous injection; up to 5 g 8-hourly by infusion
8	Flucloxacillin: oral 500–1000 mg 6-hourly
9	Co-amoxiclav: oral 1 tablet 250 mg amoxicillin, 125 mg clavulanic acid-1 tablet 500 mg amoxicillin, 125 mg clavulinic acid, 8-hourly or 1.2 g 8 hourly by intravenous injection

meningitis. Giving large frequent doses (or continuous infusion) when treating meningitis also increases CSF delivery.

Elimination

Penicillins undergo enterohepatic circulation: drug is excreted via bile and reabsorbed. The major route of elimination after reabsorption is active secretion in the renal tubules. This tubular secretion can be blocked by probenecid with doubling of penicillin blood levels, commonly utilised in the treatment of tertiary syphilis. Dose reduction is necessary in severe renal failure (Table 9.5).

Adverse effects

Immediate hypersensitivity

This occurs in 0.05% of patients with manifestations ranging from urticaria or wheezing to a life-threatening anaphylactic response.

Delayed hypersensitivity

This occurs in <5% of patients, mainly as rashes. Rare manifestations are hemolytic anaemia, interstitial nephritis and leucopenia. Cross-sensitivity with cephalosporins occurs in around 10% of patients.

Toxicity

Convulsions may follow intrathecal or very high intravenous doses of penicillin. Patients with renal insufficiency can develop cation overload following large doses of potassium penicillin or sodium carbenicillin. Diarrhoea is commonly reported, particularly with ampicillin (20%). Ampicillin and amoxicillin are associated with a characteristic rash in up to 90% of patients with infectious mononucleosis or chronic lymphocytic leukaemia.

Drug interactions

Ampicillin can lead to oral contraceptive failure. This is probably because of diminished enterohepatic circulation. The anticoagulant effect of warfarin is potentiated.

Antibacterial spectrum

The major factor limiting efficacy is the production by certain organisms of enzymes (β-lactamases or penicillinases) that destroy the β-lactam ring of the penicillin molecule. This structure is essential to the antibacterial action of penicillins. Several synthetic penicillins incorporate side chains that protect the β-lactam ring against these enzymes. An alternative approach has been to combine amoxicillin with clavulanic acid, which itself has very little antibacterial activity but inhibits β-lactamase activity.

Penicillinase-sensitive penicillins

Benzylpenicillin and phenoxypenicillins are active against streptococci, pneumococci, gonococci and meningococci, *Treponema pallidum*, *Actinomyces israelii* and most anaerobic organisms that are found in the mouth and upper gastrointestinal tract, but not below the diaphragm such as *Bacteroides fragilis*.

Amoxicillin has a broader spectrum and is effective against some strains of *Escherichia coli*, *Proteus mirabilis*, *Shigella*, *Salmonella*, *Haemophilus influenzae* and various enterococci The main indications are acute exacerbations of chronic obstructive airways disease, acute bronchitis and pneumonia.

Examples of adult doses see Table 9.5.

Carbenicillin and ticarcillin are active against *Pseudomonas aeruginosa* and *Proteus* sp. At least in vitro, ticarcillin is more effective than carbenicillin and azlocillin is more effective than ticarcillin against *P. aeruginosa*. All three drugs must be given parenterally. Drug resistance is encountered in some strains.

Penicillinase-resistant penicillins

Cloxacillin and flucloxacillin are indicated in the treatment of infections caused by penicillinase-producing staphylococci and are also effective against most beta-haemolytic streptococci. Flucloxacillin is better absorbed from the gut than cloxacillin. Meticillin is confined to nasal Staphylococcal decolonisation.

Examples of adult doses see table 9.5

Co-amoxiclav

The amoxicillin/clavulanic acid combination is used in treating severe pneumonia, infected human or animal bites, spontaneous bacterial peritonitis and some urinary tract infections caused by β-lactamase-producing coliforms. It may also be useful in intra-abdominal sepsis.

Examples of adult doses

625 mg 8-hourly oral or 1.2 g 8-hourly i.v.

Piperacillin-tazobactam

This combination is used mainly in the treatment of patients with impaired host defences (e.g. following chemotherapy or bone marrow trans-

plantation) where infection with β-lactamase-producing coliforms is suspected. It is also used extensively in severely ill patients in intensive care units. It is inactivated by extended spectrum beta-lactamase producing coliforms.

Dose

4.5 g 6–8-hourly.

Carbapenems

These β-lactams are closely related to the penicillins and all require intravenous administration. Imipenem has a very broad spectrum of activity against many Gram-negative, Gram-positive and anaerobic organisms. It is partially inactivated within the kidney and is thus co-formulated with cilastatin, which blocks this renal metabolism. It is indicated for the treatment of severe multi-resistant infections.s. In addition to the side effects of all penicillin-like drugs, imipenem does lower seizure threshold. The closely related drug meropenem is thus preferred in patients with epilepsy. Doripenem has a very similar spectrum to imipenem and meropenem. Ertapenem is a once daily carbapenem with similar spectrum but lacks activity versus Pseudomonas. Carbapenemase producing coliforms will inactivate all the carbapenems.

Dose

Meropenem 500 mg–1 g 8-hourly
Ertapenem 1 g daily

Cephalosporins

Mechanism

Cephalosporins are bactericidal. They contain a β-lactam ring and their mechanism of action is similar to penicillins.

Pharmacokinetics

Six cephalosporins are effective orally: cefalexin, cefradine (cephradine), cefaclor, cefixime, cefadroxil and cefuroxime. They distribute widely. A range of intravenous cephalosporins is also available, such as cefotaxime and ceftriaxone. This latter agent has a long half-life allowing once-daily dosing, of considerable benefit in managing administration of a parenteral antibiotic to outpatients. The drugs are eliminated renally, partly by glomerular filtration and partly by tubular secretion, with the contribution of each route varying with individual cephalosporins.

Adverse effects

Hypersensitivity occurs with 10% cross-reactivity with penicillin-sensitive patients. Cephalosporins can reduce prothrombin concentration and bleeding has been described. Several cephalosporins, including those commonly used orally, cause false positive urinalysis tests for glucose, as measured by reducing substances. Cephaloridine can cause renal tubular necrosis, particularly in doses above 6 g/day. The main adverse effects of cephalosporins are related to the effect on normal flora with a strong association with *C. difficile*, Meticillin-resistant *Staphylococcus aureus* and the development of extended spectrum beta-lactamase producing coliform organisms.

Drug interactions

The nephrotoxicity of cephaloridine is potentiated by loop diuretics and aminoglycoside antibiotics.

Antibacterial spectrum

The early cephalosporins were broad spectrum but with limited activity against Gram-negative organisms. Cephamandole and cefuroxime are more resistant to β-lactamases and are effective against a number of Gram-negative bacilli. Cefotaxime is more effective than cephamandole or cefuroxime against Gram-negative bacilli but less effective against Gram-positive organisms. Ceftazidime is active against *P. aeruginosa*. Cefoxitin is closely related to the basic cephalosporin structure and is active against Gram-negative and anaerobic bacteria. Ceftriaxone provides Gram-negative cover as well as modest anti-staphylococcal activity.

Example of adult dose

Ceftriaxone 1 g 12 to 24-hourly

Comment. Intravenous cephalosporins are commonly used in many hospitals for both prophylaxis and treatment. Oral agents (e.g. cephalexin) are used primarily in urinary tract infection complicating pregnancy in general practice. Their indiscriminant use is discouraged as a consequence of their adverse ecological effects. They should be particularly avoided in the elderly and those with a prior history of *C. difficile*.

Aminoglycosides

Mechanism

Aminoglycosides are bactericidal. They bind to the 30S subunit of bacterial ribosomes, leading to misreading of mRNA codons.

Pharmacokinetics

Oral absorption is negligible. They have poor penetration into CSF and only moderate penetration into bile. Otherwise, there is good entry to inflamed tissue. Elimination is mainly by glomerular filtration. Gentamicin is usually administered via intermittent infusion of 5 or 7 mg/kg daily or less frequently or at a lower twice/thrice daily synergistic dose with bet-lactams in the treatment of endocarditis. Bacterial eradication is enhanced and resistance minimised with higher peak blood concentration, Gentamicin dosing regimens are individualised to the patient and reflect ideal body weight, age and renal function. Initial dose and interval should be adjusted following concentration measurement taken 6–14 hours after the first dose and cross referencing with the appropriate nomogram. Gentamicin guidelines vary between institutions so up to date local guidelines should always be consulted.

Adverse effects

There are two major adverse reactions, both concentration related: nephrotoxicity and ototoxicity.

The renal lesion consists of tubular destruction. Eighth nerve damage can be mainly vestibular (streptomycin, gentamicin) or mainly auditory (kanamycin). The severity of these reactions is related to aminoglycoside serum concentration, which in turn is related to dose, duration and rate of elimination. Accumulation of drug occurs when glomerular filtration is decreased by renal disease or at the extremes of age. Doses must be modified in these situations and drug concentration monitoring is mandatory. Oto- and vestibular-toxicity are unusual in patients who have received short term therapy as this adverse event is dependent on accumulation within the inner ear. It is important to note that toxicity may occur despite well maintained therapeutic concentration measurements. Aminoglycosides should be discontinued at the earliest signs of auditory or vestibular dysfunction as side-effects may be irreversible. Aminoglycosides cross the placenta and can cause eighth nerve damage in the fetus. An uncommon effect of aminoglycosides is neuromuscular blockade occurring after rapid intravenous injection; this is marked in patients with myasthenia gravis.

Drug interactions

Nephrotoxicity is enhanced by co-administration with other nephrotoxins. Similarly, ototoxicity is enhanced by loop diuretics. The neuromuscular blockade of curare-like drugs can be prolonged by aminoglycosides.

Antibacterial spectrum

Gentamicin is the most widely used aminoglycoside and is active against most aerobic Gram-negative rods, including *Pseudomonas* and *Proteus* spp., and also against staphylococci. Most streptococci are resistant because gentamicin cannot penetrate the cell. However, penicillin and aminoglycosides have synergistic effect against some streptococci. All anaerobic organisms are resistant. Tobramycin is two to four times more active against pseudomonas but is otherwise very similar to gentamicin. Amikacin is resistant to most of the bacterial enzymes that inactivate gentamicin,

but is more toxic than gentamicin and is thus only indicated for infections caused by aerobic Gram-negative rods against which gentamicin is no longer effective. Netilmicin has a similar antibacterial spectrum to gentamicin, but is claimed to be less ototoxic: confirmatory evidence is limited. Neomycin is given orally to decrease the bacterial content of the colon in liver failure or before bowel surgery. If there is severe liver or renal failure or inflammatory bowel disease, sufficient neomycin can be absorbed to cause ototoxicity. Streptomycin (and amikacin) are effective against tubercle bacilli and is discussed later.

Comment. The major role of aminoglycosides is the parenteral treatment of serious infection caused by sensitive Gram-negative organisms. These drugs are popular for the initial management of life-threatening sepsis of uncertain aetiology. In this situation an aminoglycoside is usually combined with extended-spectrum penicillin.

Sulphonamide–trimethoprim combinations

Mechanism

These drugs are bactericidal. Co-trimoxazole contains a sulphonamide, sulphamethoxazole (sulfamethoxazole), and trimethoprim in the ratio 5:1. The basis of the action of sulphonamides is that bacterial cells are impermeable to folic acid and so they must synthesise their own from ρ-aminobenzoic acid, with which sulphonamides have a strong similarity. Thus, competitive inhibition of folic acid synthesis occurs. Trimethoprim blocks the next synthetic step, from folic acid to tetrahydrofolate, by inhibiting the enzyme dihydrofolate reductase.

Pharmacokinetics

Co-trimoxazole is well absorbed following oral administration and is also available for intravenous use. There is wide tissue distribution and elimination is by renal excretion.

Adverse effects

The sulphonamide component can cause rashes and, much less commonly, Stevens–Johnson syndrome, renal failure and blood dyscrasias. Trimethoprim can also cause rashes and impaired haemopoiesis and can produce gastrointestinal symptoms. There is a theoretical risk of teratogenesis in malnourished pregnant patients treated with trimethoprim in the first trimester. In the newborn, sulphonamides can displace bilirubin from protein-binding sites and cause kernicterus.

Drug interactions

The sulphonamide component competes for hepatic enzyme-binding sites and can decrease the clearance of phenytoin, tolbutamide and warfarin sufficiently to produce phenytoin toxicity, hypoglycaemia and enhanced anticoagulation, respectively. Displacement of methotrexate from protein-binding sites can also lead to toxicity.

Antibacterial spectrum

These drugs have a broad spectrum, including Gram-positive cocci, *Neisseria gonorrhoeae*, *H. influenzae*, *E. coli*, *P. mirabilis*, Shigella sp., Salmonella sp., *Pneumocystis carinii* and Brucella sp.

Dose

Co-trimoxazole: 960 mg (two tablets of 400 mg sulphamethoxazole, 80 mg trimethoprim) 12-hourly for oral or intravenous administration (children, 120–480 mg 12-hourly depending on age). For prophylaxis against PCP 480–960 mg daily is used whilst for treatment 120 mg/kg daily in 2–4 divided doses is recommended.

Comment. Although an effective antibiotic, the risk of severe reactions such as Stevens–Johnson syndrome has previously limited the use of this drug. Its use is again increasing an alternative for urinary and respiratory tract infection particularly in patients at higher risk of *C. difficile*. It remains the drug of choice in treating pneumonia caused by the opportunist pathogen *P. carinii* (now renamed *P. jiroveci*), a common infection in patients with AIDS.

Trimethoprim

Trimethoprim alone is also used in treating sensitive lower urinary tract infections. Dose: 200 mg bd.

Tetracyclines

Mechanism

Tetracyclines are bacteriostatic, binding to the 30S ribosomal subunit with consequent misreading of information needed for protein synthesis.

Pharmacokinetics

Tetracyclines are adequately absorbed following oral administration. Tissue distribution is good and the drugs are eliminated mainly unmetabolised by biliary excretion. Doxycycline has a long half-life and can be administered once daily.

Adverse effects

Tetracyclines bind to calcium in bones and teeth, leading to impaired bone growth and discoloration of teeth during active mineralisation (up to 7 years). Tetracyclines cross the placenta and are contraindicated in pregnancy. Following large doses, both hepatic necrosis and renal failure have been reported. Except for doxycycline and minocycline, these drugs are contraindicated in renal failure because they impair protein synthesis and so enhance the effects of catabolism. Many patients develop nausea, reflux, diarrhoea or candidiasis on tetracycline therapy and a photosensitive rash may occur.

Drug interactions

Milk, antacids, calcium, magnesium and iron form insoluble complexes with tetracyclines in the gut lumen, leading to treatment failure, the exception being minocycline.

Antibacterial spectrum

The tetracyclines are effective against a wide range of bacteria and resistance rates are variable. They remain useful in many countries for the treatment of respiratory tract infections including infection with Pneumococcus and Haemophilus species as well as the atypical pathogens such as Chlamydia, Mycoplasma and Coxiella burnettii. They are also active against other less common organisms such as the rickettsiae, Brucella cholera and Lyme Borrelia. Tetracyclines are also useful adjuncts to the treatment of acne by preventing the growth of *Propionibacterium acnes* in the blocked sebaceous ducts.

Dose

Tetracycline and oxytetracycline: 250–500 mg 6-hourly. Minocycline: 200 mg, then 100 mg 12-hourly. Doxycycline: 200 mg loading dose, then 100 mg daily.

Other antibacterial drugs

Metronidazole

Metronidazole was initially used in protozoal infections, but was later found to be very effective against anaerobic bacteria, including *B. fragilis* and *C. difficile*. It is currently popular in treating serious anaerobic infections including *C. difficile* associated diarrhoea. In addition, metronidazole is often combined with gentamicin and amoxicillin in treating intra-abdominal sepsis. The other major uses are in treating trichomonal vaginitis, amoebiasis and giardiasis. Metronidazole is often combined with gentamicin as prophylaxis in abdominal surgery. The only major adverse effects are peripheral neuropathy following prolonged therapy and seizures following high doses.

Dose

For severe infections, intravenous infusion of metronidazole is given at the rate of 500 mg every 8 hours in adults.

Oral: 400 mg orally 8-hourly for serious bacterial infections. 200 mg 8-hourly for 7 days for trichomoniasis and 2 g daily for 3 days in amoebiasis and giardiasis. If appropriate, suppositories can be used in circumstances where intravenous infusion

might be considered: similar blood levels but much cheaper. Dose: 1 g 8-hourly.

Macrolides

Erythromycin was the first of these drugs to be used; newer agents include clarithromycin and azithromycin. They have an antibacterial spectrum similar to penicillin and often are suitable second-line drugs for patients allergic to penicillin. The use of erythromycin is frequently associated with nausea and vomiting; these side effects are much less prominent with clarithromycin and azithromycin. Clarithromycin is currently the drug of choice for *Legionella pneumophilia* and *mycoplasma* infections. Azithromycin has an extremely long half-life of 68 hours allowing once-daily dosing and short courses of treatment. It has a broader spectrum of activity than erythromycin, including enhanced activity against *H. influenzae*, a common pathogen in infectious exacerbations of chronic pulmonary disease. It is useful in the treatment of gonococcal and non-gonococcal urethritis, and pelvic inflammatory disease, where single-dose therapy ensures complete patient compliance. It will treat effectively community-acquired pneumonia in patients with previously normal lung function as well as those with chronic pulmonary disease; cheaper alternatives for both are available.

Dose

Erythromycin:
Oral: 250–500 mg 6-hourly for adults. Intravenous: 500 mg–1 g by infusion 6-hourly for adults.
Clarithromycin:
Oral: 500 mg 12-hourly for adults. Intravenous: 500 mg 12-hourly.
Azithromycin: For non-gonococcal urethritis/ cervicitis 1 g single dose.

Sodium fucidate

This drug has a narrow spectrum and is indicated only in combination with another anti-staphylococcal drug for the treatment of penicillin-resistant staphylococcal infections, e.g. those of bone.

Dose

Sodium fucidate is given at a dose of 500 mg 8-hourly by intravenous infusion or orally.

Clindamycin

Clindamycin is effective against penicillin-resistant staphylococci and many anaerobic organisms. It is well absorbed by mouth and penetrates into tissues such as bone. It is indicated in serious conditions where other agents are contraindicated, or ineffective, notably staphylococcal bone and joint infections or serious soft tissue infections. It has a particular utility in life-threatening Group A beta-haemolytic streptococcal infections, e.g. necrotising fasciitis and Streptococcal toxic shock syndrome where it reduces toxin production. Clindamycin was one of the first antibiotics to be associated with *C. difficile*-associated diarrhoea. In current practice, this complication is common with the use of many widely used broad-spectrum antibiotics.

Dose

Oral: 300–600 mg every 6 hours in adults. Intravenous: 2.4 g clindamycin daily is given in four divided doses by slow intravenous infusion in adults.

Nitrofurantoin

Nitrofurantoin, an orally administered drug that achieves antibacterial concentrations only in urine, is effective against many organisms infecting the urinary tract. Adverse effects include gastrointestinal symptoms and rashes. It precipitates haemolytic anaemia in glucose-6-phosphate deficiency and can cause peripheral neuropathy and pulmonary fibrosis when used for prolonged periods, e.g. for long-term UTI prophylaxis.

Glycopeptides (vancomycin and teicoplanin)

Vancomycin and teicoplanin are used intravenously in the treatment of wound infection, cellulitis, bacteraemia, vascular catheter-related infections and endocarditis caused by meticillin-resistant Gram-positive cocci (particularly MRSA infection) or in patients with penicillin allergy. Both teicoplanin and vancomycin are also useful in surgical prophylaxis in penicillin allergic patients. Vancomycin is also effective against *C. difficile* when given orally and is preferred in severe infections. Because of possible nephrotoxicity, serum levels need to be monitored.

Dose

Intravenous Vancomycin: Average adult dose is 1 g 12-hourly but varies depending on weight, age and renal function. Oral vancomycin (for treatment of *C. difficile*) 125 mg qds.

Teicoplanin

Teicoplanin is an alternative to vancomycin. Serum levels need not be monitored.

Quinolones

Nalidixic acid, the first quinolone, has been available for 30 years. Administered orally, it achieves low tissue concentrations and its use is restricted to the treatment of uncomplicated urinary tract infections. Chemical modifications have produced a series of improved drugs and the most recent are the 4-fluoroquinolones; ciprofloxacin was the first agent in this group available in the United Kingdom.

Ciprofloxacin

Mechanism

Bactericidal in action, ciprofloxacin inhibits DNA-gyrase activity by binding to chromosomal DNA strands. This interferes with DNA replication and prevents supercoiling within the chromosome.

Pharmacokinetics

It is well absorbed after oral administration and is distributed rapidly into body tissues. Most of the drug is eliminated unaltered by the kidneys; the remainder is excreted by hepatic metabolism or unchanged in the faeces.

Adverse effects

The most frequently reported side effects are minor gastrointestinal upsets; severe systemic adverse reactions are rare. However, central nervous system disturbances such as insomnia, confusion and convulsions have been reported. As it can cause damage to cartilage in young animals, ciprofloxacin is contraindicated in children and growing adolescents.

Drug interactions

Its absorption is reduced significantly by the co-administration of aluminium and magnesium antacids. It interferes with the metabolism of theophylline, caffeine and warfarin and so the toxic effects of these drugs may be encountered if they are given along with ciprofloxacin.

Antibacterial spectrum

It is active against aerobic Gram-negative bacteria, including *P. aeruginosa*, and less active against Gram-positive bacteria: staphylococci are more sensitive than streptococci. Anaerobes, in general, are resistant. Ciprofloxacin is particularly useful for pseudomonas infections where oral therapy is preferred, such as respiratory tract infection in patients with cystic fibrosis. It is very effective in gastrointestinal infections ranging from traveller's diarrhoea to typhoid fever.

Dose

Oral: 250–750 mg 12-hourly; intravenous: 200–400 mg 12-hourly.

Levofloxacin

Similar spectrum to ciprofloxacin but with much greater activity against *Streptococcus pneumoniae*.

Dose

Oral and intravenous: 500–750 mg once daily.

Quinupristin-dalfopristin

Mechanism

Quinupristin-dalfopristin is a streptogramin antibiotic. It combines both bacteriocidal and bacteriostatic properties. Bacterial synthesis is inhibited by binding to different sites on the 50S bacterial ribosomal subunit to form a stable quinupristin-ribosome-dalfopristin tertiary complex.

Pharmacokinetics

Quinupristin-dalfopristin is not absorbed and is administered via intravenous infusion. It is 10–20% protein bound and is excreted in bile. It achieves high intracellular concentrations.

Adverse events

Thrombophlebitis is common following infusion. Nausea, myositis and anaemia are notable side effects.

Drug interactions

Quinupristin-dalfopristin could alter the metabolism of agents metabolised via Cytochrome P450 enzyme pathway therefore such agents should be avoided or used with caution.

Antibacterial spectrum

Broad Gram-positive spectrum including MRSA and *Enterococcus faecium*. No activity however versus *Enterococcus faecalis*. May be used in skin and soft tissue infections and other resistant Gram-positive infections where other agents have failed or were not tolerated.

Dosage

7.5 mg/kg 8-hourly.

Pristinamycin

An oral streptogrammin with similar activity and to Quinupristin-dalfopristin. May be useful in skin and soft tissue and some deep-seated Gram-positive infections.

Linezolide

Mechanism

Linezolid is the first oxaozolidinone antibiotic. It is bacteriostatic, inhibiting protein synthesis by binding to a site on the bacterial 23S ribosomal RNA of the 50S subunit, preventing formation of a functional 70S initiation complex, an essential component of bacterial translocations.

Pharmacokinetics

Well absorbed, minimally protein bound and has a wide distribution amongst body tissues, including lung, skin, bone and CSF. It is mainly non-renally excreted.

Adverse events

Prolonged linezolid use is associated with myelotoxicity, notably anaemia and thrombocytopenia. Mitochondrial toxicity may occur with peripheral neuropathy, lactic acidosis and rarely optic neuropathy.

Drug interactions

Linezolid is a weak monoamine-oxidase inhibitor so should not be co-administered with many antidepressants and tyramine-containing foods should be avoided.

Antibacterial spectrum

Broad Gram-positive spectrum of activity including vancomycin resistant *Enterococci* and MRSA. Also has activity against *Mycobacterium tuberculosis*. Most commonly used in health care associated Gram-positive infections resistant to glycopeptides particularly pneumonia and skin and soft tissue infections.

Dosage

600 mg 12-hourly (oral or intravenous).

Daptomycin

Mechanism

Daptomycin is the first lipopeptide antibiotic. It inserts its lipophilic tail into the cell membrane leading to potassium efflux and cell death. It is rapidly bacteriocidal.

Pharmacokinetics

Not absorbed from the gastrointestinal tract, highly protein bound and excreted via the renal tract.

Adverse events

Myotoxicity may occur in approximately 2.5%. Creatinine phosphokinase should be monitored weekly.

Drug interactions

Caution with other agents which may elevate muscle enzymes.

Antibacterial spectrum

Broad Gram-positive spectrum of activity including vancomycin resistant *Enterococci* and MRSA. Most commonly used in skin and soft tissue infections and Staphylococcal bacteraemia. Daptomycin is inactivated by surfactant and so should not be used in the treatment of pneumonia.

Dosage

4 mg/kg (actual body weight) for skin and soft tissue infections. 6 mg/kg for bacteraemia and more complex infections.

Tigecycline

Mechanism

Tigecycline is the first semi-synthetic glycylcycline antibiotic. Antibacterial action is bacteriostatic by binding to a single high affinity intracellular site on the bacterial 30S-ribosome so blocking entry of amino-acyl transfer molecules and preventing protein synthesis.

Pharmacokinetics

Tigecycline is not absorbed from the gastrointestinal tract. It is highly protein bound, has a half-life of about 36 hours and distributes rapidly, concentrating in tissues. It is mainly excreted via the biliary tree.

Adverse events

Main side effects are nausea and vomiting in 25–40% of patients.

Drug interactions

May interact with warfarin although the mechanism is not known.

Antibacterial spectrum

Broad activity against Gram-positive, Gram-negative and anaerobic organisms. Spectrum of activity includes MRSA, Enterococcal species and extended spectrum beta-lactamase producing Gram-negatives. Tigecycline is less active against non-fermentative Gram-negatives (e.g. pseudomonal species) than antipseudomonal penicillins and carbapenems. Tigecycline is reserved for skin and soft tissue and intra-abdominal infections caused by resistant organisms and caution should be used in bacteraemia tissue distribution is rapid.

Dosage

100 mg loading dose followed by 50 mg 12 hourly.

Antituberculous drugs

Mycobacterium tuberculosis multiplies slowly and the long periods of treatment required encourage the emergence of resistant strains. Combination chemotherapy is thus the basis of treatment. Because of increasing drug resistance (usually as a consequence of poor adherence), initial treatment is with four drugs: isoniazid, rifampicin, ethambutol and pyrazinamide, administered for 8 weeks. Co-formulation of rifampicin, isoniazid and pyrazinamide allows for simplification of therapy. Subsequently, isoniazid and rifampicin are given (again usually co-formulated), as long as cultures indicate that the organism is susceptible, or, if the organism is not grown, that drug resistance is considered unlikely. Six months of treatment with this regimen is adequate for pulmonary TB. If other drugs are used, 9 months of therapy is necessary. In central nervous system TB and in selected other extra-pulmonary cases, therapy in excess of nine months will be required. In patients at risk of poor adherence 'directly observed therapy' on a thrice weekly basis is preferred.

Isoniazid

Mechanism

Isoniazid inhibits a step in the biosynthesis of essential fatty acids within mycobacteria.

Pharmacokinetics

Isoniazid is well absorbed following oral administration and is widely distributed throughout the body, including the CSF where concentrations equal those in blood. Isoniazid is inactivated in the liver by pathways including genetically dependent acetylation. The same metabolic pathway is involved in the acetylation of hydralazine, procainamide and dapsone (see 'Principles of drug elimination', Chapter 1). About 50% of Caucasians are slow acetylators but the proportion varies widely in other populations, and slow acetylation is very uncommon in people of Asian ethnic origin.

Adverse effects

Peripheral neuropathy occurs mainly in slow acetylators and can be prevented by co-administration of pyridoxine (20 mg/day). Hepatotoxicity occasionally occurs and is more frequent in the elderly and those with a large alcohol intake. Very high doses of isoniazid can lead to psychosis, convulsions or coma.

Drug interactions

Isoniazid inhibits enzymes that metabolise phenytoin and warfarin; thus, phenytoin concentrations and anticoagulation level should be carefully monitored.

Dose

Oral: 3 mg/kg adults or 6 mg/kg daily in children, i.e. children require more on a weight basis; for tuberculous meningitis, 10 mg/kg daily. Also available for parenteral use.

Rifampicin

Mechanism

It is bactericidal, and inhibits the DNA-dependent RNA polymerase of *Mycobacterium* sp.

Pharmacokinetics

Rifampicin is well absorbed following oral administration and widely distributed, including the CSF. It is deacetylated in the liver and eliminated by biliary excretion.

Adverse effects

There is often a transient elevation of liver enzymes but serious hepatotoxicity is uncommon. The risk of liver damage is increased by alcoholism and pre-existing liver disease. Intermittent treatment is associated with more frequent and serious adverse effects, including renal failure and thrombocytopaenia. Rifampicin causes red urine, tears and sputum.

Drug interactions

Rifampicin induces hepatic enzymes and hence, because of increased clearance, can cause treatment failure with oral contraceptives, sulphonylureas, warfarin, steroids and barbiturates. There are significant drug interactions with many antiretroviral agents.

Dose
Rifampicin is given at a dose of 10 mg/kg daily one to 2 hours before breakfast. An intravenous formulation is also available.

Ethambutol

Mechanism

The mechanism is uncertain but bacteriostatic.

Pharmacokinetics

Ethambutol is well absorbed following oral administration. It has poor penetration of CSF but otherwise is adequately distributed. Excretion of unchanged drug is mainly renal.

Adverse effects

The most important reaction is retrobulbar neuritis with loss of visual acuity and colour vision. This is largely preventable by using doses below 25 mg/kg daily. The visual defect usually reverses over several months after stopping the drug.

Drug interactions

Aluminium hydroxide can decrease absorption.

Dose
A daily dose of 15 mg/kg is given.

Pyrazinamide

Mechanism

Pyrazinamide is bactericidal and is an essential component of the initial 2-month phase in short course (6 months) anti-TB therapy.

Pharmacokinetics

It is well absorbed following oral administration and has good penetration to CSF. It is eliminated by renal excretion.

Adverse effects

Pyrazinamide causes hepatotoxicity and arthralgia. Dose modification is required in patients with renal impairment.

Dose
A daily dose of 1.5 g (<50 kg) to 2 g (>50 kg).

Second-line drugs
Streptomycin is now infrequently used. It is an aminoglycoside that is eliminated by the kidneys.

Ototoxicity is the main adverse reaction. Streptomycin could particularly be considered for use in patients with liver disease. Several other agents are available for use in situations of bacterial resistance or adverse reactions to first-line drugs, e.g. capreomycin, cycloserine, prothionamide, p-aminosalicylic acid, amikacin, thiacatezone and linezolid.

Comment. Multi-drug resistant TB is defined as resistance to both isoniazid and rifampicin. It is increasingly recognised in the former Soviet Union and in several developing countries. Treatment is usually with as many susceptible agents as tolerated for at least 18 months.

Antifungal drugs

Amphotericin B

Mechanism

Amphotericin B combines with sterols in the plasma membrane, with a resulting increase in permeability and cell death.

Pharmacokinetics

Absorption is negligible following oral administration. In practice it is usually given intravenously. It is highly protein-bound with apparently poor penetration to tissues and body fluids. It is not removed by haemodialysis. The mode of elimination is unknown but it is not influenced by renal function. Newer formulations consist of liposomal amphotericin. These formulations are largely replacing standard amphoteracin as toxicity is lessened.

Adverse effects

These are very common. Most patients develop fever, chills and nausea. Nephrotoxicity (distal tubular destruction and calcification) usually occurs during prolonged treatment at or above 1 mg/kg daily and manifests as hypokalaemia, hypomagnesaemia, loss of concentrating ability and renal tubular acidosis; nephrotoxicity may reverse if detected early. Liposomal amphotericin has much less renal toxicity but cost is increased considerably.

Drug interaction

It is additive with other nephrotoxic drugs. Concurrent digoxin therapy can become toxic if hypokalaemia develops.

Antifungal spectrum

It is currently the drug of choice for most systemic mycoses: active against *Cryptococcus*, *Candida* and other yeasts, *Aspergillus*, *Coccidioides* and other fungi.

Dose

A dose of 1.0–1.5 mg/kg daily depending on disease severity and appearance of nephrotoxicity, infused over 2–4 hours. Hydrocortisone or chlorpheniramine can reduce febrile reactions and chlorpromazine can reduce nausea. Loading the patient with normal saline before administering the drug may limit nephrotoxicity.

Liposomal amphotericin requires higher doses of 3–6 mg/kg.

Comment. Amphotericin B is an example of the need to carefully weigh the risks and benefits of treatment. It is highly toxic but untreated systemic mycoses are invariably fatal.

Flucytosine

Mechanism

It is deaminated inside the fungal cell to 5-fluorouracil, which inhibits nucleic acid synthesis with cell death.

Pharmacokinetics

It is well absorbed following oral administration and is widely distributed, including the CSF. Elimination is mainly renal. Clearance is decreased in patients with renal impairment.

Adverse effects

Concentration-related bone marrow suppression is the only major problem. This can usually be avoided by drug level monitoring.

Antifungal spectrum

It is only active against yeasts; efficacy is limited by rapid emergence of resistance.

Dose

A dose of 150–200 mg flucytosine is given daily in divided doses.

Comment. Although much less toxic than amphotericin, flucytosine is of limited value because of its narrow spectrum and the existence of resistant organisms. It is usually administered together with amphotericin B. This combination is the therapy of choice for cryptococcal meningitis.

Imidazoles and related compounds

Mechanism

Imidazoles increase permeability by preventing ergosterol formation in cell membranes. They also produce cell necrosis by inhibiting peroxidative enzymes.

Miconazole, clotrimazole, econazole

Pharmacokinetics
These drugs are poorly absorbed following oral administration and are usually restricted for topical use.

Antifungal spectrum
They are active against a wide range of yeasts and fungi. Their main use is topical, e.g. athlete's foot or vaginal candidiasis.

Fluconazole, itraconazole, ketoconazole, voriconazole

Pharmacokinetics
Following oral administration these drugs are widely distributed; adequate CSF levels are ob-

tained with the exception of ketoconazole. Fluconazole is eliminated by the kidneys; itraconazole, ketoconazole and voriconazole are metabolised by the liver.

Antifungal spectrum
They are active against a wide range of yeasts and fungi; fluconazole is particularly effective against yeasts and itraconazole and voriconazole additionally against filamentous fungi, e.g. *Aspergillus*.

Adverse effects
Hepatotoxicity is associated particularly with ketoconazole, which requires monitoring of liver function. Voriconazole commonly produces a number of reversible visual disturbances that do not require cessation of the drug.

Drug interactions

These agents have many drug-drug interactions. They may be substrates for or may be metabolised via Cytochrome P450 pathways. Caution therefore should be employed when co-administered with other agents and up to date texts should be consulted.

Doses
Fluconazole: 100–400 mg orally or by i.v. infusion, daily single dose.
Itraconazole: 100–200 mg orally, daily single dose.
Ketoconazole: 200–400 mg orally, daily single dose.
Voriconazole: 200 mg orally b.d. An i.v. preparation is also available.

Nystatin

Nystatin is used topically in the treatment of yeast infections of the skin and mucous membranes. It is not used parenterally because of high toxicity.

Griseofulvin

Griseofulvin is active only against dermatophytes and is given orally in the treatment of skin or nail infections. It is fungistatic and so must be given for weeks or months. It diminishes the anticoagulant effect by enzyme induction. Barbiturates lead to griseofulvin treatment failure by enzyme induction. Griseofulvin can precipitate porphyria.

Caspofungin

Caspofungin is a member of a novel family of antifungal drugs, the echinocandins. It acts as a non-competitive inhibitor of the synthesis of 1,3-ß-glucan, a polysaccharide in the cell wall of many pathogenic fungi. Glucans are essential in maintaining osmotic integrity of the fungal cell wall, and hence inhibition of their synthesis leads to fungal cell death. Caspafungin is highly active against many *Candida* sp. and *Aspergillus* spp. It is available as an intravenous formulation for the treatment of serious infections caused by these organisms.

Antiviral drugs

These are the least developed as a group of antimicrobial agents: viruses use the biochemical system of their host cells, and it is therefore difficult to prevent viral multiplication without seriously damaging the patient. However, effective therapy is now available for a number of virus infections of clinical importance.

Aciclovir, valaciclovir and famciclovir

Mechanism

The pharmacological effect of aciclovir depends on its conversion to an active metabolite by a herpes simplex coded enzyme, thymidine kinase. It is phosphorylated only in herpes-infected cells and normal cellular processes are unaffected. The resulting aciclovir triphosphate inhibits herpes-specified DNA polymerase, preventing further viral DNA synthesis. The herpes genome in latently (non-replicating) infected cells is not altered during antiviral therapy. Aciclovir is active against herpes simplex virus 1 and 2 as well as varicella zoster. Valaciclovir is an orally administered prodrug of aciclovir, which is much

better absorbed than aciclovir and is converted into aciclovir by first-pass metabolism in the liver. Famciclovir is a prodrug of penciclovir, an agent with very similar structure and antiviral activity to aciclovir.

Pharmacokinetics

Aciclovir is absorbed orally in patients with normal gut function, but with a bioavailability of only 15–30%. It is eliminated by renal clearance involving glomerular filtration and tubular secretion. Aciclovir penetrates the blood–brain barrier passively to enter CSF. The prodrugs valaciclovir and famciclovir have a much higher oral bioavailability of 50–80%, and are thus preferred for oral therapy.

Adverse effects

Renal impairment occasionally follows intravenous administration.

Drug interactions

No clinically important interactions have been observed yet.

Clinical use

Aciclovir is indicated for herpes simplex and varicella zoster infections of the skin and mucous membranes, the brain and in lung disease and in prophylaxis against herpes infections in immunocompromised hosts. An intravenous route is required for serious disease manifestations and in immunocompromised patients.

Dose
Aciclovir

For herpes simplex: oral, 200 mg five times per day for 5 days; intravenous, 5 mg/kg over 1 hour, repeated every 8 hour (10 mg/kg in herpes encephalitis). A dose modification is necessary in renal failure. For varicella zoster: oral, 800 mg five times per day for 7 days; intravenous, 10 mg/kg 8-hourly.

Valaciclovir

For herpes simplex: oral, 500 mg b.d. for 5 days.

Famciclovir

For herpes simplex: oral, 750 mg once daily for 7 days.

Idoxuridine

Idoxuridine is a thymidine analogue that inhibits DNA synthesis. It is highly toxic when given systemically and is therefore only used topically in the treatment of herpes simplex infections of the eye, as an aqueous solution.

Amantadine

Amantadine (including its analogue, rimantadine) prevents entry of influenza A to host cells and is used predominantly in prophylaxis and also in the treatment of infections caused by this virus. Influenza B virus is not susceptible. Amantadine can produce neurological side effects but usually only if high concentrations are achieved, e.g. in renal failure.

Zanamivir and Oseltamivir

Zanamivir and oseltamivir are sialic acid analogues that potently inhibit influenza A and B neuraminidases, an activity that is essential for viral release and spread within the respiratory tract. These drugs shorten the clinical symptoms in influenza infection when administered within 2 days of onset. However, they only shorten the disease by about 1 day. They are also effective in prophylaxis of infection, for example in susceptible high-risk patients such as nursing home residents exposed to infection. Routine immunisation of such populations is, however, more cost-effective.

Ribavirin

Ribavirin inhibits a number of DNA and RNA viruses. Its antiviral action has been demonstrated in vitro and in vivo against a number of important viruses, including respiratory syncytial virus (RSV), influenza A and B viruses, parainfluenza 1 and 3 Lassa fever virus and hepatitis C. The mechanism of action is not completely understood but involves the action of ribavirin triphosphate interfering with the binding of viral messenger RNA to ribosomes. It is predominantly used in the form of a nebulised aerosol in the treatment of bronchitis in infancy as a consequence of RSV infection and in combination with α-interferon in the treatment of chronic hepatitis C.

Interferon-α

Interferons are natural antiviral proteins produced by humans in response to viral infection. They are active in vitro against a wide range of viruses, but their main clinical use is in the treatment of chronic hepatitis B and C, the latter in combination with ribavirin. Interferons have numerous side effects, including an 'influenza-like' syndrome, leucopenia, thrombocytopenia, depression, renal impairment, arrhythmias and thyroiditis. They are only active when administered parenterally, usually by subcutaneous injection. Modification of interferons by addition of a polyethylene glycol side chain, 'pegylation', prolongs the half-life significantly without altering the antiviral activity, and is the preferred form for treatment of chronic hepatitis.

Anti-retroviral agents

These are discussed in Chapter 10

Key points – general principles of antimicrobial therapy

Patient	Microbiology	Drug
Risk of infection: Susceptibility to particular infection based on immunocompromise, age, comorbidity, pregnancy, occupation, genetic and other factors	Awareness of likely organism(s), site of infection (e.g. intra or extra-cellular, biofilm), potential complications of infection (e.g. suppuration) and antimicrobial sensitivity patterns for common organisms	Pharmacokinetics (absorption, distribution, protein binding, clearance)
Clinical examination: Identify and document clinical signs of infection, assess severity and assess for most appropriate route of administration	Investigations: Take appropriate samples for diagnosis (microscopy, culture, serology, polymerase chain reaction). Confirmation of organism(s) and antimicrobial susceptibility	Pharmacodynamics: Mode and site of action including rate of killing (cidality) and mode of killing (concentration or time dependent)
Factors altering kinetics: age, renal/hepatic function, pregnancy, burns	Interpretation of microbiological results: False negative and false positive results. Differences between colonisation and infection. Does the organism fit the clinical syndrome? Effect of prior antimicrobial therapy	Spectrum of activity of the agent
Contraindications: Clarify and document any drug sensitivity, previous toxicity, pregnancy, breast feeding, comorbidity, etc.		Therapeutic drug monitoring
		Drug interactions Side effects Ecological impact

Chapter 10

HIV and antiretroviral treatment

Clinical scenario

A 37-year-old man was found to be HIV positive. He does not know when he was infected and is entirely asymptomatic. He has a CD4 count of 310 cells/mm³ with a viral load of 87500 copies/mL. He has a history of previous episodes of recurrent, severe depression, requiring inpatient admission on three occasions. What HIV therapy should he be offered? Are there any drugs that should be avoided?

Key points

In chronic HIV infection the aim of therapy is to:
- Fully suppress HIV replication using antiretroviral combination therapy, with the aim of achieving persistently undetectable levels of virus in the plasma
- Allow immune recovery, through the suppression of HIV replication, thus preventing HIV/AIDS associated morbidity and mortality
- Prevent drug resistant HIV from emerging
- Minimise drug toxicity

Introduction

The first cases of AIDS were reported from the United States in 1981. Over the next 15 years HIV-1 infection (subsequently referred to simply as 'HIV' in this chapter unless otherwise stated) spread globally. During this period HIV infection led inexorably to increasingly severe immunosuppression, AIDS and eventually death. Although zidovudine – a nucleoside reverse transcriptase inhibitor – and a small number of other antiretroviral drugs became available in the late 1980s and early 1990s, resistance to these drugs developed rapidly when they were given by themselves as monotherapy, so treatment had little durable impact on HIV viral suppression and disease progression.

The revolution in HIV therapy came in 1995–1996, with the advent of highly active antiretroviral therapy (HAART). HAART refers to combination antiretroviral therapy using three or more agents, with the aim of fully suppressing the HIV virus to undetectable levels in the blood. This, in turn, results in less viral resistance developing, significant immune recovery and a greatly improved prognosis.

Although the therapeutic advances have been tremendous, HIV therapy remains a difficult and complex area. Lifelong treatment, the requirement for a high level of treatment adherence, food interactions, extensive drug interactions and the potential for short- and long-term toxicity remain challenging issues.

Lecture Notes: Clinical Pharmacology and Therapeutics, 8th edition. By Gerard McKay, John Reid and Matthew Walters. Published 2010 by Blackwell Publishing Ltd.

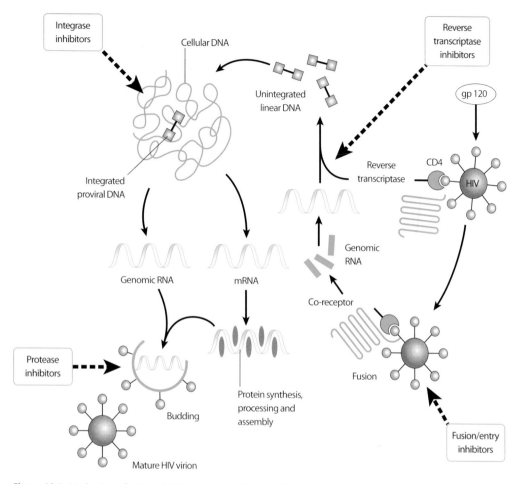

Figure 10.1 Mechanism of action of HIV drugs. (From Fauci, 2007).

Overview of mechanisms of drug action

The HIV virus is a single stranded RNA virus belonging to the retrovirus family. During its replication cycle it uses the enzyme reverse transcriptase (RT) to convert RNA to dsDNA, which is then incorporated into host cell DNA. Zidovudine, the first antiretroviral drug that was discovered, acts by inhibiting RT. RT also serves as the target for many of the newer drugs. Inhibitors of other enzymes involved in the replication cycle of the HIV virus, including the protease and integrase enzymes, have also been developed, along with drugs that act by preventing the HIV virus from entering host cells (Fig. 10.1).

Drug classes and drugs

Anti-retroviral drugs are classified by their mechanism of action. At present there are five main drug classes, shown in Table 10.1. The drugs that are currently (2009) available in the UK are shown in Table 10.2, grouped by their drug class. The combination preparations available are shown in Table 10.3.

The NRTIs, NNRTIs and PIs have been in use longest and remain the most important drugs at

Table 10.1 The five main classes of antiretroviral drugs.

1 Nucleoside/nucleotide reverse transcriptase inhibitors (NRTIs).
2 Non-nucleoside reverse transcriptase inhibitors (NNRTIs).
3 Protease inhibitors (PIs).
4 Fusion and entry inhibitors.
5 Integrase inhibitors.

present. However, this is a rapidly evolving area of therapeutics. New drug classes, drugs and combination preparations will undoubtedly become available over the next few years.

Nucleoside/nucleotide reverse transcriptase inhibitors

Nucleotide reverse transcriptase inhibitors (NRTIs, also referred to as 'nucleoside/tide analogues') are small molecules with structures that closely resemble naturally occurring nucleosides (all agents other than tenofovir) or nucleotides (tenofovir). Competitive inhibition of RT and termination of the developing DNA chain are the principal mechanism of action.

Pharmacokinetics

These agents are pro-drugs that require intracellular activation, although tenofovir is less dependent on intracellular activation. They typically have long intracellular half-lives, despite having fairly short serum half-lives. NRTIs are predominantly excreted by the kidneys and dosage reduction or avoidance is therefore required in renal failure.

Food and drug interactions

Apart from didanosine, there are no food restrictions for the NRTIs (Table 10.1). Drug interactions are also infrequent compared to the PIs and NNR-TIs. Caution is required when combining NRTI drugs together in a regime as some combinations result in increased toxicity (e.g. stavudine with

didanosine). Dangerous interactions may also with some NRTIs if they are co-prescribed with some other antiviral drugs such as ganciclovir and ribavirin.

Drug resistance

Mutations in the reverse transcriptase gene can result in drug resistance. The individual drugs differ in their behaviour, with some drugs (e.g. lamivudine) being relatively 'fragile' and a single mutation may cause full resistance. Other drugs (e.g. abacavir) are more resilient. Certain mutations may cause multi-NRTI resistance. It is therefore important to 'protect' drugs and prevent resistance mutations from emerging by using these drugs within a fully suppressive HAART regime.

Adverse effects

Minor side effects including headache, nausea and GI upset are common during the first few weeks after starting the older NRTIs such as zidovudine. These symptoms are usually self-limiting.

NRTIs may also cause more serious side effects (Table 10.4). Lactic acidosis is a rare but life-threatening complication that is a particular concern for the NRTI class. The onset is typically insidious and may start months or years after a patient has started HIV therapy, so it is easy to miss. Routine monitoring of lactate levels is not recommended as the clinical significance of mild, asymptomatic hyperlactataemia is not established. However, lactate levels must be checked urgently in symptomatic patients.

Lipodystrophy is a complex HAART- associated disorder of fat metabolism that may be clinically evident as lipoatrophy (loss of fat of the face, limbs and buttocks), fat accumulation (abdominal, breasts, dorso-cervical or lipomas) or a combination of both. NRTI therapy with the thymidine analogues stavudine and zidovudine is particularly associated with lipoatrophy.

Metabolic abnormalities including dyslipidemia and insulin resistance/diabetes mellitus may occur in conjunction with lipodystrophy.

Table 10.2 Approved antiretroviral drugs in the UK (2009).

Drug		Usual adult dose	Food restrictions
Nucleoside/nucleotide reverse transcriptase inhibitors (NRTIs)			
	Zidovudine (AZT)	250 mg twice daily	—
	Didanosine (ddI)	250 mg once daily (wt < 60 kg)	1/2 hour before or 2 hours after a meal
		400 mg once daily (wt > 60 kg)	
	Lamivudine (3TC)	150 mg twice daily	—
		or 300 mg once daily	
	Stavudine (d4T)	30 mg twice daily (wt < 60 Kg)	—
		40 mg twice daily (wt > 60 kg)	—
	Abacavir (ABC)	300 mg once daily	—
	Tenofovir disoproxil fumarate (TDF)	245 mg once daily	—
	Emtricitabine (FTC)	200 mg once daily	—
Non-nucleoside reverse transcriptase inhibitors (NNRTIs)			
	Nevirapine (NVP)	200 mg once daily for 14 days, then 200 mg twice daily	—
	Efavirenz (EFV)	600 mg once daily	Best on an empty stomach, at bedtime.
	Etravirine (ETR)	200 mg twice daily	Take with/after food
Protease inhibitors (PIs)			
	Saquinavir (SQV)	1000 mg twice daily, with ritonavir (100 mg b.d.) boosting	Take within 2 hours of a meal
	Ritonavir (RIT)	Rarely used, other than as a booster for other drugs	Preferably with food
	Indinavir (IDV)	800 mg three times daily (boosted regimes unlicensed)	1 hour before or 2 hours after a meal
	Nelfinavir (NFV)	1250 mg twice daily	Take with food
	Fosamprenavir (FPV)	700 mg twice daily, with ritonavir (100 mg b.d.) boosting	—
	Lopinavir + ritonavir (Kaletra®) (LPV/r)	Two 200/50 mg tablets twice daily	—
	Atazanavir (ATV)	300 mg once daily, with ritonavir (100 mg o.d.) boosting	Take with food
	Tipranavir (TPV)	500 mg twice daily, with ritonavir (200 mg b.d.) boosting	—
	Darunavir (DRV)	600 mg twice daily, with ritonavir (100 mg b.d.) boosting	Take with food
Fusion and entry inhibitors			
Fusion inhibitor	Enfuvirtide (T20)	90 mg subcutaneously twice daily	—
CCR5-inhibitor	Maraviroc (MVC)	300 mg twice daily	—
Integrase inhibitors			
	Raltegravir (RAL)	400 mg twice daily	—

Table 10.3 Combination tablets available in the UK (2009).

Combination	Generic name	Trade name
	Zidovudine + lamivudine	Combivir®
2 NRTIs	Zidovudine + abacavir	Kivexa®
	Emtricitabine + tenofovir	Truvada®
3 NRTIs	Zidovudine + lamivudine + abacavir	Trizivir®
PI + low-dose ritonavir (booster)	Lopinavir + ritonavir	Kaletra®
2 NRTIs + NNRTI	Tenofovir + emtricitabine efavirenz	Atripla®

Non-nucleoside reverse transcriptase inhibitors

The non-nucleoside reverse transcriptase inhibitors (NNRTIs) mechanism of action is also to inhibit reverse transcriptase, but they do this by different mechanism from the NRTIs.

Pharmacokinetics

The NNRTIs (particularly efavirenz) have long serum half-lives, allowing for once or twice daily administration. They do not require intracellular activation. Metabolism occurs through the hepatic cytochrome p450 (CYP450) system, with complex interactions with various the CYP450 isoenzymes.

Food and drug interactions

These are more challenging than for the NRTIs. Both efavirenz and etravirine levels are increased if the drugs are taken with food. In the case of etravirine this is helpful, whilst for efavirenz the higher drug levels can increase side effects and the drug is best taken on an empty stomach.

As these drugs induce the cytochrome P-450 system, they interact with many other drugs that are metabolised through this system, including many antiretroviral drugs and a number of other antimicrobial agents. Table 10.5 shows some examples of important interactions. Many of these interactions are manageable (although potentially requiring dosage modifications), but in some cases co-administration has to be avoided altogether. The University of Liverpool online HIV drug interaction charts (www.hiv-druginteractions.org) should

be consulted before co-prescribing a drug with an NNRTI agent.

Drug resistance

One of the main drawbacks of NNRTIs is that they are relatively 'fragile' drugs with a low genetic barrier to resistance. A single mutation at a key site can confer high-level resistance, with cross-resistance between the drugs in the class. Etravirine is a newer 'second generation' NNRTI that is intended to remain active against virus that has the common efavirenz/nevirapine mutations.

Adverse effects

Table 10.4 shows the potential adverse events associated with NNRTIs. NNRTIs have a reasonably good adverse event profile, particularly with regards to long-term toxicity, but rash and hepato-toxiciy in particular (especially with nevirapine) are concerns. Transient CNS side effects are common on starting efavirenz, but usually settle down after a few weeks. Efavirenz must be avoided in pregnancy.

Protease inhibitors

The discovery of the first drugs of the protease inhibitor (PI) class was the breakthrough that led to the initial widespread introduction of HAART in the mid 1990s.

Pharmacokinetics

The PIs have very complex pharmacokinetics. Cytochrome P-450 isoenzymes such as CYP3A4

Table 10.4 Major adverse effects of HIV drugs.

Adverse effects	Associated drugs	Clinical manifestation	Risk factors	Prevention/management
Lactic acidosis/hepatic steatosis	NRTIs, especially stavudine and didanosine	Often insidious onset – nausea, vomiting, fatigue, weight loss. Can progress rapidly to multi-organ failure & death	Obesity, female gender, pregnancy, liver disease. Some drug combinations (e.g. didanosine + stavudine)	Use NRTIs (esp stavudine and didanosine) with caution if risk factors present. Discontinue NRTIs if: symptomatic hyper-lactataemia, lactic acidosis, progressive hepatomegaly or rapid LFT deterioration occurs
Lipodystrophy	Lipoatrophy: NRTIs, esp. stavudine and zidovudine, particularly if PI given in combination Lipohypertrophy: PIs in particular, but also other drugs	Lipoatrophy: fat loss from face, arms and buttocks Lipohypertrophy: abdominal fat accumulation, dorsal 'buffalo hump' fat pad	Low baseline BMI, Caucasian race, male gender	Avoid drugs associated with lipoatrophy (esp. stavudine and zidovudine) Diet & exercise may help prevent lipohypertrophy
Cardiovascular effects (MI and CVA)	PIs – use has been linked to premature CVA and MI Some NRTIs (abacavir and didanosine) – recent use associated with MI	Premature CVA, angina or MI	Other risk factors for cardiovascular disease	Assess and modify other cardiovascular risk factors Use drugs with the least potential for cardiovascular disease, where possible
Hyperlipidaemia	PIs Some NRTIs (esp. stavudine) NNRTIs (efavirenz > nevirapine)	Raised total cholesterol, LDL cholesterol and triglycerides may occur	Underlying hyperlipidaemia Certain drugs/combinations increase the risk	Consider switching to other drugs Lifestyle modification Statin therapy may be required (note potential interactions with HIV drugs)

(Continued)

Table 10.4 (Continued)

Adverse effects	Associated drugs	Clinical manifestation	Risk factors	Prevention/management
Insulin resistance/diabetes mellitus	Some PIs Some NRTIs (stavudine and zidovudine)	Impaired glucose tolerance or frank diabetes mellitus	Other risk factors for diabetes mellitus (e.g. family history)	Consider switching to other drugs Diet +/− treatment for diabetes
CNS side effects	Efavirenz	Dizziness, insomnia, vivid dreams, drowsiness, depression, psychosis	Pre-existing psychiatric illness High plasma efavirenz levels	Mild effects are common and usually disappear after 2–3 weeks Some patients may need to discontinue efavirenz
Hypersensitivity reaction	Abacavir	Malaise, rash, fever, vomiting, abdominal pain, dyspnoea Usually occurs in first 6 weeks of therapy	Associated with HLA B5701	Patients must be screened for HLA B571 prior to starting abacavir Never re-challenge after a suspected reaction (has led to deaths)
Stevens Johnson syndrome	NNRTIs (Nevirapine > efavirenz) Occasionally with other drugs	A mild self-limiting rash is common with nevirapine, but fever, malaise and mucosal involvement suggests SJS	Female gender; Black or Asian (nevirapine)	Potential culprit drugs should be stopped Supportive care, potentially including ITU
Peripheral neuropathy	Some NRTIs: stavudine, didanosine	Paraesthesia of extremities, progressing to a painful peripheral neuropathy. May become irreversible	Advanced HIV; pre-existing neuropathy Combining high-risk nucleosides	Discontinue drugs responsible and substitute with other agents gabapentin or tricyclic agent, for symptom relief
Pancreatitis	Some NRTIs: stavudine, didanosine	Often a sub-acute presentation	Excess alcohol, hyper-triglyceridaemia Certain NRTI combinations	Discontinue likely culprit drugs Symptomatic management

Hepatotoxicity	all NNRTIs (esp. nevirapine) all PIs most NRTIs maraviroc	May be asymptomatic initially Rash (nevirapine- associated cases) or lactic acidosis (NRTI-associated cases) may also be present	Pre-existing liver disease (e.g. alcohol, HBV or HCV) Nevirapine risk greatest with higher pre-treatment CD4 counts	Mild asymptomatic LFT rise often just requires monitoring If symptomatic and/or major LFT abnormality, suspend all ARVs
Anaemia and neutropenia	Zidovudine	Severe anaemia and/or neutropenia relatively uncommon	Other bone marrow suppressants	Stop other implicated drugs. Investigate and treat other causes Switch NRTI, if required
Nephrotoxicity	Tenofovir, indinavir	Severe renal impairment is rare Hypophosphataemia (usually mild) and Fanconi syndrome (rare) can occur with tenofovir	Pre-existing renal disease, advanced age and use of other nephrotoxic drugs.	Monitor urinalysis, U&Es and phosphate levels (tenofovir) Indinavir seldom used now
Renal stones	Indinavir	Loin pain	Inadequate fluid intake	Increase fluid intake (1.5 L water/day)
Osteopenia/osteoporosis	Linked to HIV and to HAART, but specific drugs not very clear Some NRTIs (e.g. tenofovir and stavudine) and ?PIs reduce bone mineral density	Usually asymptomatic; increased fracture risk in later life	Other 'traditional' risk factors for osteoporosis will increase the risk	Consider DEXA scan for assessment Consider switching HIV drug regimen if osteopenia confirmed Follow standard guidelines for osteopenia/osteoporosis.

Table 10.5 Examples of important drug interactions with NNRTIs and PIs.

Drug class	Example/comment
Antiretroviral drugs: other PIs and NNRTIs	Complex interactions occur when PI and/or NNRTI agents are used together
Anticonvulsants	Phenytoin, carbamazepine and phenobarbital in particular
Antidepressant and antipsychotic drugs	Many potential interactions. Some anti-psychotics (e.g. pimozide) cannot be safely co-prescribed
Antihistamines	Arrhythmias may occur with some (older) drugs
Antimicrobial agents	Rifampicin (cannot be given with a PI); clarithromycin; some azoles
Cardiac drugs	Anti-arrhythmic drugs such as amiodarone, flecanide and propafenone are a particular concern; interactions with calcium channel blockers
Herbal medicines	St John's wort interacts significantly with all PIs and NNRTIs
Immunosuppressants	Ciclosporin, tactolimus
Opiates	Methadone (dosages may need adjustment)
Proton pump inhibitors	Atazanavir and nelfinavir in particular – cannot be co-prescribed with PPIs
Sedatives and anxiolytics	Significant interactions with many benzodiazepines
Statins	Simvastatin and lovastatin cannot be used with PIs
Other	Ergot derivatives; erectile dysfunction, oral contraceptive and antimalarial agents

enzyme are important for PI drug metabolism and are present both in the gut wall and the liver. CYP3A4 inducers or inhibitors can therefore affect PI absorption, hepatic metabolism, or both. The PIs themselves can also act as both inducers and inhibitors for different parts of the p-450 system. To complicate matters even further, inducers or inhibitors of P-glycoprotein (P-gp), a cellular efflux pump system, can also affect PI bioavailability.

Unboosted PIs have relatively short half lives, leading to the risk of inadequate serum drug levels between doses and the potential for virological failure and resistance. PI–PI drug interactions can be used to advantage to overcome this problem, with a small dose of ritonavir now being routinely co-prescribed as a pharmacokinetic 'booster' (through p450 inhibition) to increase the levels of the main active PI agent (see Table 10.1).

Food and drug interactions

From a consideration of the pharmacokinetics it is no surprise that PIs have a lot of potential drug interactions. Several also have important food in-

teractions and must be taken either fasted or with a meal, depending on the drug in question (Table 10.1). Table 10.5 shows some examples of important drug interactions. As with NNTRIs, reactions may be manageable in some cases whilst in other cases co-administration must avoided altogether (consult online drug interaction charts (www.hiv-druginteractions.org) before co-prescribing a drug with a PI).

Drug resistance

As a class, PIs tend to be relatively robust agents that require a number of mutations in the virus before clinically significant drug resistance occurs. However, PI drug resistance is certainly still seen, with a number of mutations (e.g. the L90M mutation) conferring PI class cross-resistance. Using newer 'boosted' PI regimens ensures that suppressive drug levels are maintained at all times thus helping to prevent drug resistance from emerging and/or suppressing partial resistance. The concept of the inhibitory quotient (IQ), defined as the ratio between (trough) drug concentration and level of drug required to inhibit replication of the HIV isolate, is useful here.

Adverse effects

Adverse events associated with PIs are show in Table 10.4. Overall, the toxicity profile for PIs is somewhat worse than for NNRTIs, with concern over long-term side effects such as lipodystophy, hyperlipidaemia and vascular disease in particular.

Fusion and entry inhibitors

Enfuvirtide acts by blocking gp-41 mediated membrane fusion and viral entry. Maraviroc also blocks viral entry but through inhibition of the CCR-5 co-receptor; it is therefore only active against HIV-1 virus that expresses CCR-5 and this needs to be assayed prior maraviroc use.

Enfuvirtide has to be given by subcutaneous injection – local injection site reactions are also the principle side effect of this drug. Maraviroc, which is given orally, is a substrate of p450 CYP3 A and p-glycoprotein and consequently has a number of significant drug interactions, whilst enfuvirtide has no significant drug interactions

These drugs are still relatively infrequently used in the UK and are reserved as second- or third-line agents.

Integrase inhibitors

This is another relatively new drug class that prevents HIV replication by inhibiting the integrase enzyme (Fig. 10.1). Raltegravir, the only currently available agent in the UK, is given orally and has a reasonably favourable adverse event profile. It is metabolised by UGT1A1-mediated glucuronidation rather than via the p450 system. Drug interactions occur, but are generally not as challenging as with the PIs and NNRTIs. Raltegravir is currently still used as a second- or third-line agent in the UK.

Combination therapy using HAART

To maximise virological suppression and thus enhance immune recovery and prevent drug resistance from emerging, antiretroviral drugs are combined within 'HAART' regimens consisting of 3 or more agents. Combination preparations (Table 10.3) can help to reduce the 'pill burden' and promote treatment adherence.

For heavily immunocompromised individuals (typically where the CD4 lymphocyte count is <200 cells/mm^3), anti-microbial prophylaxis against opportunistic infections (e.g. co-trimoxazole or dapsone for *Pneumocystis jiroveci* pneumonia (PCP) prophylaxis) may be required in addition to HAART until adequate immune recovery has occurred.

Indications for HAART therapy

Patients with significant HIV-mediated immunological impairment, as judged by their CD4 lymphocyte count, are prioritised for treatment – particularly if an AIDS defining condition is present. The best time to start therapy in asymptomatic individuals is not clear and remains controversial, although the current trend is towards starting earlier rather than later. Current UK recommendations produced by the British HIV Association (BHIVA) are shown in Table 10.6.

Table 10.6 Recommendations for when to start HAART*.

Presentation	
Primary HIV infection	No treatment indicated in most cases
Established HIV infection	
CD4 count < 200	Treat
CD4 count 200–350	Treat as soon as possible – rather less urgency
CD4 count 350–500	Treat in specific situations only
3. AIDS defining illness present	Treat

*Based on BHIVA 2008 guidelines.

Antiretroviral therapy is usually life-long once started.

Preferred first-line regimens

First-line regimens typically use combinations of two NRTIs (given as a combination tablet, with Truvada® currently favoured) and either an NNRTI or a boosted PI. Currently, the NNRTI efavirenz is considered the best first line drug to use and boosted PIs are usually reserved for specific groups of patients, such as those with drug resistance, women who wish to become pregnant, and patients with psychiatric problems. These guidelines change frequently so the latest BHVIA guidance should be consulted (see www.bhiva.org).

Monitoring

The aim is to suppress the HIV viral load (VL) to undetectable levels in the blood (typically < 40 copies virus/mL). This is associated with an improvement in immune function. Regular clinic follow-up (typically 3-monthly once on treatment) with CD4 and VL monitoring is important. Clinical, biochemical and haematological drug toxicity is also assessed at visits.

Treatment adherence

High levels of treatment adherence (ideally >95% adherence) are required for durable virological suppression with HAART. This is one of the most challenging aspects of therapy for patients and medical staff alike. Adherence must be assessed at each follow-up visit. A number of strategies have been devised to help improve adherence.

Changing therapy

A change of therapy may be required if there is a sustained rebound in VL from undetectable levels, or if an undetectable VL is not obtained after 24–36 weeks of first-line therapy. Drug side effects may also necessitate treatment changes.

The possibility of sub-optimal treatment adherence should always be explored and addressed in cases of virological failure prior to considering drug regimen changes. Wherever possible, an HIV drug resistance assay should be performed to guide the change in therapy. Therapeutic drug level monitoring (TDM) may also be appropriate in some cases.

Usually, the whole regime will need to be changed in cases a virological failure: the virus will rapidly become resistant to a single new drug that is added to a failing regimen.

HIV therapy in special situations

Pregnancy

HIV drug therapy for pregnant women has an important role in the prevention of mother-to-child HIV transmission. When used in combination with appropriate obstetric management, avoidance of breastfeeding, and a 4–6 week course of HIV post-exposure prophylaxis for the infant, HIV transmission rates can be reduced from 15–25% down to <2%.

Whilst monotherapy with zidovudine is still occasionally used, HAART combination therapy is nearly always recommended now as number of HIV drugs have been found to be safe in pregnancy. A 2NRTI + PI regimen (e.g. Combivir + Kaletra) is generally used. Drug metabolism is altered in pregnancy, so TDM (PI levels) is usually undertaken.

Children

There are many differences between children and adults with regards to both immunological function and HIV drug metabolism. Furthermore, fewer drugs are available. Paediatric HIV therapy is therefore a very specialised area. The Children's HIV Association (CHIVA) website (www.chiva.org.uk) is a useful information resource.

Post-exposure prophylaxis (PEP)

A 4-week course of HAART can reduce the chances of HIV transmission in cases of per-cutaneous exposure (e.g. needle-stick injury) or unprotected sexual exposure (e.g. condom rupture) from an HIV infected individual. Treatment needs to be commenced as soon as possible. Most Emergency Medicine departments now have starter packs of the relevant HIV drugs for these situations.

HIV-2 infection

HIV-2 is much less common than HIV-1, occurring mainly in West Africa and countries with close links to West Africa. It is uncommon in the UK. Whilst many of the general principles of HAART therapy apply to HIV-2 treatment, the HIV-2 virus is resistant to the NNRTIs such as efavirenz and nevirapine that are first-line agents against HIV-1.

Chapter 11

Travel medicine and tropical disease

Introduction

Over 45 million Britons travel abroad each year. Many travelling to Europe, the United States and Australia require no special prophylaxis against infections different to those in Britain as the risks and public health are similar. However, travel to many other countries, especially in the tropics and subtropics, can expose the traveller to new health risks. Making a sound risk assessment for each traveller is the first stage of any pre-travel consultation.

It must be remembered that most illness encountered by travellers is not preventable by prophylaxis and much morbidity and mortality encountered abroad is not infection-related (e.g. sunburn, dehydration, alcohol excess and road-traffic accidents). To prevent infections it is always important to emphasise other health precautions, including care with food and water hygiene, safe sex, caution with fresh water exposure and the avoidance of mosquito bites through repellents and impregnated bed nets when appropriate.

Those planning to work or travel in Africa or Asia should be aware of the high prevalence of HIV infection in these regions and the ways in which risk of infection can be minimised. Healthcare

workers who may be carrying out exposure-prone procedures may consider a post-exposure prophylaxis pack containing three antiretroviral agents to be administered if there is mucosal exposure or a penetrating needle stick injury with HIV-infected body fluids.

There are a number of sources of continually updated information on disease prevalence within different countries combined with other information necessary to make these risk assessments. The TRAVAX (A–Z of Healthy Travel) database is provided within the National Health Service (NHS) by Health Protection Scotland (http://www.travax.scot.nhs.uk) and it is available through the NHS Net. A public site is also available (http://www.fitfortravel.scot.nhs.uk).

Key points – assessing the need for prophylaxis

- The significance to the individual traveller relates to the potential seriousness of the disease itself but it must not be forgotten that infected asymptomatic carriers can often, after the traveller returns home, transmit serious illness to other family members and close contacts (e.g. hepatitis A, HIV infection).
- The likelihood of contracting any infection depends upon multiple factors including the prevalence of the infection in the countries being visited, the length of time abroad and activities to be undertaken (e.g. rural or safari trips where malaria and rabies need to be given

Lecture Notes: Clinical Pharmacology and Therapeutics, 8th edition. By Gerard McKay, John Reid and Matthew Walters. Published 2010 by Blackwell Publishing Ltd.

extra consideration and adventure sporting activities where injury, fresh water exposure and high altitude are possible).
• The value of any immuno- or chemoprophylaxis depends upon the level of protection it provides, ease of administration (e.g. number of doses) and cost in relation to the protection provided.
• Sometimes peer pressures and less logical considerations enter into the decision-making process and these cannot be ignored. For example, there is a lot of understandable and sometimes exaggerated fear over the risk of contacting rabies, and while the risk of yellow fever in East Africa is negligible for the package tourist the vaccine is usually given in line with national directives. The media can also have a positive role to play in increasing the traveller's awareness of real risks such as the recent increase in diphtheria in countries of the former Soviet Union or the risk of food- and water-borne diseases following natural disasters such as earthquakes.

These points are shown schematically in Table 11.1. They can help the advisor and traveller make decisions only after balancing these various factors. A high score makes it likely that a particular form of prophylaxis will be worthwhile and a low score makes it questionable.

The decision whether to give a particular traveller prophylaxis should be the result of an informed decision and this may also involve the patient and when appropriate parents or other family and party members or group leaders.

Principles of immunisation

Passive immunisation

Passive immunisation uses existing antibodies in human immunoglobulin, prepared from pooled human blood donations, to provide protection.

Human normal pooled immunoglobulin (HNIG) is almost entirely IgG, and can provide pre-exposure protection against diseases prevalent in the blood-donating population such as hepatitis A.

Human-specific immunoglobulin is obtained from convalescent patient sera or taken from those recently actively immunised. This is used as post-exposure treatment for rabies, tetanus and hepatitis B to prevent or modify any subsequent illness. It should always be given as soon as possible following exposure.

Occasionally HNIG, against hepatitis A, and specific hepatitis B immunoglobulin are given to those going to be a high risk when there is no time to give effective active vaccination. However, the indications for this are now few with more rapidly effective, and often single dose, active vaccines.

Passive immunity following the administration of HNIG wanes within a few months related to the half-life of the product. Thus, it should be given close to the date of travel.

Live vaccinations should ideally be given 3 weeks before or 3 months after normal human immunoglobulin, which may contain antibodies to the relevant live vaccine, preventing an optimal vaccine response. Yellow fever vaccine is an exception to this rule, because HNIG does not contain significant specific antibodies to yellow fever.

Active immunisation

Active immunisation is achieved when the immune system is challenged by immunogens to produce humoral or cellular responses. Should infection subsequently rechallenge the immune 'memory', it will provoke a rapid and specific response to that antigen.
• Active immunisation may be induced by inactivated organisms, inactivated toxins (toxoids), immunogenic components of organisms or live attenuated organisms (Table 11.2).
• Active vaccines can be absorbed onto an adjuvant such as aluminium salts to increase their immunogenicity.
• Oral vaccines can provide gut immunity through stimulating IgA in enteral secretions.
• The length of protection of active vaccination varies but is usually longer with live vaccines.

Most active vaccines induce humoral (antibody-related) immunity; however, intradermal attenuated mycobacterium, bacillus Calmette–Guérin (BCG), provides protection against *Mycobacterium tuberculosis* infection by inducing cell-mediated immunity.

Table 11.1 Scheme for helping to make risk assessments on the need for prophylaxis for a traveller.

Grade	Qualifier	Description
1 Significance to the individual traveller		
How serious could the specific infection be for the individual if infected?		
0	Minor	Rarely a severe illness
1	Moderate	Serious illness, complete recovery usual, rare death
2	Major	Severe illness, complications and death possible
3	Critical	Severe illness, serious or long-term complications common
4	Grave	Severe illness, complications and death are usual
2 Significance to the community		
How serious are the public health implications if the traveller was to be infected?		
0	Minor	Minimal or no risk to public health
1	Moderate	Potential for spread to close contacts but usually confinable
2	Major	Potential for spread within the population
3	Critical	High probability of spread within a population
4	Grave	Certainty of spread within the exposed population
3 Likelihood of exposure		
How likely is the traveller to become infected – considering destination and intended lifestyle?		
0	Very unlikely	Disease not normally present at destination
1	Unlikely	Disease present, intended lifestyle makes infection unlikely
2	Possible	Disease widespread but traveller likely to be able to avoid infection
3	Probable	Disease widespread; traveller's lifestyle makes avoiding infection difficult
4	Almost certain	Disease widespread and highly contagious
4 Evaluation of active intervention		
How effective and practical is the available prophylaxis (vaccine or tablets) also considering side effects, cost and time available for completing optimal schedule?		
0	Passable	Marginal benefits, acceptable side effects, may be difficult to deliver
1	Satisfactory	Significant benefits, possible side effects, may be difficult to deliver
2	Useful	Useful and feasible intervention with some measurable benefits and few adverse side effects
3	Effective	Useful and feasible intervention with significant measurable benefits and few or no adverse side effects
4	Ideal	Highly effective and feasible intervention with side effects very unlikely
5 Context		
Could the 'best' decision about prophylaxis be influenced by current public concerns, peer or media pressure?		
0	Indifferent	Little public interest or likely media response
1	Unsettled	Some public or media unease. Potential for repercussions if intervention fails
2	Sensitive	A publicly sensitive issue, press interest. Risk of serious repercussions if intervention fails
3	Adverse	Considerable public concern, political and emotional pressure, unhelpful and antagonistic media reports
4	Hostile	A lot of public and media interest, political involvement. Inappropriate demands may lead to inappropriate responses

Table 11.2 Current vaccines available in Britain.

	Viral	**Bacterial**
Live attenuated vaccines	Rubella Measles Mumps Yellow fever	BCG
Inactivated organisms	Inactivated polio Hepatitis A Rabies Japanese B encephalitis (only Ixiaro® licensed in the UK) Tick-borne encephalitis (not licensed in the UK)	Pertussis Typhoid Cholera
Immunogenic components of organisms	Influenza Hepatitis B	*Haemophilus influenzae* type B Pneumococcal (polysaccharide) Quadravalent meningococcal vaccine (A, C, W135 and Y) Typhim Vi (polysaccharide)
Inactivated toxoids		Tetanus Diphtheria Cholera

Following administration of a live or inactivated vaccine, there is a primary delay before appreciable levels of antibody are manufactured by the immune system. Therefore, for maximum protection, primary active immunisation courses require to be in advance of possible exposure, and in some instances quite long periods (e.g. toxoids of diphtheria and tetanus) and with rabies (see Table 11.3).

If a definite exposure occurs before these intervals have passed, extra immediate doses of vaccine may have to be considered (e.g. following a potentially rabid bite) or a dose of specific immunoglobulin (e.g. after a tetanus-prone wound or exposure to hepatitis B).

In time, most vaccine-induced antibody responses decline and may require to be boosted. These intervals can vary greatly (e.g. 3 years with typhoid and 10 years with yellow fever). Increasingly it is being recognised that real protection can be achieved for much longer than the detectable presence of antibodies because a very rapid

Table 11.3 Approximate time interval required for maximum protection after primary course of vaccination.

Vaccine	Interval required primary course for maximum protection
Poliomyelitis (parenteral)	1–2 weeks after three doses
Tetanus	1–2 weeks after three doses
Diphtheria	1–2 weeks after three doses
BCG	6 weeks after one dose
Typhoid Vi	2 weeks after one dose
Hepatitis A	2 weeks after one dose
Immunoglobulin	Immediate
Hepatitis B	1 month after three doses
Japanese B encephalitis	1–2 weeks after three doses
Rabies intramuscular	1–2 weeks after three doses
Rabies intradermal	4 weeks after three doses
Tick-borne encephalitis	2 weeks after two doses
MMR	2 weeks after one dose
Yellow fever	10 days after one dose

anamnestic response can still occur after exposure to infection.

Boosters normally give maximum protection after a few days, although this may be longer with intradermal vaccinations. If the booster dose interval has been substantially delayed, the interval may be longer.

Live vaccines

Live vaccines are usually best stored at cool temperatures (0–5°C) and are heat- and light-labile once reconstituted. Thus, provision of a 'cold chain' of refrigeration is important but may be difficult, especially in poorer and tropical developing countries.

When more than one live vaccine is required, they are best given simultaneously or at least 3 weeks apart to prevent the interferon response from the first vaccine reducing the effectiveness of subsequent vaccines.

Vaccine contraindications

Live vaccines should usually be avoided in pregnancy and also in patients who are significantly immunosuppressed from either illness or medication. Manufacturers often also advise that inactivated vaccines are best avoided in pregnancy, although there is little evidence of them causing any harm to the fetus. They can be administered if the risk of infection is substantial. Febrile reactions can sometimes precipitate a miscarriage.

During an acute febrile illness, vaccination should be postponed, as it will be difficult to recognise a vaccine 'reaction'. Mild afebrile or non-systemic illnesses are not normally contraindications.

If there has been a severe local or systemic reaction such as anaphylaxis, to a previous dose of vaccine then further doses of that vaccine must be avoided.

Some vaccines contain traces of egg proteins or antibiotics and should be avoided in those who have serious allergy to these components.

As vaccines may induce severe allergic reactions, all vaccination centres should have facilities for dealing with anaphylaxis. Vaccinated patients should ideally be observed in the vaccination centre for 30 minutes. Vasovagal reactions are much more common and these can be quite alarming, sometimes with anoxic convulsions. A previous history of faints should alert the advisor to this possibility.

Vaccines used for preventing infection in travellers

Table 11.2 provides a list of all vaccines currently provided in the UK.

Malaria prevention and treatment

Forty per cent of the world's population is at risk of malaria and 90% of cases occur in sub-Saharan Africa. It causes an estimated 300 million clinical infections and more than 1 million deaths annually. Children and non-immune adults are at most risk of severe infection and death. In the United Kingdom, non-immune travellers to malarious areas are at great risk unless the appropriate precautions are taken and there are about 2000 cases of imported malaria each year with approximately 10 deaths.

Malaria is caused by the *Plasmodium* genus of protozoans. Four species cause disease in man:

1 *Plasmodium falciparum* is the most serious and potentially life-threatening form of malaria.

2 *P. malariae* causes quartan malaria as it may produce fever every third day. Infection is occasionally complicated by a glomerulonephritis. Relapse has been recorded in patients up to 40 years after leaving the tropics.

3 *P. vivax* and *P. ovale* are known as tertian malaria as they may give fever on alternate days after the disease has become established. These species of malaria have a hypnozoite stage, where the parasite has the ability to lie dormant in the liver for months before reactivating.

P. malariae, *P. vivax* and *P. ovale* are rarely life-threatening and are referred to as benign malaria. Co-infection with different parasites may occur.

Life cycle

Parasites are introduced into humans via the bite of the female anophiline mosquito. After an infected bite sporozoites invade hepatocytes where they undergo pre-erythrocytic shizogeny. At this stage *P. vivax* and *P. ovale* may become dormant, producing hypnozoites. Hepatocyte rupture leads to merozoite release into the circulation with subsequent erythrocyte invasion where they undergo further development into schizonts (erythrocytic shizogeny) or gametocytes, which are the sexual form. Gametocytes are taken up by the mosquito during a blood meal and further sexual reproduction of the parasites takes place in the mosquito gut. Clinical signs of malaria occur at the time of red cell invasion and rupture. In the case of *P. falciparum* sequestration in the venules of the deep organs (particularly the CNS, liver, kidneys and lungs) accounts for many of the severe features of the infection. The pathophysiology of severe malaria is complex and is dependent on a number of factors including the parasite, its interaction with endothelium and the host immunological response to the infection.

The cardinal symptom of malaria is fever often with rigors, followed by profuse sweating, headache and myalgia. Falciparum malaria may result in severe anaemia, jaundice and cerebral malaria which is manifested by confusion, coma, seizures and death if untreated. Other complications of severe malaria are renal failure and respiratory failure due to adult respiratory distress syndrome.

Disease risk areas: Malaria is endemic in the tropics and subtropics below altitudes of 2000 m (see Fig. 11.1). Optimal conditions for the vector are an ambient temperature of 16–33°C. The most serious risk areas for *P. falciparum* malaria are sub-Saharan Africa, South-east Asia (including rural Thailand, Laos, Cambodia, Burma and Vietnam) and Amazonia in South America.

Chemoprophylaxis against malaria

Malaria prevention through chemoprophylaxis is not absolute. Avoidance of mosquito bites is fundamental in preventing malaria. Therefore, long sleeves and trousers should be worn, especially after sunset when the female mosquito is most active. The importance of insect repellents and mosquito nets impregnated with an insecticide should be emphasised.

The choice of antimalarial is decided by the likelihood of exposure, the prevalent species and local resistance patterns of the parasite. Chemoprophylaxis is primarily directed against *P. falciparum* in which resistance to chloroquine is now widespread.

Prophylaxis should be commenced 1 week before travel (3 weeks for mefloquine and 1 or 2 days for malarone) to ensure adequate blood levels and to detect those likely to get side effects, during the whole time of exposure and for 4 weeks after visiting a malaria area to cover the 'incubation' phase of malignant malaria. As malarone has activity against the erythrocytic and pre-erythrocytic stages of the parasite, it can be stopped 1 week after return from travel.

Despite adequate precautions, malaria infection remains possible; thus any febrile illness should be promptly investigated and treated, sometimes empirically, within 1 year of return from a malarious area. Commonly used prophylactic agents are shown in Table 11.4.

Drug resistance

Drug resistance in *P. falciparum* occurs directly as a consequence of antimalarial drugs causing resistance in parasites. Resistance leads to delayed response to treatment of clinical infections, early recrudescence and increased transmission. This increases the parasite reservoir and leads to an increase in infections and greater use of antimalarials. Malarial prophylaxis recommendations alter as a result of changing patterns of resistance. Currently, chloroquine resistance in *P. falciparum* is widespread in Africa, Asia and much of South America. Mefloquine resistance is now well established in South-east Asia. Fansidar resistance in Africa and South-east Asia is also well established. The artemsinin derivatives (e.g. artemether) are now widely used in the treatment of severe malaria

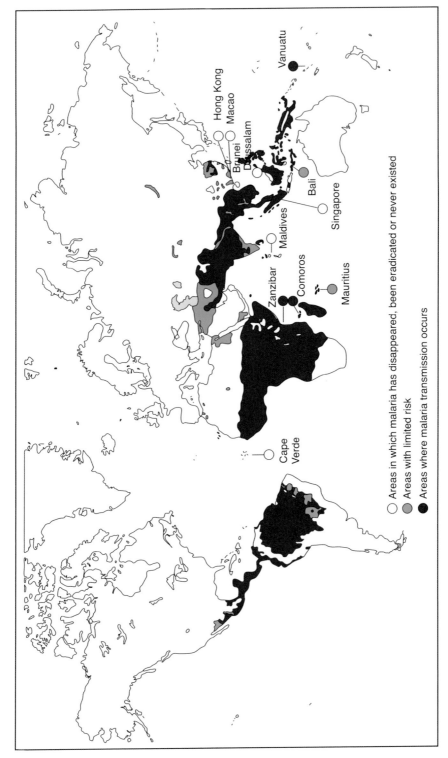

Figure 11.1 Areas requiring malaria prevention. The map has been kindly provided by *International Travel and Health* (1999, WHO, Geneva).

Table 11.4 Antimalarial drugs.

Drug	Mechanism of action	Use			Adverse effects/cautions
		Treatment	**Prophylaxis**		
Chloroquine	Inhibits erythrocytic phase of plasmodial development	Non-falciparum malaria	In combination with proguanil in some areas of the world		GI upset, rash, headaches avoid in epilepsy. Caution in renal/hepatic dysfunction. Arrhythmia, seizure, visual loss in over dose
Proguanil	Inhibits dihydrofolate reductase, preventing plasmodial tissue development	Uncomplicated falciparum combined with atovaquone (see malorone)	In combination with chloroquine or atovaquone (malorone)		GI upset, apthous ulcers Caution in severe renal failure. Folate supplements in pregnancy
Mefloquine	Unknown; quinine derivative. Destroys asexual parasites (trophozoites)	Uncomplicated falciparum in combination with artesunate derivative; effective against other species but chloroquine preferred	Yes, but resistance in SE Asia and increasing in Africa		GI upset, dizziness, erythema multiforme, cardiac conduction defects Neuropsychiatric disturbances. Contraindicated in renal and severe hepatic impairment, history of psychiatric illness, epilepsy, cardiac conduction defects, lactation and pregnancy. Avoid co-administration with other agents that may prolong the QT interval
Doxycycline	Inhibits protein synthesis	In combination with quinine in *P. falciparum*	Chloroquine/mefloquine resistance or when contra-indicated		GI upset, photosensitivity, interactions with warfarin Contraindicated in pregnancy, lactation and in children under 12 years of age
Atovaquone with proguanil (Malarone)	Interferes with pyrimidine biosynthesis. Acts on pre-erythrocytic stage of development	Initial treatment of uncomplicated falciparum malaria	Start 1–2 days prior to travel and can be stopped one week following return.		Nausea, mouth ulceration, hyponatraemia Contraindicated in pregnancy and lactation

(Continued)

Table 11.4 (*Continued*)

Drug	Mechanism of action	Treatment	Use Prophylaxis	Adverse effects/cautions
Pyrimethamine/ dapsone (Maloprim)	Dapsone is a sulphone with antifolate activity	No	No longer used as prophylaxis as more efficacious alternatives available	Haemolytic anaemia, bone marrow suppression, haemolysis in those with G6PD deficiency
Pyrimethamine/ sulphadoxine (Fansidar)	Pyrimethamine inhibits Plasmodium folate metabolism; sulphadoxine also interferes with microbial folate synthesis	Yes; adjunctive therapy of *P. falciparum* malaria that has some quinine resistance	No	Severe drug rash including Stevens–Johnson syndrome, but very rare when given as single dose
Primaquine	Inhibits plasmodium mitochondrial transport	Used to eradicate liver forms of *P. ovale* and *P. vivax*	No	Nausea, vomiting, methaemoglobinaemia and haemolytic anaemia. Contraindicated in G6PD deficiency, pregnancy and lactation
Quinine	Cidal vs. all four asexual parasite species. Mode of action not understood	Treatment of *P. falciparum* in combination with doxycline or with a single dose of Fansidar	No	Ventricular arrhythmias (avoid with other agents that prolong QT interval), hypoglycaemia, blurring of vision, tinnitus, deafness and rarely haemolysis
Artemesinin derivatives (artemether, artemesinin, artesunate)	Rapidly cidal vs. young trophozoites	Use oral forms alone or in combination with mefloquine or lumefantrine (Riamet) in uncomplicated falciparum. i.m. or i.v. forms used in severe falciparum	No	Well tolerated; serious adverse effects rare Neurotoxicity in animals not demonstrated in man Lumefantrine may cause arrhythmias

Table 11.5 Selected parasitic infections of medical importance.

Parasite	Disease	Antimicrobial therapy	Alternative (Alt) or Adjunct (Adj) therapy
Protozoa			
Entamoeba histolytica	Amoebic colitis and liver abscess	Metronidazole	Diloxanide fumarate (Adj)
Giardia lamblia	Giardiasis	Metronidazole	Tinidazole (Alt)
Leishmania sp.	Visceral leishmaniasis and New world cutaneous leishmanisis	Sodium Stibogluconate	Amphotericin B (Alt), Miltefosine (Alt)
Trypanosome sp.	African Trypanosomiasis		
	Early	Suramin (rhodesiense)	Pentamidine (gambiense)
	Late	Melarsoprol	Eflornithine (Alt)
	South American T. (Chaga's)	Nifurtimox	Benzidazole (Alt)
Helminths			
(i) Nematodes			
Strongyloides	Strongyloidiasis	Albendazole	
Ancylostoma caninum and *Necator americanis*	Cutaneous larva migrans	Mebendezole	Albendazole (Alt)
Ascaris lumbricoides Wuchereria bancrofti,	Ascariasis	Mebendazole	
Brugia malayi	Lymphatic filariasis	Diethylcarbamazine (DEC)	Albendazole (Alt), Ivermectin (Adj)
Onchocerca volvulus	River blindness, skin nodules	Ivermectin	Doxycycline (Adj)
(ii) Trematodes			
Schistosome sp.	Schistosomiasis	Praziquantil	Artemesinin (Alt)
(iii) Cestodes			
Taenia solium (pork tape worm)	Neurocystercicosis	Albendazole	Praziquantel (Alt) Steroids (Adj)
Echinococcus granulosus (canine tape worm)	Hydatid disease	Albendazole	Surgical excision

and in combination in non-severe *P. falciparum* in South-east Asia particularly. They are not advised for use in prophylaxis. Resistance to these compounds has been described. When deciding on suitable prophylaxis for travellers, up-to-date advice should always be sought from specialist centres or continually updated on-line databases such as TRAVAX (described above) or recently published guidelines such as those produced by the Health Protection Agency's advisory committee on malaria prevention.

Treatment of malaria

Malaria treatment should be considered in the context of the infecting species, the severity of the infection and the healthcare setting in which the patient is being managed. The emergence of drug resistance impacts on treatment options as well as on prophylaxis. The benign forms of malaria (*P. vivax*, *P. ovale* and *P. malariae*) can be treated with short-course chloroquine. *P. vivax* and *P. ovale* require an additional 2-week course of primaquine (assuming G6PD status is normal and patient is not pregnant) to eradicate hypnozoites from the hepatocytes.

Non-severe *P. falciparum* can be treated with either oral quinine plus doxycycline, atovaquone/proguanil (malarone), mefloquine or artesunate (an artemesinin derivative). In patients with partial immunity in endemic areas pyrimethamine/sulphadoxine (Fansidar) is still frequently used. There is increasing interest in combination therapy with artesunate and mefloquine. This strategy appears to rapidly destroy the parasites and may reduce the risk of resistance emerging. Co-formulated artemether and lumefantrine (Riamet) is available in the United Kingdom for the treatment of uncomplicated falciparum malaria.

Severe *P. falciparum* malaria should be treated with intravenous quinine. A loading dose of 20 mg/kg (maximum 1400 mg) should be given unless the patient has previously received mefloquine. Subsequent dosing is 10 mg/kg 8-hourly. Doxycycline should also be given in case of quinine resistance. An alternative to quinine is intramuscular artemether or intravenous artemisinin. These agents are derived from sweet wormwood, a ubiquitous weed, used for centuries in China in the treatment of fever. The artemsinin derivatives are associated with a more rapid drop in parasitaemia than quinine and have no recognisable serious adverse effects in comparison. Neurotoxicity found in animals following high dosing has not been observed in clinical trials in man. Recent studies have demonstrated an improved survival in severe malaria with intravenous artesunate when compared to quinine. The artemisinin derivatives are also useful in quinine resistance or intolerance. Drug therapy of *P. falciparum* malaria is usually 7 days. Drugs used in the treatment of malaria are outlined in Table 11.4.

Severe malaria is a multi-system disorder and close attention should be paid to adjunctive measures, including intravenous rehydration, blood transfusion and correction of hypoglycaemia and acidosis. Co-existent bacterial sepsis should also be sought and managed with parenteral antibiotic therapy.

Treatment of other common imported parasitic infections

There are a great variety of other parasitic infections (protozoal and helminthic) which may affect any organ system. The most common or serious parasitic infections in the returning traveller include (by system) gastrointestinal (giardiasis, amoebiasis, schistosomiasis, strongyloidiasis and ascariasis), genitourinary (schistosomiasis), cutaneous (cutanous larva migrans, onchocerciasis, leishmaniasis), lymphatic (filariasis), multisystem (malaria, leishmaniasis) and neurological (cystercicosis, trypanosomiasis). An overview of treatment of the more common or important infections is given in Table 11.5.

Chapter 12

Drugs and endocrine disease

Diabetes mellitus

Clinical scenario

A 55-year-old man presents with symptoms of thirst nocturia (2–3 times nightly) and polyuria. His blood sugar is 17 mmol/L and HbA1c 11% (97 mmol/mol). Body mass index is 36 kg/m². There is a family history of a paternal grandfather with type 2 diabetes. He has no other medical history of note. He is diagnosed with diabetes. No complications of diabetes are observed. He is given lifestyle and started on metformin increased to a dose of 500 mg tds. At 6 months HbA1c is 8.0% (64 mmol/mol) and BMI 35 kg/m². Does he require further pharmacological intervention?

If so, what would be the best next agent in the management of his diabetes and obesity?

Introduction

Pathophysiology

Diabetes mellitus is a group of metabolic disorders characterised by hyperglycaemia. This can be due to abnormalities of insulin secretion, insulin action or both. Diabetes mellitus causes increased morbidity and premature mortality. Sustained hyperglycaemia is associated with both microvascular complications (retinopathy, nephropathy and neuropathy) and macrovascular complications especially coronary heart disease, stroke and peripheral vascular disease.

Type 1 diabetes mellitus (previously known as insulin-dependent diabetes mellitus or juvenile onset diabetes mellitus) accounts for approximately 5% of cases. It usually presents in childhood or adolescence but can occur at any age. The majority of cases arise through a cellular-mediated autoimmune destruction of pancreatic β-cells. The resulting insulinopenia results in hyperglycaemia and ketoacidosis. Patients depend on exogenous insulin for survival.

Type 2 diabetes mellitus (previously referred to as non-insulin-dependent diabetes mellitus or maturity onset diabetes) accounts for approximately 95% of cases. It usually presents in later adult life, most cases are obese and there is a strong genetic predisposition. Weight loss improves the metabolic abnormalities but the disease is progressive and patients usually need to be treated with a combination of one or more oral hypoglycaemic agent, and ultimately insulin treatment may become necessary.

Diabetes may also occur secondary to other pancreatic diseases (for example pancreatitis) and secondary to a range of other endocrine conditions including acromegaly and Cushing's syndrome. Autosmal dominant forms of diabetes (Maturity Onset Diabetes of the Young) are also increasingly

Lecture Notes: Clinical Pharmacology and Therapeutics, 8th edition. By Gerard McKay, John Reid and Matthew Walters. Published 2010 by Blackwell Publishing Ltd.

recognised and may account for up to 1% of cases while other genetic conditions notably haemocromatosis may also be associated with diabetes.

Aims of treatment

The aims of treatment are the relief of the symptoms of hyperglycaemia and the prevention of diabetic complications. Strict glycaemic control in both type 1 and type 2 diabetes mellitus has been shown to reduce the onset and progression of diabetic complications in the Diabetes Control and Complications Trial and UK Prospective Diabetes Study. Glycaemic control is monitored by measuring glycated haemoglobin levels (usually HbA_{1c}). A target HbA_{1c} level of less than 7% (53 mmol/mol) is usually set but this should be adjusted to individual patient circumstances and may be different for example in pregnancy, in the elderly and if frequent hypoglycaemia or hypoglycaemia unawareness is present.

There is also good evidence supporting aggressive treatment of hypertension. Angiotensin-converting enzyme (ACE) inhibitors or angiotensin receptor antagonists should be considered as first-line treatment, especially in those with microalbuminuria or proteinuria. Other aspects for consideration in the management of diabetes are summarised in Table 12.1.

Non-pharmacological therapy

In type 2 diabetes mellitus, weight loss, nutrition and exercise should be used as first-line management. In type 1 diabetes, nutrition and exercise should be used as an adjunct to insulin therapy.

Table 12.1 Aspects for consideration in the management of diabetes.

Glycaemic control optimisation
Blood pressure management
Weight loss/treatment of obesity
Smoking cessation
Treatment of hyperlipidaemia
Anti-platelet agents

Table 12.2 Drug treatment of diabetes mellitus.

Class of diabetes	Drug
Type 2	Oral hypoglycaemic agents
	Biguanides
	Sulphonylureas
	Meglitinide analogues
	Thiozolidinediones
	Glucosidase inhibitors
	Glucagon like peptide 1 agonists
	Dipeptidyl peptidase 4 inhibitors
Type 1 and type 2	Insulin

Drug treatments in diabetes mellitus

Pharmacological therapies used in the treatment of diabetes mellitus are shown in Table 12.2.

Insulin

Mechanism

Insulin is a peptide hormone. Endogenous insulin is synthesised in the pancreatic β-cells and secreted into the portal circulation. The main actions of insulin are shown in Table 12.3.

Pharmacokinetics and insulin preparations

Insulin is destroyed in the gastrointestinal tract and must be given parenterally. Once absorbed it is inactivated enzymically in the liver and kidney and has a half-life of approximately 9 minutes. Therapeutic insulin (subcutaneous or intravenous) is delivered into the systemic circulation, resulting

Table 12.3 Main actions of insulin.

1 Glucose transport into muscle and fat cells
2 Increased glycogen synthesis
3 Inhibition of gluconeogenesis
4 Inhibition of lipolysis and increased formation of triglycerides
5 Stimulation of membrane-bound energy-dependent ion transporters (e.g. sodium/potassium ATPase)
6 Stimulation of cell growth

Table 12.4 Insulin formulations.

Type of insulin	Examples	Peak activity (hour)	Duration of action (hour)
Rapid-acting analogue	Insulin lispro (Humalog) Insulin aspart (Novorapid) Insulin glulisine (Apidra)	0.5–1.5	3–5
Short acting (soluble)	Human Actrapid Humulin S	1–3	4–8
Intermediate acting (isophane)	Human Insulatard Humulin I	4–8	12–18
Long acting Long-acting analogue	Human Ultratard Insulin glargine Insulin detemir	6–16 Smooth profile	24–30 18–26
Mixed short/rapid with intermediate acting	A variety of combinations using insulin lispro, aspart and human sequence insulin now available	Biphasic profile	12–18

in an unphysiological situation with high insulin levels in both the systemic and the portal circulation, rather than in the portal circulation alone.

Therapeutic insulin is usually human insulin synthesised using recombinant DNA technology or genetically engineered insulin analogues in which the human amino acid sequence is altered to modify its properties. Animal insulin extracted from bovine or porcine pancreas is still available but is rarely used.

Subcutaneous injection of insulin slows its rate of delivery to the circulation, and different insulin formulations are available with varying onset and duration of action. Insulin is usually broadly classified into five categories based on these properties: rapid, short, intermediate, long and mixed (Table 12.4). Precipitating insulin with protamine (a basic protein), zinc or both slows absorption by the formation of amorphous solid or relatively insoluble crystals. In the rapid-acting insulin analogues, insulin lispro and aspart, one or two amino acid substitutions reduce the tendency of the molecules to form dimers and hexamers and speed absorption from the subcutaneous tissue.

Two long-acting soluble insulin analogues have become available. The first, insulin glargine, has an altered isoelectric point, which causes insulin to precipitate on injection into the subcutaneous tissue. This forms a depot from which insulin is slowly released. In the second, insulin detemir, the addition of a fatty acyl chain promotes the formation of insulin hexamers and its binding to albumin prolongs the duration of action.

Dose and regimes

In the United Kingdom, all insulin preparations are available in a uniform strength of 100 units/mL. The dose and insulin regime should be tailored to the individual. It can be monitored and adjusted by the patient, if educated, on a daily basis according to capillary blood glucose levels.

An ideal regimen would mimic physiological insulin secretion, with low, basal level between meals and increased secretion at meal times. Regimens in common use include injection of a short- or rapid-acting insulin with meals and a longer acting insulin once or twice daily (basal-bolus regime); alternatively, a twice daily injection of an intermediate acting or a mixed insulin might be appropriate.

Insulin delivery can be via needle and syringe, using pen injector devices or, in selected patients, by continuous subcutaneous infusion.

Adverse effects

1 Hypoglycaemia is a common side effect. It is usually a result of decreased carbohydrate intake, unaccustomed exercise, administration of too much insulin or ingestion of alcohol. Symptoms and signs are those of adrenergic activation (sweating, tachycardia, systolic hypertension and hunger) and of neuroglycopaenia (visual disturbance, drowsiness, seizures and coma). The patient is usually alerted by the adrenergic symptoms and can take corrective action before neuroglycopaenic symptoms ensue.

2 Weight gain is commonly seen on insulin initiation. This is a particular problem in patients with type 2 diabetes mellitus in whom weight loss is recommended. It is thought to be due to reduced urine glucose loss and the general anabolic effects of insulin.

3 Local effects of subcutaneous insulin injection are hypertrophy of fat (lipohypertrophy) or loss of fat (lipoatrophy). Injection into areas of lipohypertrophy increases the variability of insulin absorption. Lipoatrophy is uncommon since the advent of human or highly purified animal insulins.

4 Antibodies may develop to insulin, resulting in prolongation or attenuation of the action of insulin. They are not usually seen with human insulin.

Oral hypoglycaemic agents

Biguanides

Mechanism

Biguanides have many metabolic effects, including reduced hepatic glucose production (gluconeogenesis) and increased glucose uptake and oxidation by skeletal muscle. They reduce insulin resistance. The mechanism of action is not completely understood but recent evidence shows that metformin activates AMP-activated protein kinase (AMP kinase) a key regulator of cellular lipid and glucose metabolism.

Pharmacokinetics

Metformin is rapidly absorbed and has a half-life of 2–5 hours. It is excreted unchanged by the kidney.

Clinical use and dose

Metformin is considered the drug of first choice in overweight or obese patients with type 2 diabetes. It is also used extensively as first-line monotherapy in patients of normal weight. The dose should be titrated up from a starting dose of 500 mg daily to a maximum dose of 3000 mg/day in divided doses although in most cases 2000–2500 mg/day are used and evidence of increased efficacy at higher doses limited. Metformin does not lead to weight gain or hypoglycaemia. Metformin can be used in combination with all other classes of oral hypoglycaemic agents and with insulin.

Adverse effects

The most frequent adverse effects are abdominal discomfort and gastrointestinal upset (e.g. nausea, diarrhoea, anorexia). It is dose related and can be minimised by gradual dose titration. Lactic acidosis is the most serious adverse event. It is rare but carries a high mortality, and metformin should not be given to patients with renal, hepatic, hypoxic respiratory or cardiac disease, or who are shocked. Metformin should be withdrawn before use of iodine containing X-ray contrast media. The use of metformin in patients with stable cardiac failure is currently under review with some evidence of benefits in this group.

Sulphonylureas

Mechanism

Sulphonylureas stimulate insulin secretion by a direct effect on pancreatic β-cells. They bind to sulphonylurea receptors on these cells, resulting in release of insulin granules. Functioning pancreatic tissue is therefore necessary for their action.

Pharmacokinetics

All sulphonylureas are well absorbed and reach peak plasma concentrations within 2–4 hours. Their duration of action is variable (Table 12.5). The main one used in clinical practice is gliclazide All are metabolised by the liver but routes of

Table 12.5 Sulphonylureas – pharmacokinetic properties of selected few.

Drug	Daily dose (mg)	Duration of action (half-life) in hours	Metabolites
Gliclazide	40–320	up to 24 (12)	Inactive
Glipizide	2.5–20.0	6–12 (3)	Inactive
Glimepiride	1–6	up to 24 (9)	Active

elimination differ. All bind strongly to albumin and can interact with other highly protein-bound drugs (e.g. warfarin, sulphonamides).

Clinical use and dose
Sulphonylureas are used as first-line agents in patients who are not overweight, or in patients who have contraindications or intolerance to other agents. Patients should start at a low dose, which should be gradually titrated up. A sulphonylurea with a shorter duration of action and without active metabolites (e.g. glipizide or tolbutamine) should be used in the elderly or those with renal or hepatic impairment to reduce risk of hypoglycaemia. Sulphonylureas can be combined with metformin, acarbose, thiazolidinediones or insulin to optimise glycaemic control.

Adverse effects
All sulphonylureas can cause hypoglycaemia which can be severe and prolonged. It is more likely with the long-acting agents and chlorpropamide is no longer recommended for this reason. Sulphonylurea therapy is also associated with weight gain. Other adverse effects include allergic reactions (mainly rashes), gastrointestinal symptoms and, rarely, bone marrow suppression or cholestatic jaundice.

Glucosidase inhibitors (acarbose)

Inhibition of α-glucosidase activity in the gastrointestinal tract reduces breakdown of more complex sugars to glucose. This reduces post-prandial hyperglycaemia. Acarbose can be given as monotherapy or in combination with other oral hypoglycaemic agents or insulin. Unfortunately, failure to adequately digest carbohydrate results in bacterial fermentation within the gut, resulting in excessive flatus production, and many patients do not tolerate the treatment. The α-glucosidase inhibitors do not cause weight gain and are unlikely to cause hypoglycaemia.

Meglitinide analogues (repaglinide and nateglinide)

Mechanism
The meglitinides are rapid-acting insulin secretagogues. Like sulphonylureas they act at the sulphonylurea receptor of pancreatic β-cells but they bind at a different site.

Pharmacokinetics
They are rapidly absorbed and eliminated, peak plasma concentrations are reached within 1 hour and the half-life is approximately 3 hours.

Clinical use and dose
The meglitinides should be given 30 minutes before meals and started at a low dose. The indications and adverse event profile are similar to the sulphonylureas. They have a lower risk of hypoglycaemia and potentially cause less weight gain. They may suit individuals with an irregular lifestyle (e.g. shift workers).

Thiazolidinediones (glitazones)

Mechanism
Two thiazolidinediones, rosiglitazone and pioglitazone, are currently marketed. Troglitazone was withdrawn following reports of idiosyncratic hepatotoxicity. They are insulin-sensitising drugs. They activate nuclear receptors (peroxisome proliferator-activated receptor-γ or PPARγ) that increase the transcription of insulin-sensitive genes.

Drug	Half-life parent drug (hour)	Half-life metabolite (hour)	Elimination
Rosiglitazone	3.5	100–150	Mainly urine
Pioglitazone	3–7	16–24	Mainly bile

Table 12.6 Thiazolidinediones – pharmacokinetic properties.

PPARγ is predominantly expressed in adipose tissue and also in skeletal muscle and liver. The effect of thiazolidinediones on glucose lowering is slow and maximal effect may be achieved only after 2–3 months.

Pharmacokinetics
Both rosiglitazone and pioglitazone are rapidly and almost completely absorbed (Table 12.6). They are highly protein bound but their concentrations are generally low. Both agents undergo extensive hepatic metabolism. Rosiglitazone is excreted mainly in urine and pioglitazone mainly in bile. No significant drug interactions have been reported.

Clinical use and dose
Rosiglitazone has a starting dose of 4 mg/day (maximum 8 mg/day) and pioglitazone 15–30 mg/day (maximum 45 mg/day). The dose should be titrated gradually. They can be used as monotherapy or in combination with metformin or a sulphonylurea. In the United Kingdom, combination with insulin therapy is contraindicated due to concerns about fluid retention; however, this combination is being widely used in the United States.

Adverse effects
The commonest adverse effects are weight gain, fluid retention, increased plasma volume and a reduced haematocrit. Contraindications are heart failure and hepatic impairment. Precautionary monitoring of liver function is currently recommended, although to date the hepatotoxicity seen with troglitazone has not been observed. There is controversy over the cardiovascular safety of rosiglitazone, while data are conflicting it is recommended that rosiglitazone is not used in pa-

tients with acute coronary syndrome. Recent data suggests that thiazolidinediones may be associated with reduction in bone mineral density and both of the thiazolidonediones have been associated with an increase in predominantly distal fractures. The absolute increase in fracture risk appears to be small and overall significance of these findings remain under review.

Glucagon like peptide 1 agonists (exenatide)
Mechanism
Glucagon like peptide 1 (GLP-1) is secreted by L cells of the small intestine in response to food ingestion. Along with glucose dependent insulinotropic polypeptide (GIP) it is believed to be responsible for the incretin effect: the increased secretion of insulin in response to oral as opposed to intravenous administration of glucose. GLP-1 is rapidly broken down by the enzyme dipeptidyl peptidase 4 (DPP-4) limiting therapeutic use of the native molecule. Exenatide is a synthetic GLP-1 agonist based on exendin-4 -a component of Gila monster venom. Exenatide is resistant to degradation by DPP-4 and acts to promote glucose-dependent insulin secretion by direct action on the pancreatic beta cell. A number of longer acting GLP-1 analogues may become clinically available in the near future.

Pharmacokinetics
Exenatide is given by subcutaneous injection and has a half life of 2.4 hours. It is given by twice daily subcutaneous injection.

Clinical use and dose
Exenatide is started at 5 mcg twice daily and increasing to 10 mcg twice daily. As monotherapy it is associated with a reduction HbA1c of around 0.6%. Importantly exenatide is also associated

with significant reduction in weight (1.6–2.8 kg at 30 weeks of treatment) with some evidence that weight loss continues with longer term use. For this reason exenatide may find a clinical role in patients failing to control body weight on current therapy. In 2008 NICE suggested that exenatide might be considered where BMI was >35 kg/m^2 and additional glucose lowering therapy was required. The most significant side effect of exenatide is nausea which may be found in up to 40–50% of those on exenatide, declines with time and appears more common in combination with metformin. Pancreatitis is reported as a rare association with exenatide and it remains unclear as yet whether this is a causative association.

Dipeptidyl peptidase 4 inhibitors (sitagliptin, vildagliptin)

Mechanism

DPP-4 inhibitors act to increase naturally occurring levels of the incretin hormone Glucagon like peptide 1 (GLP-1 see above) and thus increase postprandial insulin secretion and decrease glucogon secretion. The class includes both sitigliptin and vildagliptin although several others are expected to become available in the future.

Pharmacokinetics

Clinical use and dose. Sitagliptin is given as a single tablet of 100 mg once daily and vildagliptin 50 mg once or twice daily. At present these agents are approved for use in addition to other oral agents (metformin, thiazolidinediones or sulphonylureas). Side effects include nausea, peripheral oedema, headaches and rarely nasopharyngitis. DPP-4 inhibitors are weight neutral, offering no additional weight loss unlike the GLP1 agonists. HbA1c is reduced by 0.6–0.9% (~7–10 mmol/mol). DPP-4 inhibitors appear to be associated with lower rates of hypoglycaemic compared to sulphonylureas and are used clinically in combination with others agents such as metformin where avoidance of hypoglycaemia is a primary therapeutic aim. Hypoglycaemia may still occur, however, commonly when used in combination with sulphonylureas where a lower dose is recommended.

Diabetic emergencies in adults

Clinical scenario

A 23-year-old is admitted with a 2 day history of vomiting. He has become more unwell and becomes unconscious. His family report that he has been unwell for some weeks with weight loss, lethargy and complaining of thirst and polyuria. He has a raised blood glucose, a metabolic acidosis and ketones in his urine. What is the diagnosis and how should this patient be managed?

Ketoacidosis

Causes

Infections are the most common identifiable cause. Myocardial infarction, trauma and inadequate insulin dosage are other causes.

Clinical features

Typically these patients are dehydrated, hyperventilating and may have impaired consciousness. Blood glucose is usually markedly elevated, ketones are present (measured in the urine or blood) and there is acidosis. Venous bicarbonate measurement is used to assess severity. Total body potassium stores are always depleted largely due to the osmotic diuresis. However, the plasma potassium is usually high normal or slightly elevated because insulin deficiency prevents entry of potassium into cells and there is extracellular potassium shift in response to the acidosis.

Treatment

This is based on replacement of fluid, electrolytes and insulin.

1 Fluid replacement. The free water deficit averages 5–7 L in diabetic ketoacidosis (DKA). Isotonic saline should be used in most cases. A suggested regime over the first hours of treatment is shown below.

1000 mL isotonic saline in 30 minutes

1000 mL isotonic saline in 1 hour (with added potassium, see Table 12.7)

1000 mL isotonic saline in 2 hour (with added potassium, see Table 12.7)

Subsequent fluid should be tailored to the patient, e.g. 1000 mL isotonic saline 4- to 8-hourly

Table 12.7 Suggested potassium regimen in patients with diabetic ketoacidosis.

Plasma potassium (mmol/L)	Potassium added (mmol/L)
>5.5	None
3.5–5.5	20
<3.5	40

until the fluid deficit is corrected. Use a central venous pressure line in the elderly or those with cardiac disease. If serum sodium rises above 150 mmol/L (mEq/L), use half normal saline instead.

2 Insulin. In DKA, insulin is given intravenously and the infusion rate adjusted according to blood glucose. A typical starting rate is 5–6 units/hour. An initial dose of 10 units of soluble insulin can be given intramuscularly if there is a delay in initiating intravenous treatment.

When blood glucose is <15 mmol/L (270 mg/100 mL), change the infusion fluid to 5% glucose with potassium replacement and continue the insulin infusion.

3 Potassium replacement. The total body potassium deficit ranges from 3 to 12 mmol/kg (mEq/kg). With insulin and fluid replacement, serum potassium concentrations fall and early potassium replacement is vital. Replacement should begin with the second and subsequent bags of fluid, adjusting as shown in Table 12.7.

The use of sodium bicarbonate in treating acidosis in DKA is controversial. It has been associated with serious fluid disequilibrium and development of cerebral oedema. The use of bicarbonate is therefore not routinely recommended. The majority of cases respond to the treatments above and bicarbonate should be considered only in patients who remain hypotensive and have severe acidosis (pH <6.9).

Key points

• Patients require frequent observations and glucose and electrolyte monitoring. Remember that there is often an underlying cause.

• If you suspect infection, treat with antibiotics after relevant culture specimens have been obtained.

Hyperosmolar, non-ketotic hyperglycaemic coma

Cause
It usually occurs in patients older than 60 years and may be the first presentation of type 2 diabetes mellitus. The cause is obscure.

Features
The patient is often drowsy and is dehydrated. Typical laboratory findings are very high blood glucose, raised urea, raised sodium and a high plasma osmolality.

Treatment
Isotonic saline is given, or half normal if plasma sodium is >150 mmol (mEq)/L. Fluid replacement is otherwise similar to DKA, and a central venous pressure line may be required. Intravenous insulin is given; insulin sensitivity is greater in these patients due to lack of severe acidosis. Patients are at risk of thrombosis, and unless contraindicated, full anticoagulation with heparin should be given.

Hypoglycaemic coma

Causes
Coma is usually precipitated by missing a meal, unaccustomed exercise or taking too much insulin or sulphonylurea.

Clinical features
Coma can present with a wide range of neurological signs. Every medical emergency arriving with mental impairment, coma or other neurological signs must have capillary glucose checked on arrival.

Treatment
Intravenous glucose should be used, i.e. 50 mL of a 20% solution. The dose may need to be repeated. This is irritant and should only be given into a large vein and through a large gauge needle. Higher osmolarity solutions such as 50% dextrose

are very irritant and should be avoided if possible. Alternatively, 1-mg glucagon is given intravenously or intramuscularly, which is useful if the patient is difficult to restrain. Glucagon may be given to patients for administration by relatives as emergency treatment for hypoglycaemia.

Thyroid disease

Thyrotoxicosis (hyperthyroidism)

Clinical scenario

A 28-year-old woman presents with heat intolerance, sweats palpitations and 3 kg weight loss. She has a strong family history of thyroid disease with mother, maternal grandmother having had thyrotoxicosis and a maternal aunt with hypothyroidism. On examination she is tachycardic (120 bpm) has a large goitre with bruit and no signs of dysthyroid eye disease. Thyroid function tests reveal raised total T3 = 4 nmol/L (0.8–2.5 nmol/l), free thyroxine (FT4) = 35 pmol/L (9–21 pmol/L) and suppressed thyroid stimulating hormone <0.04 mU/L (TSH 0.35–5 mU/L). She has two small children at home aged 2 and 4 years. What is the likely diagnosis? What would be the best form of initial management?

Pathophysiology

Thyrotoxicosis results from the actions of excess thyroid hormone on target tissue. Typical features are caused by stimulation of metabolism and effects on catecholamines. They include weight loss with increased appetite and heat intolerance, palpitations, tremor, nervousness. It is more common in females.

Hyperfunction of the thyroid gland can be caused by
1 Graves' disease
2 Toxic multi-nodular goitre
3 Toxic solitary nodule.
Graves' disease is an organ-specific autoimmune disease. Stimulating antibodies to the thyroid-stimulating hormone (TSH) receptor can be detected in the majority of cases. The disease can relapse and remit. Following a course of anti-thyroid drugs, 30–40% of cases enter long-term remission.

Patients with toxic multi-nodular goitres or a toxic solitary nodule do not enter remission with anti-thyroid drugs, and definitive treatment is with radioiodine or surgery.

Aims of treatment

Treatment of thyrotoxicosis is dependent upon the underlying aetiology and is summarised in Table 12.8. In general, the aims of treatment are symptom relief, control of the disease and if appropriate definitive treatment with radioiodine or surgery. Thiourylene anti-thyroid drugs are often used to achieve a euthyroid status prior to definitive treatment.

Table 12.8 Treatments used in the management of thyrotoxicosis.

Treatment	Example	Indication
β-Adrenoreceptor blockade	Propanolol	Symptom relief only
Thiourylene antithyroid drugs	Carbimazole, methimazole, propylthiouracil	Control of throtoxicosis, induction of remission in Graves' disease
Radioactive iodine	Iodine-131	Definitive treatment of relapsed Graves' disease, toxic multi-nodular goitre and toxic solitary nodule
Potassium iodide		Preparation for surgery and treatment of thyrotoxic crisis (thyroid storm)
Surgery	Total or subtotal thyroidectomy	Definitive treatment as per radioactive iodine. Often reserved for cases with local compressive symptoms

Drug treatments in thyrotoxicosis

Thionamide (thiourylene) anti-thyroid drugs

Mechanism

These drugs (carbimazole, methimazole, propylthiouracil) all share a similar chemical structure. Methimazole is a product of carbimazole metabolism and is the active compound. Methimazole is widely used in the United States and Europe, while carbimazole is available in the United Kingdom.

Their exact mode of action is unclear but is thought to involve reduced thyroid hormone synthesis by:

1 Inhibition of iodide oxidation.

2 Inhibition of iodination of tyrosine.

3 Inhibition of coupling of iodotyrosines.

Propylthiouracil also reduces the conversion of T_4 to T_3 in the peripheral tissues, which may have additional therapeutic benefit.

As anti-thyroid drugs do not alter the secretion of pre-formed thyroid hormone, the effects on circulating thyroid hormone levels and on the symptoms of thyrotoxicosis are not apparent for some time (2–4 weeks).

Pharmacokinetics

The thionamides are given orally. Carbimazole is rapidly hydrolysed in plasma to methimazole. Methimazole has a plasma half-life of 12–15 hours.

Clinical use and dose

Carbimazole: A starting dose of 20–40 mg daily is normally used in adults. Once a euthyroid state has been achieved, one of two regimes to prevent hypothyroidism can be used – either dose titration or a block and replace regime. In the dose titration regime the dose of carbimazole is gradually reduced to reach a maintenance (usually 5–10 mg/day). In the block and replace regime, carbimazole is continued at 40 mg daily together with levothyroxine sodium (100–150 μg).

Propylthiouracil: A starting dose of 200–400 mg daily is used in adults. Once euthyroid, the dose is gradually reduced to a maintenance of 50–100 mg.

Patients with Graves' disease who may enter remission are often given anti-thyroid drugs for up to 18 months. If remission seems likely at that point, treatment may be withdrawn and the patients monitored to detect relapse. This approach is not appropriate for patients whose disease will not enter remission (e.g. multi-nodular goitre).

Adverse effects

1 All the drugs will cause hypothyroidism and goitre enlargement, when given chronically. This can be prevented by using the dosing regimes described above.

2 Agranulocytosis is the most serious side effect. It is rare and generally resolves on stopping therapy. Patients should be given a written warning at the start of treatment about this and should be instructed to report any sore throat or fever immediately.

3 The most common side effects are skin rashes and pruritus. A substantial proportion of patients who develop a rash when on carbimazole will also do so on propylthiouracil.

4 Arthralgia, hepatitis and serum sickness type reactions are all rarely seen with these drugs.

5 Carbimazole/methimazole and propylthiouracil cross the placenta and can cause fetal hypothyroidism and goitre. Pregnant patients should therefore be given the lowest possible dose to control the disease. Use of carbimazole in pregnancy has been associated with a very rare occurrence of aplasia cutis, a congenital abnormality of scalp skin development although whether this is a causative relationship remains disputed. The drugs are secreted in breast milk (propylthiouracil to a lesser extent than carbimazole/methimazole), and this can result in neonatal hypothyroidism. Propylthiouracil is considered the drug of choice during pregnancy and lactation.

Radioactive iodine

The indications for using radioiodine are shown in Table 12.8. It is well absorbed orally and is given as a single dose. It is taken up by the thyroid where it causes localised destruction by a radiation thyroiditis. There is little radiation dose to other tissues. The iodine-131 has a half-life of 8 days. The effects on the thyroid take several weeks with the maximal effect occurring approximately 2 months later.

The advantages of radioactive iodine are its simplicity, low cost and safety. The major disadvantage is the occurrence of hypothyroidism. Early hypothyroidism (within a few months) is a dose-related phenomenon. Thereafter, late hypothyroidism will affect between 2 and 4% of patients per year. This is an inexorable phenomenon and the incidence of hypothyroidism is approximately 50% at 10 years.

There is no evidence of any carcinogenic risk following radioactive iodine treatment. There is no evidence of any harm to germinal tissue; however, women are advised to avoid conception for a minimum of 6 months following radioactive iodine therapy (male patients are advised not to father children for 4 months after treatment).

Potassium iodide

Iodide has multiple actions on the thyroid. The most important is an immediate reduction in thyroid hormone release and for this reason potassium iodide is used in thyroid crisis. The drug will also inhibit thyroid hormone formation and iodide trapping and reduces gland vascularity. With regular dosing it has a maximal effect at 10–15 days, its effects then diminish because of loss of its inhibitory effects on the thyroid.

β-Adrenoreceptor blockade

Propranolol reduces peripheral conversion of T_4 to T_3, and also provides some symptomatic relief. It should be emphasised that beta-blockers have no effect on the underlying process of Graves' disease or on thyroid hormone secretion.

Thyroid crisis

This condition has a high mortality and is characterised by fever, tachycardia, dehydration and confusion. It is treated with potassium iodide and carbimazole. Patients also require general supportive measures, including rehydration, intravenous beta-blocker therapy and steroids.

Hypothyroidism

Clinical scenario

An elderly lady has been treated by her GP for depression. She has gained weight despite poor appetite. She is found at home unkempt with coarse hair facially, brady cardia and a slow relaxation phase of deep tendon reflexes. On admission she is given some fluids. Thyroid stimulating hormone has come back >100. What is the diagnosis and how should she be treated?

Pathophysiology

Hypothyroidism results from insufficient secretion of thyroid hormones; classical features include lethargy, weight gain, dry skin and cold intolerance. It is most commonly due to an autoimmune thyroiditis (Hashimoto's thyroiditis) but has a variety of other causes including congenital dysfunction, iodine deficiency and following treatment of thyrotoxicosis.

Treatment – thyroid replacement therapy

Treatment is directed at replacing thyroid hormone levels in the circulation. Two thyroid hormone preparations are available: levothyroxine sodium (thyroxine, T_4) and liothyronine sodium (T_3), although the latter is rarely used.

Mechanism

T_4 is converted to T_3 in cells by a deiodinase enzyme. T_3 binds to nuclear receptors and regulates gene transcription. This leads to multiple metabolic actions. In some tissue (e.g. the pituitary) there is an obligatory requirement for a high percentage of T_3 to be derived from intracellular T_4 conversion. For this reason, T_4 is a more effective hormone in suppression of TSH than is T_3 and is therefore the preferred thyroid hormone for replacement.

Pharmacokinetics

Both T_4 and T_3 are adequately absorbed following oral administration. T_4 has a half-life of about a week and T_3 about 2 days. Both undergo conjugation in the liver and enterohepatic circulation.

Clinical use and dose

The doses of thyroid hormone required for adequate replacement are assessed by measurement of serum TSH concentrations unless there is underlying pituitary disease. Levothyroxine sodium is started at a dose of 50–100 μg/day (starting dose 25 μg/day if elderly or with heart disease), with dose increments every 4 weeks, depending on thyroid function. The usual maintenance dose is 100–200 μg/day. Liothyronine sodium can be used to achieve a more rapid response and is given intravenously in hypothyroid coma; 20 μg is equivalent to 100 μg of levothyroxine.

Levothyroxine sodium is also used postoperatively in thyroid carcinoma to replace endogenous thyroxine and to suppress TSH, as many tumours are TSH dependent. The dose of levothyroxine used under these circumstances is higher than that given as replacement therapy, and is normally in the region of 200 μg/day.

Adverse effects

These are related to the physiological and pharmacological actions of thyroid hormone. Elderly patients, or those known to have ischaemic heart disease, are given low initial doses with slow increments because angina or myocardial infarction can be precipitated. Thyroid hormone excess produces the usual clinical features of thyrotoxicosis.

Obesity

Clinical scenario

A 34-year-old female has made an appointment to discuss her weight problem with her GP. She has always been 'heavy boned' but put on a lot of weight following the birth of her second child 5 years previously. She has tried various diets without success and was keen to try drug treatment or indeed be considered for gastric band surgery if all else fails. What drug treatment options are available?

Pathophysiology

Obesity is increasing in prevalence amongst both the developed and the developing world. In Europe, approximately 15–20% of the middle-aged population are obese. Obesity is a risk factor for serious diseases including ischaemic heart disease, hypertension, type 2 diabetes mellitus, stroke and certain malignancies (e.g. breast, ovary, colon, prostate, endometrial). It is also associated with obstructive sleep apnoea, osteoarthritis, gallstones and varicose veins.

Most patients have 'simple' obesity although it is a feature of certain conditions, e.g. Prader–Willi syndrome. It results from energy intake in excess of energy expenditure over a prolonged period of time. Genetic factors, environmental change (sedentary lifestyle with an abundance of energy-rich foods) and potentially, alterations in neurotransmitters that influence appetite, e.g. leptin, contribute to the tendency to develop obesity.

Aims of treatment

Treatment should aim for realistic weight loss (e.g. 0.5–1 kg/week) which is then maintained. A 10% weight loss is a reasonable initial aim and is associated with a reduction in mortality and morbidity.

Non-pharmacological therapy

A reduction in dietary calorie intake, increased energy expenditure through exercise and behavioural modification are fundamental aspects of obesity management.

Drug treatments of obesity

Drug treatment can be used as an adjunct to diet and exercise in patients who are obese or overweight with significant co-morbidity.

Pancreatic lipase inhibitors (Orlistat)

Mechanism
Orlistat binds to the active site of pancreatic lipases and slows the breakdown of dietary fat in the gastrointestinal tract. It can reduce the amount of fat absorbed by up to 30%.

Pharmacokinetics

Orlistat is given orally, has it's effect locally in the gut and is excreted in the faeces.

Clinical use and dose

When used as part of a weight-control program, average weight loss of 10% in a year has been observed. A dose of 120 mg is taken immediately before or within an hour of each main meal (up to a maximum of 360 mg daily). It is contraindicated in patients with chronic malabsorption and cholestasis.

Adverse effects

The most frequent adverse effects are loose oily stools and faecal urgency, and oily rectal discharge. The potential for impaired absorption of fat-soluble vitamins and concomitant medications, e.g. oral contraceptive pills, should be considered.

Sibutramine

Mechanism

Sibutramine is a centrally acting anti-obesity drug. It blocks the re-uptake of noradrenaline and serotonin. It causes dose-dependent weight loss by reduced food intake and increased satiety.

Pharmacokinetics

Sibutramine is well absorbed after oral administration. It undergoes extensive first-pass metabolism and the metabolites are pharmacologically active. The active metabolites are inactivated in the liver and are excreted in the urine and faeces.

Clinical use and dose

The starting daily dose is 10 mg; this can be increased up to 15 mg if target weight loss is not achieved.

Adverse effects

In some individuals, sibutramine may cause a rise in blood pressure and pulse rate, and its use is contraindicated in patients with uncontrolled hypertension and cardiovascular disease. Dry mouth, constipation and insomnia are common adverse effects.

Bone metabolism

Clinical scenario

A 60-year-old post menopausal women attends a well women clinic. She is a long term smoker with no other health problems until she fractured her scaphoid three months previously. A bone densitometry test was done showing that she has moderately severe osteporosis. What treatment should be prescribed?

Introduction

The drugs described in this section are used in the management of disorders of bone structure, e.g. osteoporosis and osteomalacia, and disorders of calcium metabolism, e.g. hypoparathyroidism and hyperparathyroidism.

Calcium salts

Calcium salts are used in the management of
1 Dietary deficiency
2 Prevention and treatment of osteoporosis
3 Hypocalcaemia due to malabsorption or hypoparathyroidism
4 Hyperphosphataemia
5 Cardiac dysrhythmias associated with hyperkalaemia.
Dietary deficiency is more likely during childhood, pregnancy and breast feeding, due to increased demand, and in the elderly, due to reduced absorption.

Calcium preparations

Calcium salts are given orally in divided doses. Calcium salts used include calcium gluconate, calcium lactate and calcium carbonate. A daily calcium dose of 1000–1500 mg is recommended in osteoporosis. The main adverse effect is gastrointestinal disturbance. Calcium carbonate binds phosphate in the gut and is used to treat the hyperphosphataemia seen in renal failure. Calcium gluconate is given intravenously in the treatment of hypocalcaemic tetany and in the treatment of cardiac dysrhythmias caused by severe hyperkalaemia.

	Ergocalciferol, calciferol (IU/day)	Alfacacidol (μg/day)	Calcitriol (μg/day)
Vitamin D deficiency			
Dietary deficiency	400–5000		
Malabsorption			
Chronic liver disease	Up to 40,000		
Hypoparathyroidism	25,000–100,000	0.5–2.0	0.25–1.00
Renal osteodystrophy		0.5–2.0	0.25–1.00
Osteoporosis			0.5

Table 12.9 Vitamin D preparations and their use.

Vitamin D compounds

Vitamin D is a prehormone. In humans, the main source of vitamin D (cholecalciferol/calciferol) is from the photoactivation of 7-dehydrocholesterol in the skin. This undergoes hydroxylation in the liver to 25-hydroxycholecalciferol and in the kidneys to the active metabolite 1,25-dihydroxycholecaciferol (calcitriol). Some vitamin D (ergocalciferol) is derived from the diet.

A range of vitamin D compounds are available for therapeutic use, including ergocalciferol, calciferol, alfacalcidol (1α-hydroxycholecalciferol) and calcitriol (1,25-dihydroxycholecalciferol).

Mechanism

The main action of vitamin D compounds is to facilitate intestinal absorption of calcium and phosphate. They also promote calcium mobilisation from bone and increase calcium reabsorption in the kidney tubules.

Pharmacokinetics

All vitamin D compounds are given orally and are well absorbed. Vitamin D is fat soluble and bile is necessary for absorption. Vitamin D undergoes enterohepatic circulation and is largely eliminated in the faeces.

Clinical use and dose

The indications and dosages of the commonly used vitamin D compounds are shown in Table 12.9.

Adverse effects

Hypercalcaemia is the main complication of vitamin D therapy. All patients receiving pharmacological doses should have monitoring of their serum calcium. Some anti-convulsants induce the enzymes that metabolise vitamin D and cause increased requirements.

Bisphosphonates

Mechanism

Bisphosphonates are a family of carbon-substituted pyrophosphates that bind avidly to bone. They have an inhibitory action on osteoclasts and therefore reduce bone resorption. Substitution of different chemical moieties at the carbon atom produces compounds with differing potencies (Table 12.10).

Pharmacokinetics

When administered orally, bisphosphonates are poorly absorbed. Between 20 and 50% of the absorbed drug binds to bone within 24 hours where it remains for many months, possibly years, until the bone is resorbed. Unbound (free) drug is excreted unchanged by the kidneys. Calcium and other chelating agents reduce the absorption of bisphosphonates from the gastrointestinal tract. Bisphosphonates should be taken with plain water on an empty stomach first thing in the morning at least 30 minutes before breakfast or, if taken at any other time of day, food and drink should be avoided for 2 hours before and after the dose.

Table 12.10 Bisphosphonates.

Drug	Relative potency	Indications (*current licensed indications in the United Kingdom*)
First generation (short alkyl or halide side chain)		
Etidronate	1	Osteoporosis, Paget's disease
Clodronate	10	Hypercalcaemia, metastatic bone disease
Second generation (generally with amino terminal group)		
Tiludronate	10	Paget's disease
Pamidronate	100	Paget's disease, hypercalcaemia, metastatic bone disease
Alendronate	100–1000	Osteoporosis
Third generation (cyclic side chain)		
Risendronate	1000–10,000	Osteoporosis, Paget's disease
Ibandronate	1000–10,000	Hypercalcaemia, metastatic bone disease
Zolendronate	10,000+	Hypercalcaemia, metastatic bone disease

Clinical use and dose

The indications are summarised in Table 12.10.

1 *Treatment and prevention of osteoporosis.* Bisphosphonates are associated with an increase in bone mineral density and a significant reduction in risk of vertebral fractures (etidronate, alendronate, risedronate, ibandronate) and hip and other fractures (alendronate, risedronate, ibandronate) when given orally in association with calcium supplementation. Etidronate is given in 14-day cycles followed by 76 days of calcium carbonate. Alendronate and risedronate are given as a once-daily or once-weekly regimen and oral ibandronate has a daily or monthly dosing schedule.

2 *Paget's disease.* In Paget's disease, bisphosphonates are used to suppress disease activity, aiming for an alkaline phosphatase in the normal range, and in the treatment of bone pain.

3 *Hypercalcaemia.* Intravenous bisphosphonates (pamidronate, clodronate and zolendronate) are used in the treatment of severe hypercalcaemia. They should not be used until there has been adequate intravenous saline rehydration (with furosemide diuresis if salt and water retention occurs). The dose should be reduced if there is renal impairment. Plasma calcium usually falls by 72 hours.

4 *Metastatic bone disease.* Bisphosphonates have been found to reduce complications (including pathological fracture) associated with advanced multiple myeloma and metastatic bone disease (e.g. breast cancer).

Adverse effects

Bisphosphonates are generally well tolerated. They have a number of gastrointestinal side effects including nausea, diarrhoea, and oesophageal irritation and ulceration. Intravenous use of bisphosphonates can be associated with transient pyrexia and flu-like symptoms.

Hormone replacement therapy

Mechanism

Oestrogen suppresses osteoclast-mediated bone resorption. Hormone replacement therapy (HRT) prevents menopause-associated bone loss, and an increase in bone mineral density is seen. HRT use is associated with a reduction in hip, vertebral and forearm fractures.

Pharmacokinetics

Orally administered oestrogens undergo extensive first-pass metabolism by the liver. They have a half-life of 10–18 hours.

Clinical use

Due to the risk of serious adverse events (see below), HRT is no longer recommended as first line in the prevention and treatment of post-menopausal osteoporosis. Short-term use of HRT is still appropriate for women with menopausal symptoms, e.g. vasomotor instability, where benefits outweigh the risks.

Adverse effects

HRT is associated with a slight increase in stroke and an increase in thromboembolic disease, breast cancer and endometrial cancer. HRT does not prevent coronary heart disease. Common side effects include breast tenderness, fluid retention and weight gain.

Selective oestrogen-receptor modulators

Mechanism

Selective oestrogen-receptor modulators (SERMS) are non-hormonal agents that bind to oestrogen receptors. Raloxifene is the only SERM currently available. Depending on the target tissue, SERMS have agonist or antagonist action. Raloxifene has agonist action on bone and cardiovascular system and antagonist action on mammary tissue and the uterus. Their action on bone causes a reduction in osteoclast activity and an increase in bone mineral density.

Pharmacokinetics

Approximately 60% of an oral dose is absorbed. Raloxifene undergoes extensive first-pass metabolism and has a bioavailability of around 2%. It has a half-life of approximately 32 hours and after metabolism is excreted in the faeces. Cholestyramine reduces its absorption due to reduced enterohepatic cycling.

Clinical use and dose

Raloxifene is used in the treatment and prevention of post-menopausal osteoporosis at a daily dose of 60 mg. Raloxifene does not reduce menopausal vasomotor symptoms.

Adverse effects

Hot flushes and leg cramps are common side effects. SERMS are associated with an increased risk of thromboembolic disease similar to that observed with HRT.

Calcitonin

Mechanism

Calcitonin is a peptide hormone synthesised by the parafollicular cells within the thyroid gland. Synthetic forms (salmon, porcine) are available for therapeutic use. Calcitonin reduces bone resorption by decreasing the number and activity of osteoclasts.

Pharmacokinetics

Administration is by subcutaneous or intramuscular injection or nasal spray (licensed for osteoporosis in the United Kingdom). Calcitonin has a short half-life (4–40 minutes according to preparation) but its duration of action is several hours. It is metabolised by the kidneys.

Clinical use and dose

1 *Treatment and prevention of osteoporosis:* Calcitonin is associated with a reduction in the incidence of osteoporotic vertebral fractures. It is less efficacious than bisphosphonates and HRT. Patients should also be prescribed calcium and vitamin D supplements. A daily dose of 100 units (subcutaneous or intramuscular injection) or 200 units (intranasally) is used. Calcitonin has potent analgesic properties and can be used in the management of acute fracture pain.

2 *Paget's disease:* Calcitonin is effective in relieving bone pain in Paget's disease and can suppress disease activity. The dose ranges from 50 units three times weekly to 100 units daily.

3 *Hypercalcaemia:* Calcitonin can be used to treat severe hypercalcaemia following saline

rehydration and furosemide diuresis. High doses are required (up to 400 units 6 hourly). It is usually reserved for cases who have not responded to intravenous bisphosphonates.

4 *Bony metastases:* Bone pain in neoplastic disease can be treated with 200 units of calcitonin 6 hourly or 400 units 12 hourly.

Adverse effects

Nausea, vomiting and flushing are common side effects. Local discomfort can occur at injection sites. Nasal spray can cause local irritation and ulceration. Antibodies may develop with long-term use, which attenuate its action. Allergic reactions rarely occur.

Teriparatide

Mechanism

Teriparatide is a recombinant peptide composed of 34 amino acids identical to the active region of parathyroid hormone. It stimulates osteoblasts, and increased bone formation and improved bone architecture are seen. A reduction in fractures has been demonstrated in post-menopausal patients with established osteoporosis.

Pharmacokinetics

It is given by daily subcutaneous injection. It has a half-life of approximately 1 hour and is thought to be metabolised by the liver and excreted by the kidneys.

Clinical use and dose

Teriparatide is used in the treatment of established osteoporosis. A daily dose of 20 μg is given by subcutaneous injection.

Adverse effects

Teriparatide is generally well tolerated. A transient increase in serum calcium is seen. Pre-clinical toxicology data showed a high incidence of osteosarcoma in rats given high doses of the drug. To date, development of osteosarcoma has not been reported in the clinical trials of teriparatide.

Strontium ranelate

Strontium ranelate promotes bone formation by stimulating osteoblast activity and inhibiting osteoclasts. It is associated with a reduction in vertebral and non-vertebral fractures in established osteoporosis. An oral daily dose of 2 g is used in the treatment of osteoporosis.

Pituitary and adrenal cortex disease

Hypopituitarism

Partial or complete deficiency of anterior pituitary hormones arises from conditions including pituitary tumours, pituitary infarction and radiotherapy. It can result in inadequate production of thyroid hormones, adrenal steroids, sex steroids and growth hormone.

Treatment is with hormone replacement. Replacement of thyroid hormone, adrenal and sex steroids is considered elsewhere. Treatment of growth hormone deficiency depends on whether it is of childhood or adult onset. In childhood, growth hormone deficiency requires replacement. In adults, there is evidence that replacement improves quality of life and has favourable effects on lipid profile, bone mineral density and lean body mass. Growth hormone replacement for adults has now been approved in many countries. Synthetic human growth hormone, manufactured using recombinant DNA technology, is given by daily subcutaneous injection. In childhood, the dose is determined by body weight and surface area. Adults are started at a dose of 100–300 μg daily, which is titrated up to a usual maintenance dose of 200–600 μg.

Cranial diabetes insipidus

Cranial diabetes insipidus is due to deficiency of circulating arginine vasopressin (anti-diuretic hormone). It arises due to hypothalamic or posterior pituitary dysfunction. In patients with an intact thirst mechanism, it presents with polyuria and polydipsia. In patients with an absent thirst mechanism (sometimes seen in head injury and hypothalamic syndromes) polyuria is seen without polydipsia, which can result in severe hypernatraemia.

Treatment is with synthetic vasopressin analogue (desmopressin). Treatment is given in divided doses, intranasally (10–40 μg/day), by parenteral injection (1–4 μg/day) or orally (100–1000 μg/day). There is wide variation in the doses required, and monitoring of the serum sodium and osmolality is essential. Desmopressin is broken down by vasopressinase. The activity of this enzyme increases during pregnancy and dose requirements increase in pregnancy.

Drug treatment of pituitary tumours

Dopamine agonists

Mechanism

Dopamine agonists cause activation of D2 receptors. Bromocriptine is short acting and is taken daily. Cabergoline is long acting and is taken once or twice weekly.

Clinical use

1 Hyperprolactinaemia/prolactinoma – D2 receptor stimulation inhibits prolactin secretion and leads to tumour shrinkage.
2 Growth-hormone-secreting tumours – A fall in growth hormone is seen in approximately half of patients with growth-hormone-secreting tumours given dopamine agonists. Dopamine acts directly on the tumours to inhibit growth hormone release. Tumour shrinkage can be seen and is more likely if the tumour co-secretes prolactin.

Adverse effects

Nausea and postural hypotension are common side effects. They may be minimised by slow initiation of therapy. Cabergoline is often better tolerated than bromocriptine.

Somatostatin analogues

Mechanism

Somatostatin is released from the hypothalamus and inhibits the secretion of growth hormone and TSH. It is also produced in neuroendocrine cells in the gastrointestinal tract where it inhibits the release of numerous gut peptides including gastrin, glucagon and insulin. Ocreotide and lanreotide are synthetic analogues of somatostatin.

Clinical use

1 Growth-hormone-secreting tumours – somatostatin analogues can be used as initial therapy or as an adjunct to surgery and radiotherapy. A reduction in growth hormone is seen in approximately 60% of patients and tumour shrinkage can occur.
2 Neuroendocrine tumours – somatostatin analogues are used in the treatment of several neuroendocrine tumours including glucagonomas and VIPomas. They are also used in the management of carcinoid syndrome.

Octreotide is a short-acting formulation that is given by subcutaneous injection (50–100 μg three times a day). Long-acting preparations of lanreotide and octreotide are available, which are given by intramuscular injection on a 1–6 weekly regime dependent on the preparation and response.

Adverse effects

Gastrointestinal side effects are common and include nausea, abdominal pain and mild steatorrhoea. Gallstones have been reported after long-term treatment. Pain may occur at injection sites.

Adrenal steroid replacement

Adrenal steroid deficiency occurs in primary adrenal failure (Addison's disease) or can be secondary to adrenocorticotropic hormone (ACTH) deficiency in pituitary disease. In primary adrenal failure there is deficiency of the glucocorticoid, cortisol and also the mineralocorticoid, aldosterone. In secondary adrenal failure there is only glucocorticoid deficiency because aldosterone secretion is regulated by the renin–angiotensin system.

Glucocorticoid replacement is usually with hydrocortisone although prednisolone or dexamethasone can be used. The replacement dose of hydrocortisone is usually 15–25 mg/day. The dose is divided to mimic the normal diurnal pattern of cortisol production; a typical regimen would be 10 mg on waking, 5 mg at midday and 5 mg at 6 p.m. The replacement dose needs to be increased during times of intercurrent illness, surgery or major physiological stress. All patients taking steroid replacement should carry a form of identification (e.g. medic alert) that gives details of their medical condition and current therapy.

Mineralocorticoid replacement is with fludrocortisone. Fludrocortisone is a synthetic steroid that has high affinity for the mineralocorticoid receptor. The usual dose is 100 µg/day (range 50–300 µg): the dose is titrated against blood pressure and plasma electrolytes.

Chapter 13

Drugs and the reproductive system

Hormonal contraception

Clinical scenario

A 25-year-old female attends her GP requesting contraception. She is in a stable relationship with her partner. She has had no previous pregnancies, but would like to start a family before she is 30. She has a regular menstrual cycle of 28 days. She is generally well, and has a blood pressure measurement of 115/73 mmHg. However she smokes 4–5 cigarettes a day, has a body mass index (BMI) of 28.4 and her father (aged 55 years) currently takes anti-hypertensive medication. What options are available for use in this patient?

Introduction

Hormonal contraception offers the most effective method of reversible fertility control available to women of childbearing age. This is most commonly provided by either a combination of oestrogen and progesterone or by progesterone alone. Combined oestrogen and progesterone hormonal contraception can be administered orally as the combined oral contraceptive (COC) pill, transdermally via a patch or intravaginally as a vaginal ring. Progesterone-only methods can be administered as an oral progesterone only pill (POP), an intramuscular depot-injection, subcutaneous implant or as an intrauterine system (IUS). Progesterone only emergency contraception is also available as a one dose tablet.

Composition

Both of the naturally occurring steroids, oestradiol (estradiol) and progesterone, are ineffective if taken orally because of extensive first-pass metabolism; thus, synthetic compounds are used in hormonal contraception. Combined hormonal contraception (pills, patch, vaginal ring) usually contains a synthetic oestrogen (ethinyloestradiol, EE). An alternative to EE, mestranol, is found in the COC (Norinyl-1) but its bioavailability compared to EE is unknown. Synthetic progesterones (called a progestogen) are mainly derivatives of 19-nortestosterone. Progestogens have androgenic, estrogenic as well as progestogenic properties. Progestogens have been described as 'first-generation' (norethynodrel), 'second-generation' (levonorgestrel and norethisterone), 'third-generation' (desogestrel and gestodene) and 'fourth-generation' (drospirenone).

Mechanism

The COC is taken for 21 consecutive days and primarily inhibits ovulation by acting on

Lecture Notes: Clinical Pharmacology and Therapeutics, 8th edition. By Gerard McKay, John Reid and Matthew Walters. Published 2010 by Blackwell Publishing Ltd.

the hypothalamo-pituitary-ovarian axis to reduce luteinising hormone (LH) and follicle-stimulating hormone (FSH). It also has contraceptive actions on cervical mucus preventing sperm entry and endometrium making it inhospitable to implantation. Usually, women use the hormone tablets, patches or ring for 21 days followed by a 7-day hormone-free interval. Some women use every day pills that have seven placebo hormone-free pills which are taken in week 4. During this hormone-free week a withdrawal bleed usually occurs due to the withdrawal of EE and progestogen. Contraceptive protection is maintained during the hormone-free interval as long as the previous and subsequent pills or patches are taken consistently and correctly.

The POP works by thickening cervical mucus so that it inhibits sperm penetration into the upper reproductive tract. With traditional POPs ovulation is inhibited in up to 60% of cycles. The newer desogestrel-containing POP (Cerazette) has been shown in randomised controlled trials to inhibit ovulation in up to 97% of cycles. All POPs should be taken every day without a pill-free interval. The progestogen-only injectables (depot medroxyprogesterone acetate [DMPA] and norethisterone enanthate [NET-EN]) and the progestogen-only implant [Implanon] work by inhibition of ovulation in all women. The levonorgestrel-releasing intrauterine system (LNG-IUS) works by preventing endometrial proliferation, and in around 25% of women ovulation is also inhibited. Due to its actions on the endometrium, the LNG-IUS is also used in the treatment of primary menorrhagia.

The mode of action of levonorgestrel when used as a single dose for emergency contraception is not fully understood. In the follicular phase of the cycle it is thought to postpone ovulation for 5–7 days in 80% of women, however, its mode of action in preventing pregnancy after ovulation has occurred is unclear.

Pharmacokinetics

Oral progestogens and EE are primarily absorbed from the small intestine and undergo extensive first pass metabolism in the small intestine and the liver. This absorption and first pass metabolism affects the bioavailability of the active hormones in the circulation, and levels can be affected by conditions involving the small intestine or the liver. After metabolism, liver conjugates of EE, unaltered EE and progestogens are excreted into the bile and subsequently into the small intestine. In the large intestine, hydrolytic enzymes released from colonic bacteria break down inactive conjugates of EE, into active metabolites which can be reabsorbed and eventually excreted in the urine. This is called the *enterohepatic circulation*, and contributes to the bioavailability of EE in the circulation. There is no enterohepatic circulation for progestogens and metabolites are excreted in bile and by the kidneys.

Parenteral administration of EE and progestagens allows direct absorption into the circulation thereby bypassing the first pass metabolism in the small intestine and liver. However, subsequent metabolism will still occur within the liver.

Adverse effects

The use of hormonal contraception is safe for the majority of women, but can be associated with rare but serious harm.

Venous thromboembolic disease

Among users of COC, there is an increased risk of venous thromboembolism (VTE) including deep vein thrombosis and pulmonary embolism. However, in absolute terms, the risk is still very small. The level of risk in women not using COC and not pregnant is 5 per 100 000 woman years, increasing to 15–25 per 100,000 woman years with COC use. In pregnancy VTE risk increases further to 60 per 100,000 woman years.

1 The risk is increased by:
   - High EE content of pill preparation. EE is known to be thrombogenic, and risk is increased where EE content is ≥ 50 μg. Women using liver enzyme-inducing drugs may use a 50-μg COC; however, due to increased liver metabolism, this is clinically comparable to lower doses of EE.
   - The progestagen component influences VTE risk; different preparations are thought to

counteract the thrombogenic effect of EE to a different extent. The relative risk is increased 3 fold with levonorgesteral and norethisterone containing COCs, whereas with third generation progestogens, desogestrel and gestodene the relative risk is increased 5 fold.

- Obesity is associated with increased VTE risk, with the risk increasing 2 fold for those taking COC with a BMI > 30 kg/m^2, and a 4 fold increased risk in COC users with a BMI > 35 kg/m^2.
- Major surgical procedures or travel associated with immobilisation.
- Factor V Leiden and other hereditary thrombophilias.

2 The increased risk is confined to those actually taking the pill:

- Develops within first month
- Remains constant during use
- Returns to normal within 1 month of stopping.

3 Pathogenesis:

- Decreased antithrombin III
- Decreased plasminogen activator in endothelium.

Arterial disease (myocardial infarction and stroke)

1 The risk is increased by:

- Age
- Cigarette smoking
- High oestrogen content in COC
- Obesity

Age and cigarette smoking multiply, rather than add to, the risks of the COC with regard to myocardial infarction and stroke. Most cases occur in women aged over 35 years who smoke. The risk is also enhanced by hypertension, diabetes and hypercholesterolemia.

2 The risk is not confined to those currently taking the pill, but persists after stopping.

3 Pathogenesis:

- Acceleration of platelet aggregation
- Decreased antithrombin III
- Decreased plasminogen activator.

Hypertension

1 Blood pressure rises by a small amount in all women using COC. In most cases, this increase in pressure is small and of little clinical significance. Less frequently there is a rise to levels at which treatment might ordinarily be considered. In these cases to the pill should be stopped and blood pressure monitored. Rarely, malignant hypertension occurs and should be treated as a medical emergency. Blood pressure should be checked before prescribing combined hormonal contraception and at each return clinic visit.

2 Blood pressure usually returns to normal 3–6 months after stopping the contraceptive pill.

3 Pathogenesis:

- Oestrogen stimulation of synthesis of angiotensinogen in the liver.

Oral contraceptives and cancer

The role of oral contraceptives in cancer risk is controversial, and recently a large UK cohort suggested no overall increase in cancer rates among pill users. Use of COC reduces the risk of ovarian and endometrial cancer by 50%, and also reduces the risk of colorectal cancer. Cervical cancer has been identified more frequently in pill users; however a causal relationship has been questioned in view of confounding risk factors including age at first intercourse and number of sexual partners. Current UK advice is that use of COC <10 years is associated with a negligible risk of cervical cancer. In terms of breast cancer risk, current evidence suggests that the use of hormonal contraception is associated with very small increase in the risk of breast cancer. This increased risk is unrelated to duration of use and risk decreases over a period of 10 years after cessation after which time the risk is the same as for non-COC users.

Glucose tolerance and lipid metabolism

There is a small decrease in glucose tolerance. Oestrogens increase, and progestogens decrease, high-density lipoproteins. The clinical relevance of these observations is unknown.

Focal migraine

Ischaemic stroke is increased in migraine suffers and is further increased in migraine suffers who are COC users, in particular those who experience focal migraine with aura (which indicates is-chaemia).

Bone mineral density
Progestogen only injectable contraceptives have been associated with a small loss of bone mineral density (BMD); however, there is usually recovery after discontinuation.

Irregular bleeding patterns and return to fertility
Irregular bleeding is a particular problem with progesterone-only methods (pill, injectable and implants), however COC and LNG-IUS are used in the treatment of menorrhagia and dysmenor-rhoea. There is no evidence of a delay in return to fertility with COC or POP, however with injectable progesterone preparations there may be a delay of up to 1 year.

Other adverse effects
1 Skin disorders
2 Change in libido
3 Headaches
4 Mood swings.
  Less commonly, subjects may be affected by:
1 Cholestatic jaundice
2 Increased incidence of gallstones
3 Systemic lupus erythematosus
4 Precipitation of porphyria.

Hormonal contraception and breastfeeding

There is no good evidence that oral contracep-tives containing low doses of oestrogen reduce the quality of breast milk, but since there is a suggestion that milk quantity may be decreased by oestrogen particularly in the first 6 weeks postpartum, the COC is not generally recom-mended if breastfeeding and less than 6 months postpartum. Progesterone only contraceptives do not affect breastfeeding, milk quantity or infant growth.

Drug interactions

The efficacy of hormonal contraception is reduced by the co-administration of drugs which induce cytochrome P450 enzymes (see Chapter 1). This results in an increased metabolism of EE and progestogens and ultimately a reduction in the bioavailability of the active compounds.

This applies to oestrogen-containing and some progestogen-only contraceptives (POP and im-plants but not injectables or the LNG-IUS). If long-term treatment with liver enzyme-inducing drugs is necessary (e.g. treatment of epilepsy) then a higher dose of COC should be used (at least 50 μg of EE) or an alternative method should be found.

Re-absorption of EE via the enterohepatic cir-culation contributes to its bioavailability. The importance of this re-absorption in terms of contraceptive efficiency is not clear. Neverthe-less, the administration of antibiotics that alter colonic bacteria may reduce re-absorption of EE and potentially reduce contraceptive efficacy. The mechanism depends on the fact that oestrogens undergo conjugation in the liver, but hydrolytic enzymes produced by gut bacteria cleave these conjugates and release free hormone, which is then reabsorbed. Broad-spectrum antimicrobials prevent this process by altering gut flora, and hor-mone absorption is decreased. When a non-liver enzyme-inducing antibiotic such as ampicillin is prescribed for a woman who is also taking a COC she should be advised to use additional contra-ception while taking the antibiotic and for at least 7 days after their discontinuation. Progestagens do not undergo secondary reabsorption in the entero-hepatic circulation, and therefore efficacy is not reduced by the use of non liver enzyme-inducing antibiotics.

Clinical use and administration

The dose of both oestrogen and progestogen should be kept as low as possible. Combined prepa-rations are taken to mimic a 28-day cycle, proges-terone only preparations are taken continuously.
1 COCP: One tablet is taken daily for 21 days with a 7-day pill free break. The initial pill is usually

started on day 1 of the menstrual cycle. Monophasic preparations have a fixed amount of hormone in each tablet. Biphasic and triphasic preparations have varying amounts of each hormone throughout the pill packet. Theoretically, these formulations should minimise deviations from normal metabolism, however, there are no proven benefits of biphasic and triphasic preparations compared to monophasic regimens. Current UK advice suggests an initial prescription of a monophasic COC containing 30 μg of EE with norethisterone or levonorgesteral, thereby choosing a low VTE risk progesterone with a effective dose of oestrogen with a lesser chance of breakthrough bleeding.

2 Combined contraceptive patch: Wear one patch for 7 days and replace every week for 3 weeks followed by a patch-free week.

3 Combined contraceptive vaginal ring: One ring inserted vaginally for 3 weeks of use per cycle with a new ring inserted after a 7-day ring free break.

4 Traditional POP: Continuous administration of one tablet daily starting on the first day of menstruation and taking the dose at the same time each day. A delay of more than 3 hours risks loss of efficacy.

5 Desogestrel-only POP: Continuous administration of one tablet daily starting on the first day of menstruation and taking the dose at the same time each day. A delay of more than 12 hours risks loss of efficacy.

6 Intramuscular progesterone depot injections:
- Depot medroxyprogesterone acetate (DMPA) Injections are given every 12 weeks.
- Norethisterone enanthate (NET-EN) is given every 8 weeks.

7 Progestogen-only implants: These implants provide a low daily etonorgestrel released from a rod placed in the subcutaneous tissue of the upper inner arm. They provide effective contraception for 3 years.

8 The levonorgestrel-releasing intrauterine system (LNG-IUS): It provides a high intrauterine dose of levonorgestrel with minimal systemic absorption. It can provide effective contraception for 5 years.

9 The levonorgestrel emergency contraception is taken as a single dose within 72 hours of unprotected intercourse. Its efficacy is highest in the first 12 hours and diminishes with time.

10 Hormonal methods of contraception are effective if taken consistently and correctly. True method failures are low but user failure (due to missed pills) varies. Methods of hormonal contraception that avoid daily pill taking, such as the progestogen-only implant, are among the most effective methods of female contraception.

Contraindications

When prescribing hormonal contraceptives, a balance between the risk that the hormones pose to the women and risk of unwanted pregnancy must be balanced. Ideally, where hormonal contraceptive use is not recommended, it should not be used. However, in some circumstances, where alternative methods are not suitable, hormonal contraception may be used with specialist advice and counselling about risks for the woman. Situations where the use of combined hormonal contraceptive is not recommended are summarised in Table 13.1. Of note progesterone only preparations may be suitable where combined are not recommended.

Table 13.1 Combined hormonal contraception not recommended.

Smokers aged ≥35 years
Migraine with aura any age Migraine without aura aged ≥35 years Hypertension consistently >140 mmHg systolic and/or > 90 mmHg diastolic
Personal history VTE or thrombogenic mutation Personal history cardiovascular disease or stroke Active liver disease Current breast cancer Impending major surgery Porphyria Obesity BMI ≥40 kg/m² Diabetes with disease complications or >20 years duration

Hormone replacement therapy

Clinical scenario

A 53-year-old female presents with a several-month history of hot flushes. Her menses had become increasingly irregular. She reports irritability and loss of libido. Recognising she is going through the menopause she would like hormone replacement therapy (HRT). What drugs can be used to treat this condition?

Introduction

With the onset of the menopause, oestrogen levels fall and this can give rise to menopausal vasomotor symptoms ('hot flushes') and symptoms related to tissue atrophy (e.g. discomfort secondary to vaginal atrophy). HRT aims to alleviate symptoms by giving low doses of oestrogen either alone or in combination with progesterone in women with an intact uterus. There is also good evidence that oestrogen administration will reduce postmenopausal osteoporosis, but other drugs should be considered if bone density is the main concern. In women who have had a surgical menopause with bilateral removal of ovaries or premature menopause, HRT replaces the endogenous hormone they would normally have until the approximate age of natural menopause (i.e. until aged 50 years).

Current recommendations suggest that the minimum effective dose of HRT should be used for the shortest duration. It must be acknowledged that HRT does not provide contraceptive cover, and a women is still considered potentially fertile for 2 years after her LMP if <50 years, and 1 year if >50 years of age.

Natural oestrogens (estradiol, oestrone [estrone] and oestriol [estriol]) provide a more physiological effect for HRT than synthetic oestrogens (ethinylestradiol and mestranol). Oestrogen may be administered in various ways, for example tablet, transdermal patch, cream, gel, subdermal implant or intrauterine system. Oral oestrogens are subject to first-pass metabolism; therefore, subcutaneous or transdermal administration is more representative of endogenous hormone activity than other preparations. HRT can also be given locally as vaginal pessaries, cream or rings to treat local symptoms.

HRT and cancer risk

HRT increases the risk of endometrial cancer, breast cancer and ovarian cancer. The endometrium proliferates under the stimulus of oestrogen, if this is unopposed there is an increased risk of malignancy. Therefore, a woman with a uterus should also be given one progestogen for at least 10–14 days of her cycle. Some HRT preparations contain cyclical progestogens and women have a regular withdrawal bleeding following the progestogen administration. Other HRT preparations have continuous combined oestrogen and progestogen and in women over 54 years, they can be used to prevent a cyclical bleed. The LNG-IUS may also be used to provide the progesterone component of HRT.

All types of HRT are associated with an increased risk of breast cancer. Risk is related to duration of treatment and is considered to only increase from age 50 years. Within 5 years of stopping HRT, risk reverts to the women's background risk. The risk is higher in those taking combined HRT compared with oestrogen alone; in women aged 50–59 using therapy for 5 years combined HRT gave 6 extra cases per 1000 women (24 extra cases over 10 years) whereas with oestrogen only therapy the risk increases by two extra cases per 1000 women (6 extra cases over 10 years). Long term use of HRT is associated with a small increase in the risk of ovarian cancer with between one and two extra cases per 1000 women with 10 years of HRT.

HRT, cardiovascular disease and venous thrombotic disease

Large trials have clarified the relationship between HRT and cardiovascular disease indicating that it does not protect against coronary heart disease and there is actually an increased risk if HRT is started more that 10 years after the menopause. The risk of stroke increases by between 1 and 3 extra cases per 1000 women. The risk of VTE increases with

HRT use, with an extra 2 women per 1000 affected if taking oestrogen only, with a higher risk of 7–10 extra women per 1000 where combined oestrogen and progesterone therapy is used.

Progestogens – non-contraceptive uses

1 Dysfunctional uterine bleeding (DUB). Cyclical progestogen is used to treat DUB secondary to anovulation. Side effects are mild but may include nausea, fluid retention and weight gain. The COC pill is also useful.

2 Progestogens are also used in the treatment of endometrial carcinoma only if unfit for surgery.

Anti-progestogen

Mifepristone is an anti-progesterone steroid which acts as a competitive antagonist at the progesterone receptor. It is used in termination of pregnancy, where blockage of the progesterone receptor causes endometrial decidual degeneration. It also softens and ripens the cervix and increases the sensitivity of the myometrium to prostaglandins which are then subsequently used to cause contractions of the uterus.

Drugs used to modify the pregnant uterus and cervix

Oxytocin

Mechanism

Oxytocin is a naturally occurring nonapeptide hormone which acts through a G-protein coupled cell surface receptor to stimulate contractions of the uterus. A synthetic version of this hormone is used to induce contractions of the uterus which are indistinguishable from spontaneous labour.

Pharmacokinetics

Oxytocin is administered as a slow intravenous infusion (to induce or augment labour), or as a single intramuscular or intravenous injection to help prevent and treat uterine atony and postpartum haemorrhage. In pregnant women, oxytocin is metabolised very quickly in the maternal circulation by an aminopeptidase enzyme which cleaves the protein leaving it without biological function. This oxytocinase activity is also seen within the placenta and uterine tissue, and activity increases throughout pregnancy where at term the half-life of oxytocin is between 2 and 20 minutes.

Adverse effects

The main side effects are related to overstimulation of the uterus which can compromise the placental blood supply and fetal well-being, and can also contribute to rupture of the uterus especially in women who have had a previous caesarean delivery. Oxytocin is similar in structure to Vasopressin which is also produced by the posterior pituitary, and prolonged administration with intravenous fluids may lead to fluid overload, pulmonary oedema and water intoxication.

Prostaglandins

Mechanism

Prostaglandin (PG) $F_{2\alpha}$, PGE_2 and PGI_2 (prostacyclin) are made endogenously by the uterus. They have a vasoactive role and in addition $PGF_{2\alpha}$ and PGE_2 are involved in cervical relaxation and myometrial contractions of the non-pregnant and pregnant uterus. Four main prostaglandins are used to affect the reproductive system; misoprostol, gemeprost, dinoprostone and carboprost. Prostaglandins are commonly used to stimulate contractions of the myometrium to induce medical termination of pregnancy after pre-treatment with mifepristone (misoprostol vaginal pessary) or to prime the cervix prior to surgical termination of pregnancy (gemeprost vaginal pessary). They are also used for cervical priming in the induction of labour (dinoprostone vaginal pessary) and in the treatment of post-partum haemorrhage (carboprost intramuscular injection).

Pharmacokinetics

Misoprostol is a synthetic PGE1 analogue which is taken orally and is rapidly metabolised to the active free acid. Gemeprost (PGE1 analogue) and dinoprostone (PGE2) are both administered vaginally and release the hormone locally, minimal systemic absorption occurs. Carboprost (PGF2 analogue) is administered as an intramuscular injection and does not require to be metabolised to exert an effect.

Adverse effects

The main side effects are seen in the GI tract; nausea, vomiting, diarrhoea. Others include brochospasm, flushing, fever, headache and in the extreme cardiovascular collapse.

Tocolytics

Pre-term labour (prior to 37 weeks gestation) is associated with high rates of perinatal morbidity and mortality. The aim of tocolysis is to stop uterine contractions, postpone delivery of the infant and additionally allow sufficient time to administer corticosteroids (betamethasone) to promote lung maturation in the baby. However, tocolysis is controversial since there is no clear evidence relating to improved long term outcomes for the child.

Tocolytic methods currently used include:

1 Atociban (oxytocin antagonist) – blocks the stimulatory effect of oxytocin on the myometrium, given as an intravenous infusion. Adverse effects include nausea, tachycardia, hypotension, hot flushes and hyperglycaemia.

2 β_2-adrenoreceptor agonist (ritodrine, salbutamol) – these bind to the β_2-receptor on the myometrial cell membrane, this activates adenylate cyclase, increases the level of cAMP which decreases intracellular calcium thereby leading to relaxation of the uterus. These drugs have the highest adverse effects profile, especially concerning effects on the cardiovascular system (tachycardia, arrhythmias, myocardial ischaemia, vasodilation) and are contra-indicated in those with cardiac disease.

3 Calcium channel blocker – nifedipine (not licenced in UK) – this inhibits the entry of the calcium into the cells through the slow channels in the cell membrane, and thus decreases contractile activity. Nifedipine is primarily used in the treatment of angina and hypertension (predominate effect on vasculature) hence side effects include hypotension and headache.

4 Cyclo-oxygenase inhibitor – indomethacin (not licenced in UK) – this works to reduce the production of prostaglandins thereby reducing uterine contractility. Particular adverse effects of these drugs in pregnancy are the potential neonatal complications including impairment of renal function and premature closure of the ductus arteriosus.

Ovulation induction agents

Anti-oestrogens

Mechanism

Clomiphene (clomifene) and tamoxifen are oestrogen receptor antagonists that prevent negative feedback of oestrogen at the hypothalamus, leading to increased secretion of FSH and LH.

Clinical use and dose

Female subfertility

Clomiphene taken once a day for 5 days starting within 5 days of the onset of menstruation. An important 'side effect' is the increased risk of multiple pregnancy due to multiple ovulation; 7% twins, 0.5% triplets. The association between clomiphene and ovarian cancer is not proven however it is advised that clomiphene should not normally be used for more than six treatment cycles.

Tamoxifen: once a day on days 2, 3, 4, and 5 of the cycle.

Breast cancer

Tamoxifen competes with oestrogen at binding sites on oestrogen-dependent breast tumours in pre-menopausal women. Remission occurs in about 40% of patients (see 'Cytotoxic drugs and cancer chemotherapy', Chapter 15). Tamoxifen can cause hot flushes and uterine bleeding secondary to endometrial hyperplasia.

Metformin

Metformin is a biguanide and exerts its effect mainly by decreasing gluconeogenesis and by increasing peripheral utilisation of glucose. Metformin use in obese insulin-resistant women with polycystic ovarian syndrome (PCOS) have shown significant improvements in insulin sensitivity and hyperinsulinaemia. The use of metformin in women with PCOS has also been shown to improve ovulation, however, pregnancy rates with metformin alone are no higher than with placebo. Additionally, the response to clomiphene is not enhanced by concomitant use of metformin in the majority of women.

Danazol

Mechanism

Danazol inhibits pituitary gonadotrophin release, thereby reducing ovarian function and producing atrophy of the endometrium. It also blocks oestrogen and progesterone receptors but has some androgenic activity.

Adverse effects

Avoid danazol during pregnancy; virilisation of female fetus has been reported. Danazol is not an effective contraceptive and non-hormonal methods should be used during treatment. Acne, hirsutism and voice changes occasionally occur.

Drug interactions

Danazol potentiates the action of carbamazepine and anticoagulants.

Clinical use

Endometriosis, menorrhagia and pain from benign fibrocystic breast disease.

Gonadotrophin-releasing hormone analogues

Mechanism

Gonadotrophin-releasing hormone (GnRH) is a decapeptide and was isolated and characterised in 1971. GnRH analogues are produced by altering the amino acids in positions 6 and/or 10, resulting in compounds with high affinity for the GnRH receptor, and a long half-life as a result of their resistance to cleavage by endopeptidases. After an initial brief stimulation, the GnRH analogues paradoxically result in the suppression of the pituitary, a decrease in FSH and LH levels and a subsequent suppression of ovarian function to menopausal levels. Their short-term use is of proven benefit in assisted reproduction and prior to endometrial resection or ablation. Long-term applications range from shrinking fibroids before surgery to the management of endometriosis, oestrogen receptor positive breast cancer and prostate cancer.

Adverse effects

The main disadvantages of GnRH analogues are related to induced hypo-oestrogenic state of a pseudomenopause, thus vasomotor 'hot flushes', vaginal dryness, and reduction in bone mineral density occur in these women. Add-back HRT using oestrogens, progestogens or both may be used to negate their side-effects.

Anti-androgens

Cyproterone acetate is a progestogen with antagonist properties at the androgen receptor. It can be used in low dose (2 mg) as part of a COC (Dianette) in the treatment of hirsutism or severe acne in women which is refractive to oral antibacterials. It has a high risk of VTE, and it should not be used solely as a contraceptive. If used, it should be discontinued 3–4 months after symptoms have improved or resolved. Higher doses (50 mg/day) can also be administered where more effective anti-androgen actions are required, for example in prostate cancer (Chapter 14).

Chapter 14

Drugs and the urological system

Drugs for bladder outlet obstruction

Clinical scenario

A 70-year-old male presents with a several-year history of worsening lower urinary tract symptoms (LUTS: reduction in urinary flow, hesitancy and nocturia). His past medical history is unremarkable. Serum PSA (Prostate Specific Antigen) is within the normal range. Rectal examination reveals an enlarged benign-feeling prostate (~60 gm in size). Clinical diagnosis of benign prostatic enlargement (BPE) is made. What drugs can be used to treat this condition?

Adrenergic alpha-antagonists (alpha-blockers)

Mechanism

Alpha-blockers (tamsulosin, alfuzosin, terazocin, doxazosin) remain the first line drug treatment of bladder outlet obstruction (BOO) secondary to BPE. Historically, they are believed to prevent noradrenaline release from the prostate smooth muscle cells by blockade of alpha-adrenoceptors, leading to reduced prostate tone and improved urinary flow. Prostatic contraction is mediated

predominantly, if not exclusively, by alpha-1 A-adrenoreceptors, and agents selective for this receptor isotype (tamsulosin, 400 µg daily) have better tolerability (but not efficacy) profile. More recently, extra-prostatic action antagonism of alpha-1 A-adrenoceptors (and other subtypes) in the bladder and spinal cord is thought to contribute to the rapid relief of LUTS following commencement of alpha-blockers.

Adverse effects

The side-effect profile of these agents relate to their action on alpha-adrenoreceptors in blood vessels, non-prostatic smooth muscle cells and central nervous system: nasal congestion, orthostatic (postural) hypotension, tachycardia, palpitations, dizziness, anxiety and retrograde ejaculation. These drugs should be used with caution in patients on antihypertensive agents, who are particularly susceptible to vasodilatory side effects. Treatment should be stopped prior to cataract surgery to reduce risk of intraoperative floppy iris syndrome.

5-alpha-reductase inhibitors

Mechanism

The two isotypes (1 and 2) of 5-α reductase convert testosterone to its active metabolite dihydrotestosterone (DHT), which potently activates the androgen receptor (AR) (Fig. 14.1). Inhibition

Lecture Notes: Clinical Pharmacology and Therapeutics, 8th edition. By Gerard McKay, John Reid and Matthew Walters. Published 2010 by Blackwell Publishing Ltd.

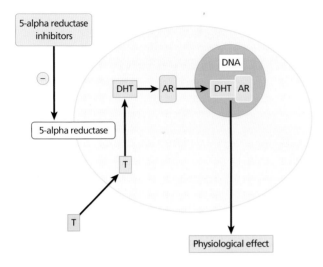

Figure 14.1 Mechanism of action – 5-alpha reductase inhibitors. In most target cells, 5-alpha-reductase converts testosterone (T) into the active metabolite dihydrotestosterone (DHT), which potently activates the androgen receptor (AR) leading to modified gene transcription and physiological influence upon secondary sex organs. Such conversion is blocked by 5-alpha-reductase inhibitors used in treatment of benign prostatic enlargement (BPE).

of the 5-alpha-reductase enzyme (finasteride 5 mg daily and dutasteride 500 μg daily) and can shrink prostate size by approximately 20%. Finasteride inhibits only one 5-alpha-reductase isotype; however dutasteride inhibits both with a similar potency and is believed to have a more rapid onset of action. Combination treatment with alpha-blockers is useful when the prostate is significantly enlarged. 5-α-reductase inhibitors also reduce bleeding during transurethral prostate surgery and may protect against prostate cancer.

Adverse effects

5-α-reductase inhibitors affect sexual function: loss of libido, impotence and abnormal ejaculation. Serum PSA levels are reduced by approximately 50%, an important consideration in the diagnosis of prostate cancer (PCa).

Drugs for overactive bladder

Clinical scenario

A 55-year-old female has a 2-year history of urinary frequency, urgency and urge incontinence. There is no history of urinary tract infections. Cystoscopy and ultrasound scan are normal. A diagnosis of over active bladder (OAB) is made. What drugs can be used to treat this condition?

Anti-cholinergic agents

Mechanism

The anti-cholinergic agents for OAB are competitive inhibitors of muscarinic acetylcholine receptors (mAchR) in the bladder. There are 5 mAchR isotypes (M1-M5) with different tissue specificities and functions, which include acting as the main end-receptor stimulated by acetylcholine released from postganglionic fibers in the parasympathetic nervous system. M2 is the most common receptor isotype within the detrusor muscle, although M3 seems to be functionally important for micturition. mChR blockade results in a reduction in detrusor overactivity, although the exact site and mechanism of action of anti-muscarinic agents for OAB is not fully understood. There are a number of agents available (tolterodine-L-tartrate, solfenacin and darifenacin) and some (oxybutinin) in immediate-release, modified-release, or topical preparations.

Adverse effects

Side effects results from extra-vesical anti-cholinergic actions and include dry mouth, blurred vision, constipation and drowsiness, which can reduce compliance. Anti-cholinergics are contraindicated in patients with closed

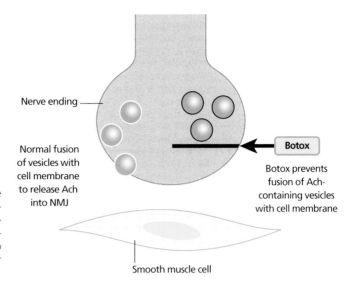

Figure 14.2 Action of Botox at the neuromuscular junction. Botox prevents fusion of acetylcholine (Ach)-containing vesicles with the cell membrane, blocking signal transmission to smooth muscle at the neuromuscular junction (NMJ).

Nerve ending

Normal fusion of vesicles with cell membrane to release Ach into NMJ

Botox

Botox prevents fusion of Ach-containing vesicles with cell membrane

Smooth muscle cell

angle glaucoma, hepatic dysfunction and renal failure. Solfenacin is metabolised in the liver by cytochrome P450 and should not be used in high doses where taken with a cytochrome P450 inhibitor. Solfenacin can also cause a prolonged QT interval.

Others

Botox (by direct injection during cystoscopy), a neurotoxic protein derived from *Clostridium botulinum*, blocks transmission at the neuromuscular junction by preventing anchoring of acetylcholine-containing vesicles to the cell membrane (Fig. 14.2). This induces flaccid muscle paralysis and dampening of detrusor muscle contractions. The initial success rate is high, but has a tendency to fall over two years. Side effects are rare, although there is a theoretical risk of systemic paralysis.

Drugs for prostate cancer

Clinical scenario

An 80-year-old male is referred with a history of urinary frequency, reduced urinary flow, nocturia and back pain. Serum PSA is 398 ng/mL. Rectal examination reveals a hard craggy (irregular) prostate. A diagnosis of prostate cancer (PCa) is made. What drugs can be used to treat this disease?

Hormone (androgen deprivation) therapy

Manipulation of the hypothalamic-pituitary-gonadal axis (Fig. 14.3) via androgen deprivation therapy (ADT) remains the treatment of choice in advanced PCa. ADT is achieved by (i) intramuscular depot injection with Gonadotrophin-releasing hormone (GnRH) analogues, (ii) surgical castration (bilateral subcapsular orchidectomy) and (iii) anti-androgens (directly blocking androgen receptor function) can be used either alone or in conjunction with GnRH analogues (short term to prevent tumour flare and long term to achieve maximal androgen blockage).

Anti-androgens

Mechanism

Anti-androgens are classified as either steroidal (cyproterone acetate) or non-steroidal (flutamide, nilutamide and bicalutamide). Both agents act by competitive binding to the androgen receptor (AR) and suppress AR-mediated gene

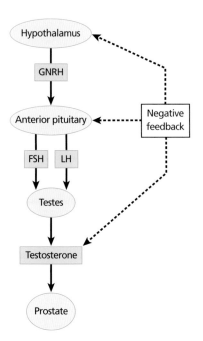

Figure 14.3 Hypothalamic-pituitary-gonadal axis. Hormonal control of the male reproductive system manipulated in treatment of prostate cancer (PCa) by androgen deprivation therapy (ADT). GnRH, gonadotrophin-releasing hormone; FSH, follicle stimulating hormone; LH, leuteinising hormone.

expression. Cyproterone acetate, derived from 17-hydroxyprogesterone, also acts on AR in the pituitary, suppressing luteinising hormone (LH)-dependent production of androgens.

Adverse effects

The main disadvantages are secondary to anti-androgenic actions and include breast tenderness, gynaecomastia, galactorrhoea, erectile dysfunction and depression. Cyproterone acetate can cause liver toxicity especially in high doses, and liver function should be monitored. Non-steroidal anti-androgens may cause gastrointestinal upset and liver dysfunction. In some PCa cells, AR genetic mutations result in anti-androgens having a paradoxically stimulatory effect on tumour growth. In such cases, withdrawal of treatment results in a reduction in cancer growth.

Gonadotrophin-releasing hormone analogues

Mechanism

Gonadotrophin-releasing hormone (GnRH), also known as luteinising-hormone releasing hormone (LHRH), is a tropic decapeptide hormone. It was isolated and characterised by Guillemin and Schally in the 1970s. Since endogenous GnRH has a short half-life due to cleavage by endopeptidases, GnRH analogues (goserelin, leuprorelin, buserelin) have been synthesised by altering the amino acids in positions 6 and/or 10, resulting in a high affinity for the GnRH receptor and a long half-life as a result of endopeptidase resistance. After an initial brief stimulation of androgen production ('flare' effect), GnRH analogues paradoxically result in the suppression gonadotropin secretion and androgen production ('downregulation') after about 10 days. While this phase is reversible it can be maintained with further GnRH agonist use for a long time.

Adverse effects

The main disadvantages are secondary to the induced hypo-oestrogenic state, including hot flushes, osteoporosis, fatigue as well as loss of libido and impotence. The initial androgen 'flare' should be covered by use of anti-androgens to prevent worsening of symptoms from metastatic disease such as bone pain.

Oestrogens

Oestrogens (ethinyl oestradiol) were once the main alternative to orchidectomy for men with advanced PCa, however have been largely replaced by GnRH analogues. They may have a role in patients with failed ADT. Side effects include venous thromboembolic and cardiovascular disease.

Other agents

Chemotherapeutic agents are used for the treatment of PCa where ADT has failed (hormone/castrate resistant prostate cancer). Anti-mitotic agents (docetaxol, paclitaxel) induce arrest of cell division by acting on microtubules within normal and cancer cells. Type II topoisomerase inhibitors (mitroxantone) disrupt separation of replicating DNA strands and prevent cell division.

Drugs for erectile dysfunction

Clinical scenario

A 55-year-old man is referred with a 2-year history of inability to maintain erections for sexual intercourse. His past medical history includes hypertension and type 2 diabetes mellitus, and he takes atenolol, lisinopril and aspirin. A diagnosis of erectile dysfunction is made. What drugs can be used to treat his condition?

Phosphodiesterase inhibitors

Mechanism

The final common pathway for sexual arousal and stimulation leading to erection is the production of cyclic guanosine monophosphate (cGMP) in cavernosal tissues, which results in smooth muscle relaxation, vasodilatation and subsequent engorgement of the corpora with blood leading to penile erection (Fig. 14.4). Phosphodiesterase inhibitors (sildenafil, tadalafil and vardenafil) inhibit cGMP-specific phosphodiesterase type 5, the isoenzyme responsible for the breakdown of cGMP in the corpus cavernosum. PDE5 inhibitors improve the rigidity and the number of erections in men with erectile dysfunction. Intracavernosal PDE inhibitors (papaverine) are thought to be more effective in cases of psychogenic or neurological impotence than that attributable to vascular aetiology.

Adverse effects

The most common side effects are headache, flushing, dyspepsia, nasal congestion and transient colour blindness. A potentially dangerous interaction caused by the potentiation of the haemodynamic effect of nitrates, is hypotension.

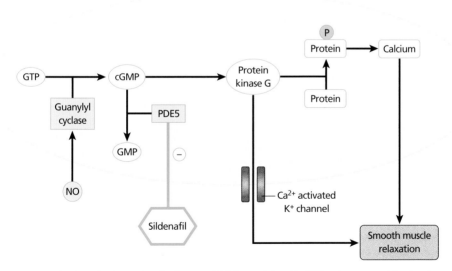

Figure 14.4 Mechanism of action – phosphodiesterase inhibitors. Nitric oxide (NO) activates guanylyl cyclase in cavernosal smooth muscle cells, causing conversion of guanosine triphosphate (GTP) to cyclic guanosine monophosphate (cGMP) and in turn activation of protein kinase G. Activated protein kinase G opens calcium-activated potassium-channels in the cell membrane resulting in smooth muscle relaxation, vasodilatation and engorgement. Phosphodiesterase inhibitors block phosphodiesterase-type 5 (PDE5) and prevent hydrolysis of cGMP to guanosine monophosphate (GMP), resulting in protein kinase G accretion.

This contraindication is important since erectile dysfunction is commonly associated with cardio-vascular disease, but also because amyl nitrates ('poppers') are recreational drugs of misuse.

Intracavernosal prostaglandins

Mechanism

Intracavernosal therapy (self-injected a maximum of three times per week) is effective in providing adequate erections within ten minutes of admin-istration. Prostaglandin E1 causes improves penile blood flow by vasodilatation and is given by intra-cavernosal injection or intraurethral suppository. Some preparations also include papaverine.

Adverse effects

Pain associated with intracavernosal injections result in poor compliance. Priapism and penile fibrosis have been reported following use of these agents.

Chapter 15

Cancer therapeutics

Clinical scenario

A 40-year-old man presented with swelling of his right testicle. Human chorionic gonadotrophin (HCG) was elevated. The patient underwent right orchidectomy and histological examination confirmed a diagnosis of malignant teratoma undifferentiated (MTU). A post-operative CT scan revealed two para-aortic lymph nodes measuring 14 mm and 12 mm respectively. Repeat HCG performed 4 weeks post-operatively had risen and on physical examination the man was found to have a 4-cm left supraclavicular fossa lymph node. How should this patient be treated?

Key points

Drug therapy can be used in cancer as:
- Radical treatment to cure disease
- Adjuvant treatment post surgery or radiotherapy
- Neo-adjuvent treatment to enable radical treatment with surgery or radiotherapy
- Palliative treatment to control symptoms

Introduction

Surgery, radiotherapy and drug therapy are the three main treatment options considered when a treatment plan is formulated for patients un-

Lecture Notes: Clinical Pharmacology and Therapeutics, 8th edition. By Gerard McKay, John Reid and Matthew Walters. Published 2010 by Blackwell Publishing Ltd.

dergoing active management of their cancer. The treatment aims are:

1 Eradicate the disease: cure the patient.

2 If eradication is not possible then control the disease: induce a remission and prolong survival.

3 If neither cure nor remission is possible, then control symptoms.

The drug therapies used to treat cancer can be classified as:

1 Chemotherapy

2 Hormone therapy

3 Biological therapy

In addition many supportive care strategies are used to control cancer related symptoms such as pain, nausea, vomiting, anorexia, bowel obstruction, raised intracranial pressure etc. These strategies are aimed at treating symptoms rather than treating the cancer directly and are beyond the scope of this chapter.

Chemotherapy

In most situations, the drugs used to treat cancer are cytotoxic agents, i.e. drugs that kill dividing cells (commonly referred to as chemotherapy). There are roughly 30–40 standard chemotherapeutic agents in common usage. They selectively damage cells that are rapidly dividing. Since tumour cells are normally in a state of rapid division, this explains the ability of these agents to reduce tumour growth and in some cases bring about tumour shrinkage. Some normal cells in the body are also dividing rapidly (for example bone marrow, gut epithelium and hair follicles). These cells are also killed by cytotoxics, which results in chemotherapy toxicity. The aim is to kill more cancer cells than normal cells. This is called the 'therapeutic window' due to the cancer cells being more sensitive to cytotoxics than the normal cells. This therapeutic window exists because:

• Cancer cells tend to be cycling more quickly than most normal cells, and are thus more susceptible to toxic agents.

• Cancer cells by their very nature have abnormal growth regulatory pathways. This makes them less able to withstand cytotoxics, and perhaps more importantly, less able to repair themselves than normal cells after exposure to cytotoxic agents.

• Some cytotoxics specifically target pathways or enzymes that are more active in cancer cells than normal cells.

Unfortunately, this therapeutic window is narrow. A way of widening it is to give the drugs repeatedly. Therefore a dose that the normal tissues (bone marrow) can recover from is administered. Just when they have recovered, another dose of chemotherapy is delivered before the cancer cells have fully recovered from the original insult.

Relevant pathophysiology

Chemotherapy, or the use of drugs in the management of cancer, was introduced in the 1890s with non-specific cell poisons. More specific agents became available with the discovery in the 1940s of nitrogen mustard, an alkylating agent, and methotrexate, an antimetabolite.

Treatment was initially restricted to patients with leukaemia and lymphomas, but then extended to drugs that are used in patients with solid tumours. Considerable progress has been made towards curative treatment of some of the childhood cancers and rarer solid tumours. Nevertheless, there are still many forms of cancer that are difficult to treat with chemotherapy. In order to obtain maximum therapeutic benefit, it is important to clearly define the aims of therapy at the outset. This often dictates the choice and duration of therapy. It may also dictate what potential adverse effects may be acceptable to patients.

Chemotherapy represents only one component of cancer management. Typically and historically, surgery has been the primary treatment modality. It is used to locally remove tumour that can be seen. Radiotherapy can also be used as primary treatment, without surgery (e.g. head and neck cancer), but more typically is used after surgery to control disease locally that cannot be seen.

Drug therapy is used in patients with cancer to:

1 Eradicate macroscopic disease: primary radical treatment (lymphoma and teratoma).

2 Eradicate microscopic disease: adjuvant treatment. Chemotherapy after surgery or radiotherapy, used to eradicate microscopic disease and increase statistical chance of cure. Adjuvant treatment significantly prolongs survival for certain groups of patients with early breast, bowel and lung cancer (Table 15.1).

3 Facilitate radical treatment: neo-adjuvant treatment. Chemotherapy before surgery or

Neo-adjuvant	Adjuvant	In combination with radiotherapy
Oesophagus	Colon	Cervix
Nasopharynx	Breast	Head and neck
Bladder	Non-small-cell lung	Oesophagus
Locally advanced breast	Ovarian	Small-cell lung
		Rectal
		Anal

Table 15.1 Chemotherapy as part of combined modality treatment of primary tumours.

Table 15.2 Chemotherapy for the management of metastatic cancer.

Curative	Prolongs survival	Useful palliation	Benefit unlikely
Testis	Ovary	Pancreas	Melanoma
Lymphoma	Small-cell lung	Cervix	Renal
Acute leukaemia	Chronic leukaemia	Head and neck	Mesothelioma
Certain childhood cancers	Myeloma	Brain: glioma	
Choriocarcinoma	Breast		
	Colon/rectum		
	Bladder		
	Non-small-cell lung		

*Although labelled as prolonging survival a small percentage of small cell lung cancers and advanced ovarian cancers are cured by chemotherapy. Additionally adjuvant chemotherapy for breast and colorectal cancer increases the percentage of patients surviving disease-free long term so although not curing the cancer as an individual treatment modality they do increase the cure rate as part of a treatment plan that also incorporates surgery.

radiotherapy to enable the radical treatment (bladder/breast/oesophageal cancer).

4 Control disease: palliative treatment: To improve survival, control symptoms and improve quality of life (most tumour types) (Table 15.2).

Patient selection

It is not always possible, appropriate or sensible to treat all patients with cytotoxics even if they have an indication for treatment. Other considerations may affect drug selection or schedule. Physiological (as opposed to chronological) age is important; however, performance status is often the most significant factor. Dose is often calculated according to body surface area. Obesity can affect planned doses as body surface area in obese patients is a less good marker for their ability to metabolise and excrete the drug. Previous chemotherapy can affect the body's capacity to tolerate further treatment. End organ function may preclude the use of certain drugs. Kidney, hepatic, bone marrow, cardiac or lung function must be checked prior to certain drugs.

Principles of drug treatment

Although cytotoxics can be given as single agents, it is more common to use a combination of two to six drugs (see below). With a few important exceptions, combinations of drugs are more effective than single agents. Drug resistance is less likely to arise when drugs with different mechanisms of action are used in combination. In addition, by using agents with different toxicities, their effects on the tumour can be additive without any individual toxicity being significantly increased. In a palliative setting, it is often more appropriate, when quality of life issues are more pressing, to use a sequence of single-agent drugs.

Most drug combinations have been developed empirically. Typically, they would have complimentary mechanisms of cytotoxicity disrupting a different point in the cell cycle or DNA synthesis. They would have different dose-limiting side effects: one might be highly myelosuppressive and the other neurotoxic so as to maximise their synergistic action. Using together two drugs that are both highly myelosuppressive means it is unlikely that they can be used at an adequate dose or frequency. When treating tumours with the aim of cure, be it in the radical or adjuvant setting, it is very important to attempt to maintain dose intensity (the frequency of administration of the chemotherapy).

Myelosuppression is the commonest dose-limiting toxicity of most cytotoxic agents. When chemotherapy is given at standard doses, treatment is usually given intermittently as pulses administered at 3- to 4-weekly intervals, allowing time for marrow recovery. The co-administration of haemopoetic growth factors (e.g. granulocyte colony-stimulating factor [G-CSF]) allows drugs to be given at significantly higher doses, or more frequently, by reducing the risk of significant neutropenia. Unfortunately, there is little evidence outwith haematolological malignancies that this approach improves outcomes and so the place of growth factors in routine practice is not established.

Much higher doses of drugs such as cyclophosphamide, melphalan, etoposide and carboplatin have been used with the aim of eliminating the tumour completely. These high-dose chemotherapy regimens result in eradication of all the bone marrow's progenitor stem cells and so the patient must be rescued from total bone marrow failure by bone marrow transplantation or peripheral blood stem cell transfusion. Such treatment is used in the management of leukaemias and lymphomas. Trials into such treatment in solid tumours have so far been disappointing. When giving high-dose chemotherapy, it is essential that supportive measures, such as platelet transfusions, are available to deal with marrow failure, infection and bleeding.

Measurement of plasma concentrations (therapeutic drug monitoring) allows administration of agents at doses that could otherwise be lethal, e.g. methotrexate. Methotrexate is a potent but reversible inhibitor of the enzyme dihydrofolate reductase, a key enzyme for DNA synthesis. Enzyme inhibition and the toxic effects of methotrexate can be reversed by the subsequent administration of folinic acid. It is possible to give methotrexate in doses of 100–1000 times those used previously, to measure plasma methotrexate levels and to calculate the amount of folinic acid required for 'rescue'. This method of treatment may be of considerable therapeutic value in some situations.

Cytotoxics are mostly given intravenously; occasionally they are given orally (e.g. capecitabine, cyclophosphamide, etoposide) and rarely they can be given in other ways:

1 Intrathecally, to achieve effective concentration in the cerebrospinal fluid (e.g. intrathecal methotrexate for CNS leukaemia). Most drugs do not readily cross the blood–brain barrier. It is important to note that if the wrong chemotherapy is administered intrathecally this can have rapidly fatal consequences for the patient.

2 Intra-arterially into a limb, the head and neck or the liver (e.g isolated limb perfusion in the treatment of melanoma).

3 Intraperitoneally or intrapleurally to increase the local concentration of drug, particularly where rapidly accumulating ascites or pleural effusions present clinical problems (e.g. intraperitoneal cisplatin in the treatment of ovarian cancer).

4 Topically onto lesions of the skin, vagina or buccal mucosa (e.g. topical miltefosine for cutaneous breast cancer lesions).

If a drug requires metabolic activation by the liver, e.g. cyclophosphamide or azathioprine, it is of little value to administer it locally, intraperitoneally or intrathecally.

Chemotherapeutic agents

The majority of chemotherapy drugs act by interfering with the synthesis and replication of DNA. The molecular basis of action of some widely used agents is shown in Fig. 15.1. They can be classified as follows:

1 *Alkylating agents*. These include drugs such as nitrogen mustard, cyclophosphamide, chlorambucil and melphalan. These are highly reactive molecules when activated and bind irreversibly to macromolecules in the cell, notably DNA, RNA and proteins, thus disrupting normal growth.

2 *Antimetabolites*. These are analogues of the normal components of metabolism or DNA synthesis. They are taken up into the normal synthetic process, but then inhibit its continued normal function. These can be split into three classes: antifolates, pyrimidine analogues and purine analogues. Methotrexate inhibits folic acid metabolism, and the nucleotides (5-fluorouracil, gemcitabine, cytosine arabinoside, 6-mercaptopurine) inhibit DNA synthesis.

3 *Natural products*. A wide range of drugs has been developed from plants, bacteria, yeasts and fungi. Others inhibit DNA synthesis through intercalation into the helix itself.

- Mitosis inhibitors: During mitosis, spindles develop between the poles of the two potential

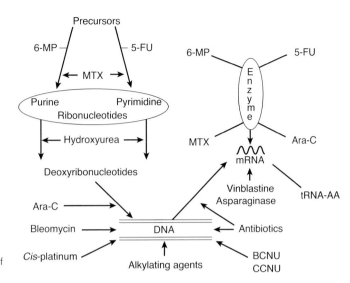

Figure 15.1 Mechanism of action of cytotoxic drugs.

new nuclei. The chromosomes move along these spindles. Stopping either spindle formation or, perhaps less obviously, their normal breakdown will prevent two new daughter cells developing during mitosis. The vinca alkaloids (vincristine, vinblastine and vindesine) stop the mitotic spindle developing. The taxanes (taxol and taxotere) inhibit mitosis by stabilising the spindle and preventing its normal breakdown.

• Topoisomerase enzyme inhibitors: These enzymes are involved in the unbinding and loosening of the DNA supercoiled double helix, as well as the cutting of DNA strands to enable access into the DNA of the enzymes required for normal DNA replication. Part of these enzymes' normal function is to cause single- or double-strand DNA breaks. Drugs that stall or disrupt this process will leave DNA uncoiled and with DNA breaks. Topoisomerase 1 and topoisomerase 2 inhibitors disrupt this process in slightly different ways. Examples of these drugs are:

  ○ Topoisomerase 1 inhibitors – the camptothecins: topotecan and irinotecan

  ○ Topoisomerase 2 inhibitors – the podophyllotoxins: etoposide and teniposide

  ○ Anthracyclines, such as doxorubicin, epirubicin and daunorubicin, intercalate into DNA and also form highly reactive free radicals.

This disrupts normal DNA synthesis. However, their principal action appears to be as inhibitors of the enzyme topoisomerase 2.

  ○ Antitumour antibiotics: Bleomycin binds to DNA to cause DNA strand breaks and may also form free radicals. Actinomycin D binds to DNA to inhibit RNA transcription.

4 *Others*. Several drugs have been identified, often by random synthesis and screening, whose mechanism of action is not fully established but are thought to interact with DNA synthesis or replication. They include the hydroxycarbamide (hydroxyurea), dacarbazine, procarbazine, cisplatin and its analogue carboplatin.

5 *Steroid hormones*. These are widely used in cancer management. They are particularly cytotoxic against lymphoid tumours but are also used in the treatment of symptoms such as anorexia and vomiting. The drug most commonly used is prednisolone.

Pharmacokinetics

Pharmacokinetic aspects of cytotoxic drugs may present drug-specific or general problems. Most cytotoxic drugs have a narrow therapeutic index: they are active only at doses close to those causing significant toxicity. This makes the administration of cytotoxics potentially lethal. The initial dose is

209

typically not the same for all patients as is the case in most other clinical scenarios (i.e. antihypertensives or antibiotics), but rather is based on body surface area (mg/m^2), calculated from the patient's height and weight. This is a concept derived from animal studies.

Individuals' normal enzyme systems function at different levels; this is called pharmacogenetics. So even in ideal circumstances, individual response to drugs may vary considerably. Some drugs are inactive on administration, but are activated in the liver or in the tumour. Cyclophosphamide is converted to an active metabolite in the liver.. If an individual's normal level of this enzyme is low, then very little of the pro-drug may be converted to active drug, thus making the process ineffective. Alternatively, body enzymes may inactivate the active drug. Drugs such as doxorubicin and vincristine are predominantly excreted via the biliary tract. In the presence of hepatic impairment, dose reduction of these drugs is recommended. Even with normal liver function, variable pharmogenetics means that active drug may be in the body longer than expected, leading to greater toxicity (e.g. patients with particular polymorphisms of the UGT1A1 gene have decreased metabolism of SN-38, the active metabolite of the drug irinotecan). Some cytotoxic drugs (cisplatin, carboplatin and methotrexate) are excreted unchanged by the kidney. When using these drugs in patients with renal impairment, dose modification is important.

There are other clinical pharmacokinetic problems with cytotoxic drugs:

1 The problem of the 'third space'. Many patients with cancer have pleural effusions or ascites. Administration of a cytotoxic drug to such a patient may result in the sequestration of the drug into this compartment, with slow release back into the circulation. This may aggravate toxicity, most classically seen with methotrexate.

2 Sanctuary sites. Often cancer can be considered to be a systemic disease. It is therefore essential that the administered drug reaches all parts of the body. Most drugs do not cross the blood–brain barrier, certainly not to therapeutic levels, and therefore may not act on tumour cells in the brain. Patients with small-cell lung cancer who respond well to chemotherapy will receive prophylactic whole-brain radiotherapy to reduce the risk of relapse in this site (and improve the chances of overall survival). Another important sanctuary site appears to be the testes; lymphomas in particular may relapse there. Clinically, perhaps the most important sanctuary site in a large tumour is the core of the tumour itself where there is poor blood supply into which the drug cannot adequately penetrate. In teratoma, an exquisitely chemosensitive disease, any residual mass post-chemotherapy will be removed surgically.

Adverse effects

Reactions to chemotherapy are secondary to cell death both in the tumour and in other rapidly dividing cells of bone marrow, gastrointestinal tract, germinal epithelium, etc. These can be divided into:

1 General adverse reactions to chemotherapy
2 Specific adverse reactions to individual agents.

General adverse reactions

1 Nausea and vomiting may be severe with many, although not all, drugs and are related to the direct actions of cytotoxic drugs on the chemoreceptor trigger zone (see 'Nausea and vomiting', Chapter 3). Anticipatory vomiting can, rarely, be a problem in patients after repeated treatments. The selective 5HT$_3$ receptor antagonists often in combination with steroids are highly effective in preventing acute emesis.

2 Alopecia is a common adverse effect of some, but not all, cytotoxic drugs. Hair re-grows after the course of chemotherapy has been completed.

3 Hyperuricaemia, with precipitation of clinical gout or renal failure, may complicate the treatment of highly chemosensitive tumours when there is rapid tumour lysis, e.g. leukaemias and lymphomas. Allopurinol, the xanthine oxidase inhibitor, may be used to prevent gout (Chapter 9) but care should be taken when azathioprine or mercaptopurine are given at the same time (see 'Drug interactions' below).

4 The gastrointestinal tract from mouth to anus has a fast turnover and thus can be susceptible to

side effects. Mucositis can occur with some drugs, causing ulceration in the mouth or oesophagus. When there is co-existent neutropenia, there is increased risk of opportunistic infections: thrush, indigestion, abdominal cramps and diarrhoea all may occur.

5 Bone marrow suppression. The bone marrow is particularly sensitive to many cytotoxic drugs (see 'Anticoagulant drugs', Chapter 14). Neutropenia is common, and opportunistic infections occur as a result of impaired humoral and cell-mediated responses. Unusual infection with fungi and protozoa, in addition to more common pathogenic bacteria and viruses, may occur. Thrombocytopenia may result in an increased risk of haemorrhage.

6 Neuropathy. Typically, the greatest effect is on the longest nerves, and thus peripheral neuropathy can occur. Classically with cisplatin and the spindle poisons (taxanes and vinca alkaloids). Most common effects are sensory, but can be motor and autonomic.

7 Infertility. Many cytotoxics cause sterility; this must be discussed prior to starting treatment and appropriate action undertaken. Conversely, treatment with chemotherapy is not a guarantee of birth control.

8 Secondary cancers. The incidence of this is hotly debated, but certainly is a real effect. Typically, they occur 10–15 years after treatment. The risks vary between agents but are the highest with alkylating agents.

Specific adverse reactions

Some of the side effects of chemotherapy have a specific pharmacological basis. Haemorrhagic cystitis with cyclophosphamide is a consequence of urinary excretion of the irritant metabolites, e.g. acrolein. Maintaining a high-fluid output can prevent this or by giving the drug mesna (mercaptoethone sulphonate) that conjugates these metabolites to promote safe excretion.

Drug interactions

Drug interactions may occur between cytotoxics but more important are interactions with non-cytotoxic agents.

Methotrexate and salicylates

As methotrexate is highly protein bound, it is readily displaced from the binding site by aspirin and other salicylates. This may increase the risk of adverse effects of methotrexate. Other acidic drugs that are highly protein bound may show similar effects.

6-Mercaptopurine and allopurinol

These two drugs are frequently used together. Allopurinol is a competitive inhibitor of xanthine oxidase (see 'Drugs used in gout', Chapter 9) and also inhibits the breakdown of 6-mercaptopurine. The dose of 6-mercaptopurine must be halved at least or toxicity ensues. Azathioprine, which is metabolised to 6-mercaptopurine, should also be given in lower doses if used with allopurinol.

Procarbazine and alcohol

Hot flushing may occur and patients should be warned of this before treatment. Procarbazine is a monoamine oxidase inhibitor, and tyramine-containing foods should be avoided (see 'Mood stabilising agents', Chapter 16).

Comment. Physicians who have experience and facilities for managing malignant disease and the problems associated with chemotherapy should give cytotoxic drugs. Haemorrhage and opportunistic infections secondary to marrow and immune suppression may shorten life rather than prolong it if they are not aggressively managed.

Hormone therapy

Oestrogens, progestogens and testosterone

Surgical removal of endocrine organs, such as the ovaries, testes, adrenals and pituitary gland, has been used for many years in the treatment of breast and prostatic cancer. These are tissues that are normally under some hormonal control. Treatment with hormones, hormone antagonists or drugs that inhibit hormone production aims to achieve the same effect by changing the hormonal environment. Hormonal effects are mediated by receptors on the cell surface or within the cell. These receptors, notably oestrogen and progesterone receptors, can be identified within tumours and allow a prediction of the response to endocrine manipulation in breast cancer. Patients whose breast cancer contains oestrogen receptors are treated with hormonal therapies. Patients whose tumour has neither oestrogen nor progesterone receptors do not receive hormonal therapies. Hormone therapy is also used (although to a lesser extent) in the treatment of relapsed ovarian cancer (tamoxifen or aromatase inhibitors), recurrent or advanced endometrial cancer (medroxyprogesterone acetate) and rare tumours such as endometrial stromal sarcomas (aromatase inhibitors). A number of different hormonal treatment strategies exist:

1 *Stop gonadal hormone production*

Ovarian or testicular ablation using surgery or radiotherapy.

2 *Stop hormone production*

LHRH (luetinising hormone-releasing hormone) agonists: Goserelin or leuprorelin. This results in the down-regulation of the hypothalamus pituitary axis.

Aromatase inhibitors: These block the production of oestrogen in the adrenals and body fat and are used in post-menopausal women only.

3 *Block the action of the hormone on hormone receptors*

SERMs (selective oestrogen receptor modifiers): Tamoxifen is widely used as an adjuvant treatment in breast cancer.

Anti-androgens: flutamide, cyproterone.

4 *Cause degradation of the hormone receptors*

Fulvestrant.

In metastatic breast and prostate cancer, first-line hormone therapies have a median duration of action of roughly 18 months.

Glucocorticoids

The corticosteroids cortisol, hydrocortisone and prednisolone are used with other drug combinations in the management of leukaemia and lymphomas. Dexamethasone is used in the management of raised intracranial pressure associated with intracerebral primary or secondary tumours, and is also a useful anti-emetic agent, often in combination with other agents.

Steroids can also be useful in stimulating appetite in patients with advanced cancer. Progestogens can also be used in this way and to improve the quality of life.

Biological therapy

Recently, there has been huge interest in the development of biological agents, which are the therapeutic fruits of 40 years of basic science research into the molecular aetiology of cancer. Rather than blindly killing rapidly dividing cancer cells these agents specifically target molecular anomalies in signal transduction pathways that exist in tumour cells (see Fig. 15.2). The molecular anomalies will differ from tumour to tumour, even within a specific cancer type. Therefore molecular testing to identify patients suitable for a particular biological therapy is crucial. As biological agents target pathways which are more critical to cancer cells than normal cells they are generally less toxic than chemotherapy and in some cases more effective (e.g. imatinib mesylate as a treatment for chronic myeloid leukaemia or gastrointestinal stromal tumours). Some cancers become highly dependent on a particular molecular pathway. This is known as oncogene addiction. Targetting of these pathways to which a cancer is so dependent (known as synthetic lethality) appears to be a particularly effective strategy and is currently being exhaustively researched.

There are a myriad of signal transduction or DNA repair pathways that are currently being targeted with therapeutic intent. For the most part therapies are either monoclonal antibodies which target growth factors/cell surface receptors or small molecules which can enter cells and inhibit signal transduction (many are tyrosine kinase inhibitors). The molecular targets and diseases treated with some of these are listed in Table 15.3. Two of the most established agents are also described below.

Imatinib mesylate

The Philadelphia chromosome is identified in 90–95% of cases of chronic myeloid leukaemia. This translocation between the long arms of

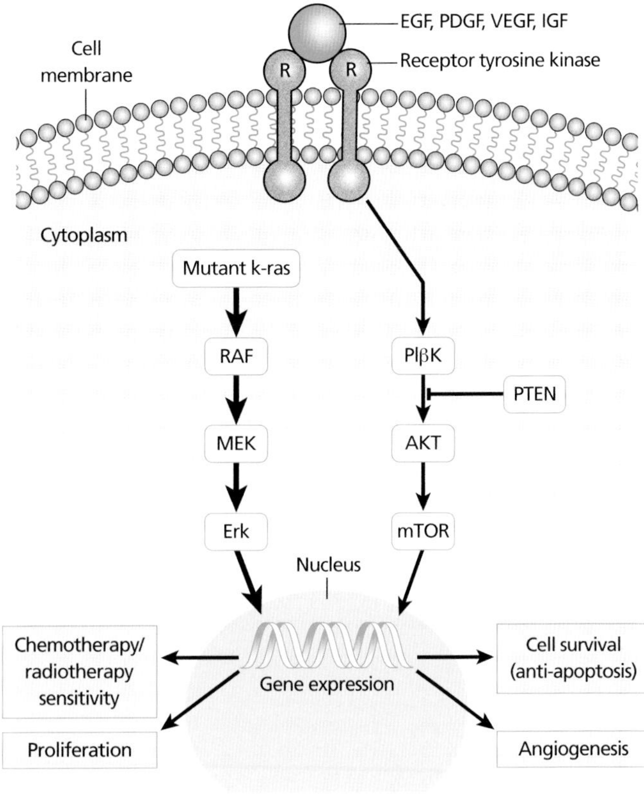

Figure 15.2 Example of a signal transduction pathway in a normal cell (a) and in a malignant cell (b). Each cell in the body reacts to signals in its environment through cell surface receptors. Through a pathway of molecular messengers this message is transduced to the cell nucleus and results in altered gene expression. This allows the cell to react normally to its environment in a particular way, e.g. proliferation, invasion (a). However, if a cell has acquired a genetic mutation in one of the messengers or genetic amplification of one of the messengers (both are frequent events in cancer) then the cell behaves as though the pathway is always being stimulated regardless of the presence of external stimuli. This can result in unchecked proliferation, invasion of adjacent tissues or other properties characteristic of the malignant phenotype.

chromosomes 9 and 22 results in the formation of a bcr-abl fusion protein that functions as a constitutively active tyrosine kinase in the cell. Medicinal chemists developed inhibitors of this tyrosine kinase activity. One of these agents (imatinib mesylate) inhibits the tyrosine kinase activity of bcr-abl, c-kit and PDGF-R (the latter two proteins being other tyroine kinases that are also important in cancer). This agent is administered orally, is well tolerated and results in a haematological complete response in 97% of patients with chronic phase CML. In terms of tolerability and efficacy this represents a considerable improvement compared to previous treatments used in the same patient group.

Imatinib has high bioavailability following oral administration. It undergoes hepatic metabolism by isoenzymes of the cytochrome p450 system, particularly CYP3A4. The drug is generally well tolerated with the main reported toxicities being oedema, nausea, rash and musculoskeletal pain.

Following the discovery that imatinib also inhibits c-kit (a cell-surface receptor that is upregulated in the inherently chemoresistant and radioresistant tumour known as a gastrointestinal stromal tumour or GIST), it was also tested in GISTs that could not be completely resected with excellent results[2]. The efficacy of the drug is much higher in patients who have activating mutations of c-kit compared to those who do not[3].

Trastuzumab

Trastuzumab is a humanised monoclonal antibody directed against HER2, which is a cell surface receptor that is overexpressed in 20–30% of breast cancers. HER2 overexpression causes increased

Table 15.3 List of established biological agents.

Name of agent	Drug type	Molecular target	Licensed disease sites*
Trasztuzumab	Monoclonal antibody	HER2	HER2 +ve breast cancer
Rituximab	Monoclonal antibody	CD20	Certain subtypes of CD20 +ve non-Hodgkin's lymphoma
Bevacizumab	Monoclonal antibody	VEGF	Colorectal cancer, breast cancer, renal cell cancer and non-small cell lung cancer
Cetuximab	Monoclonal antibody	EGFR	Colorectal cancer, head and neck cancer
Imatinib	Tyrosine kinase inhibitor	bcr-abl, c-kit and PDGFR	Chronic myeloid leukaemia, gastrointestinal stromal tumours, dermatofibrosarcoma protuberans, acute lymphoblastic leukaemia, myeloproliferative/myelodysplastic diseases associated with PDGFR gene rearrangements
Erlotinib	Tyrosine kinase inhibitor	EGFR	Pancreatic cancer, non-small cell lung cancer
Sorafenib	Tyrosine kinase inhibitor	Raf kinase, PDGFR, VEGFR, c-kit	Renal cell carcinoma, hepatocellular carcinoma
Sunitinib	Tyrosine kinase inhibitor	PDGFR, VEGFR, c-kit, RET, CSF-1R, flt3	Renal cell carcinoma, GI stromal tumours
Lapatinib	Tyrosine kinase inhibitor	EGFR and HER2	HER2 +ve breast cancer
Dasatinib	Tyrosine kinase inhibitor	bcr-abl, c-src	Chronic myeloid leukaemia, acute lymphoblastic leukaemia
Nilotinib	Tyrosine kinase inhibitor	bcr-abl	Chronic myeloid leukaemia
Temsorilimus	Tyrosine kinase inhibitor	mTOR	Renal cell carcinoma

HER2, Human epidermal growth factor receptor 2; VEGF, vascular endothelial growth factor; EGFR, epidermal growth factor receptor; PDGFR, platelet derived growth factor receptor; VEGFR, vascular endothelial growth factor receptor; mTOR, mammalian target of rapamycin.
*Note: Some licenses for these drugs specify line of therapy, disease stage, previous chemotherapy/biological therapy and chemotherapy that should be co-administered. The fact that a drug is licensed does not mean that it has been approved for use by the Scottish Medicines Consortium (SMC) or the National Institute of Clinical Excellence (NICE).

signal transduction through pathways that promote cellular proliferation, survival, invasion and angiogenesis. Trastuzumab binds to the extracellular domain of the HER2 receptor causing cell cycle arrest. Some of this effect may be mediated by disruption of heterodimerisation of HER2 and other members of the EGFR signaling pathway. Trastuzumab has demonstrated single agent activity against metastatic breast cancer when given by intravenous infusion either weekly or 3-weekly. The efficacy is increased when given in combination with chemotherapy such as docetaxel but care must be taken to monitor for cardiotoxicity. Recent studies have suggested that when Trastuzumab is given for one year as adjuvant therapy in high risk HER2 positive breast cancer the percentage of patients relapsing is reduced by up to 50%.

Cardiotoxicity is one of the main issues with trastuzumab. Any potential benefit must be weighed against the risk of significant cardiac dysfunction (occurs in up to 7% of cases). Left ventricular ejection fraction should be monitored regularly throughout treatment. Other side effects include asthenia, fever, headache, myalgia, rash, diarrhoea, nausea, nasopharyngitis, severe hypersensitivity reactions and other pulmonary events including ARDS.

Chemotherapy for metastatic testicular cancer

Clinical scenario

A 40 year-old man presented with swelling of his right testicle. Alpha fetoprotein (AFP was elevated at 37 IU/mL (normal range 0–5IU/mL). The patient underwent right orchidectomy and histological examination confirmed a diagnosis of malignant teratoma undifferentiated (MTU). A post-operative CT scan revealed two para-aortic lymph nodes measuring 14 mm and 12 mm respectively. Repeat HCG performed 4 weeks post-operatively had risen to 60 IU/mL and on physical examination the man was found to have a 4 cm left supraclavicular fossa lymph node. How was the patient treated?

The patient was treated with 4 cycles of cisplatin and etoposide chemotherapy for metastatic testicular teratoma. Just prior to his first cycle of chemotherapy his HCG level was 110 IU/mL but prior to his second cycle it had fallen to normal (<5 IU/mL). The HCG remained at this level for the rest of the patient's chemotherapy. A post-chemotherapy CT scan showed that his para-aortic and supraclavicular lymphadenopathy had changed little in size during the treatment but there was evidence of decreased density in the centre of these lesions in-keeping with necrosis. Resection of both sites of disease revealed diffentiated teratoma with no malignant elements present.

Cisplatin chemotherapy

Mechanism

Cisplatin chemotherapy causes intra-strand and inter-strand DNA crosslinks, inhibiting mitosis and resulting in apoptotic cell death.

Adverse effects

Nephrotoxicity is a common side-effect. Intra-venous pre-hydration and post-hydration as well as osmotic diuresis (if required) are used to min-imise this toxicity. Emesis is also a significant problem. This is prevented as much as possible by using prophylactic antiemetics such as granisetron and dexamethasone. Other significant toxicities include neurotoxicity, ototoxicity (eight cranial nerve damage), electrolyte disturbance, decreased fertility and myelosuppression.

Etoposide chemotherapy

Mechanism

Etoposide functions as an inhibitor of topoiso-merase II, causing DNA strand breaks and delaying the transit of cells through S phase.

Adverse effects

Common side-effects include alopecia, nausea and vomiting, decreased fertility (amenorrhoea +/− early menopause), hypotension, mucositis, abdominal pain and myelosuppression. Other significant adverse effects include secondary leukaemias.

Adjuvant chemotherapy for breast cancer

Clinical scenario

A 36-year-old woman presented with a 2 week history of a lump in the right breast which measured 18 × 7 × 12 mm on ultrasound. Fine needle aspirate (FNA) showed a grade 3 invasive ductal carcinoma ER0, HER2+++. Ultrasound of the axilla was suspicious and an FNA con-firmed metastatic carcinoma. The lady was treated with 3 cycles of FEC chemotherapy (5-fluorouracil, epirubicin and cyclophosphamide) with a view to downsising her breast cancer and facilitating breast conserving surgery. Subsequent ultrasound suggested the mass had almost completely disappeared. The lady therefore underwent wide local excision and axillary node sampling. Pathology review showed that there had been a pathological com-plete response in breast and nodes (no residual viable invasive breast cancer cells). As the original cancer was HER2 positive she was treated with 3 cycles of docetaxel chemotherapy with trastuzumab added in with the sec-ond and third cycles of docetaxel and then herceptin continued 3-weekly until one year of treatment had been completed.

5-fluorouracil chemotherapy

Mechanism

5-fluorouracil is a pyrimidine analogue that is incorporated into RNA resulting in disruption of normal RNA processing and function. It is also an inhibitor of the enzyme thymidylate synthase which converts deoxyuridine monophosphate (dUMP) to deoxythymidine monophosphate (dTMP). This reaction provides the cell with its only supply of thymidylate (necessary for DNA replication and repair) and the resultant imbalance of the deoxynucleotide pool (especially the dATP/dTTP ratio) is detrimental to DNA synthesis and repair resulting in lethal DNA damage.

Adverse effects

Side effects include mucositis, diarrhoea, palmoplantar erythrodysaesthesiae (PPE), cardiac toxicity (vasospasm) and myelosuppression.

Epirubicin chemotherapy

Mechanism

Epirubicin is an anthracycline. It has a complex mechanism of action that is not fully understood. It intercalates DNA resulting in complex formation and inhibition of DNA and RNA synthesis. It also inhibits both topoisomerase II (preventing DNA religation) and DNA helicase (interfering with replication and transcription).

Adverse effects

Side effects include alopecia, myelosuppression, emesis, extravasation, mucositis, taste disturbance, fatigue, cardiotoxicity (arrythmias or reduced ejection fraction), decreased fertility and teratogenicity.

Cyclophosphamide chemotherapy

Mechanism

Cyclophosphamide is an alkylating agent which prevents cell division by causing interstrand and intrastrand crosslinkages in DNA.

Adverse effects

Significant toxicities include emesis, alopecia, myelosuppression, decreased fertility, teratogenicity, haemorrhagic cystitis, diarrhoea, mucositis and skin rash.

Docetaxel chemotherapy

Mechanism

Microtubules form the mitotic spindle and their dynamic activity is necessary for cell division. Docetaxel binds to and stabilises these microtubules preventing their depolymerisation and thereby inhibiting cellular proliferation. This ultimately promotes apoptotic cell death of cancer cells.

Adverse effects

Side effects include alopecia, myelosuppression, neuropathy, fatigue, stomatitis, fluid retention, skin rashes, nausea, diarrhoea and hypersensitivity reactions.

Chapter 16

Immunopharmacology

Clinical scenario

A 48-year-old schoolteacher presented with a swollen tongue and lips and difficulty breathing. She has just started a course of flucloxacillin prescribed by her GP for cellulitis. The doctor seeing her in A+E makes a diagnosis of an allergic reaction and is concerned that this is anaphylaxis. How should she be treated?

Introduction

The immune system is a host-defence network of different cell types and molecules that protect against pathogens. Immune responses occur at different levels of specificity.

Innate or natural immunity

Innate immunity is mediated by phagocytic cells (neutrophils and macrophages), eosinophils and natural killer cells together with complement proteins. It is a rapid response system. It does not rely on specific recognition of organisms and has no 'memory' of previous infecting agents. Microorganisms are recognised through pattern recognition molecules, e.g. the 'toll-like' receptors. Production of cytokines, such as interleukin (IL)-12,

IL-15, IL-23 and IL-18, during innate responses is critical to efficient generation of subsequent acquired immunity.

Acquired or adaptive immunity

Acquired (adaptive) immunity is mediated by lymphocytes and their secreted products, notably cytokines and antibodies. Acquired immunity is highly specific and re-exposure to a previously encountered antigen produces a greatly augmented and more efficient immune response. T-lymphocytes are of primary importance in regulating acquired immune responses. CD4$^+$ T-inducer/helper (Th) cells initiate and define the nature of the subsequent response and as such represent important therapeutic targets. T-cells possess highly specific cell-surface receptors that recognise foreign proteins only after they have been broken into peptide antigens and attached to major histocompatibility complex (MHC) molecules expressed on the surface of specialised antigen-presenting cells, e.g. dendritic cells.

It is currently thought that Th cells may be functionally subdivided into three distinct populations – Th1 cells produce interferon γ and thereby promote a *cell-mediated immune response*; Th2 cells produce IL-4 and IL-5 and promote B-cell maturation into plasma cells, leading to antibody formation and thus *humoral responses*; and, Th17 cells, characterised by their ability to produce

Lecture Notes: Clinical Pharmacology and Therapeutics, 8th edition. By Gerard McKay, John Reid and Matthew Walters. Published 2010 by Blackwell Publishing Ltd.

IL-17, are thought to be of critical importance in the pathogenesis of a number of autoimmune conditions, notably rheumatoid arthritis. CD8$^+$ T-cells function predominantly as cytotoxic effector cells able, for example, to kill virus-infected cells or tumours. A critical role of the immune system is to distinguish self-proteins from those belonging to invading micro-organisms – this process is called *tolerance*. Tolerance is mediated via thymic selection of developing lymphocytes (*central tolerance*) or via suppression/deletion of lymphocytes post-emergence from the thymus (*peripheral tolerance*). There are a variety of immunological diseases in which the immune system inflicts damage on normal cells and body tissues, representing a 'breach' of tolerance. Immune responses have historically been classified according to the principal effector mechanism responsible.

Type I: Immediate hypersensitivity

Antigen binds to antibody (IgE) attached to mast cells or basophils and provokes release of inflammatory mediators such as vasoactive amines, proteases and prostaglandins. This results in increased vascular permeability, smooth muscle contraction and local inflammation. The clinical manifestations, especially in atopic individuals are:

1 Allergic asthma
2 Hay fever
3 Eczema

In extreme cases anaphylactic shock may result.

Type II: Antibody-mediated hypersensitivity

Autoreactive or cross-reactive antibodies (IgG and IgM) bind to antigens found on cells or tissues and cause damage by activating complement or recruiting inflammatory cells. This may result in tissue- or organ-specific autoimmune diseases (e.g. pernicious anaemia, autoimmune haemolytic anaemia or thrombocytopenic purpura and glomerulonephritis). Alternatively, antibodies directed against cell-surface receptors may either stimulate or block target cell function (e.g. anti-TSH receptor antibodies in Graves disease and anti-acetylcholine receptor antibodies in myasthenia gravis). Antibody-mediated cytotoxicity is also responsible for hyperacute (immediate) organ allo-graft rejection in sensitised renal transplant recipients who have preformed anti-donor antibodies.

Type III: Immune complex-mediated hypersensitivity

Circulating antibody–antigen complexes are deposited in tissues where they produce local activation of complement and leucocytes. Immune complex deposition occurs mainly in the glomeruli resulting in nephritis but other tissues may also be affected. Administration of large amounts of protein antigen intravenously may result in serum sickness.

Type IV: Cell-mediated hypersensitivity

CD4$^+$effector T-cells release pro-inflammatory cytokines (particularly interferon-γ, i.e. Th1 type) and recruit activated macrophages to produce a delayed-type hypersensitivity (DTH) reaction. DTH is responsible for contact sensitivity after topical exposure to chemicals. T-effector cells are suspected of causing several autoimmune diseases (e.g. insulin-dependent diabetes mellitus, multiple sclerosis and rheumatoid arthritis). This form of hypersensitivity is responsible for causing acute rejection of organ allografts and is also likely to be important in organ-specific autoimmunity.

Drugs that suppress immune responses

Excess immune activity has clinical importance in several areas, particularly transplantation and autoimmune disease. Until recently, immune suppressive drugs have comprised mainly *small chemical agents* that have been 'borrowed' from the chemotherapeutic area. Most immunosuppressive drugs currently in use are therefore relatively non-specific and therefore increase the risk of both opportunistic and conventional infections. They may also increase the risk of lymphoproliferative disorders and of solid tumours. In addition to the problem of non-specific immunosuppression, individual agents have drug-specific side effects.

The immune modulator class now also includes *biologic agents*. These represent a new class of drugs comprising either monoclonal antibodies or protein receptor complexes that are delivered by parenteral routes. They are highly specific for molecular targets in the immune system, including cytokines and cell-surface receptors.

Small chemical agents that modify immune response

A variety of small chemical drugs have been adapted to immunosuppressive use. For example, antimetabolites and alkylating agents are used as immunosuppressives but given at lower doses than when used in cancer chemotherapy. They inhibit actively dividing cells and at low doses are relatively selective for activated lymphocytes. Other agents found to be effective in treatment of inflammatory disease do so through means as yet poorly understood. The following agents are used in a variety of immunological conditions.

Azathioprine

This pro-drug is metabolised in the liver to 6-mercaptopurine, a purine nucleotide analogue, which inhibits DNA and RNA synthesis. It is widely used in organ transplantation and in several autoimmune diseases, notably systemic lupus erythematosus. Side effects include leucopenia and thrombocytopenia. Mutations in the thiopurine methyltransferase (TPMT) gene are the main cause of significant bone marrow suppression and many clinicians now screen for these prior to initiating therapy.

Mycophenolate mofetil

This drug appears more selective than azathioprine and is now commonly used in organ transplantation and in autoimmune disease; specifically there is good evidence for its efficacy in remission induction and maintenance in lupus nephritis. It inhibits inosine monophosphate dehydrogenase, the rate-limiting enzyme for the *de novo* pathway of purine synthesis. Because lymphocytes have no salvage pathway for purine synthesis, they are

selectively inhibited. Its use is most commonly limited by gastrointestinal side-effects, in which case the alternative formulation, mycophenolate sodium, may be better tolerated.

Methotrexate

Methotrexate is now widely considered to be the primary disease-modifying drug in rheumatoid arthritis and is commonly used in the treatment of psoriasis, psoriatic arthritis and Crohn's disease. It is also used as prophylaxis against graft versus host disease following bone marrow transplantation. Monthly blood samples are required to screen for marrow suppression and hepatotoxicity. A rare but notable side-effect is methotrexate-induced pneumonitis.

Clinical use and dose

Methotrexate is given by a weekly oral pulse regimen, starting at 7.5 mg and increasing by 2.5 mg every 6 weeks to 15–25 mg weekly depending on disease response. Lower doses should be used in the frail elderly or if there is significant renal impairment. Folic acid 5 mg given 3 days after each dose may reduce the incidence of toxicity, in particular oral ulceration. Cotrimoxazole should be avoided in patients taking methotrexate.

Sulfasalazine

Sulfasalazine is used in the treatment of rheumatoid arthritis, psoriatic arthritis (useful for joint but not skin disease) and inflammatory bowel disease. Its precise mechanism of action is unclear but likely includes inhibition of the pro-inflammatory transcription factor NF-$_k$B.

Hydroxycholoroquine

Originally derived as an antimalarial agent, hydroxycholoroquine is a useful disease-modifying agent used widely in the treatment of rheumatoid arthritis and systemic lupus erythematosus (SLE).

It acts in part via inhibition of phagolysosome function in macrophages and dendritic cells.

Cyclophosphamide and chlorambucil

These drugs are used to treat some types of glomerulonephritis, e.g. complicated SLE or systemic vasculitis, and occasionally other types of autoimmune disease but are not used in organ transplantation.

T-cell targeting agents

Ciclosporin

Mechanism

Ciclosporin acts predominantly on T-helper cells. It selectively impairs production of cytokines, particularly IL-2, and inhibits IL-2 receptor expression, thereby blocking T-cell growth. This prevents T-cell activation and stops the generation of the cell-mediated immune responses responsible for allograft rejection, or tissue damage in autoimmune diseases.

Pharmacokinetics

Ciclosporin is poorly absorbed following oral administration but this problem has been reduced by a new microemulsion formulation. It is a highly lipophilic compound and is distributed widely in body tissues. It is metabolised in the liver and small bowel by the cytochrome P-450 system and then excreted in the bile. Because of variation between individuals in ciclosporin pharmacokinetics, measurement of whole blood ciclosporin levels is used as a guide to dose requirements.

Side effects

Nephrotoxicity is the major drug-specific side effect of ciclosporin. Other side effects include hypertension, convulsions, mild elevation of hepatic transaminases, anorexia, nausea, vomiting, hypertrichosis, gingival hyperplasia, tremor and paraes-

thesia. Toxicity is usually managed by lowering the dose.

Drug interactions

A large number of drug interactions with ciclosporin have been reported. There are two major types:

1 Drugs that are nephrotoxic themselves. Examples are the aminoglycosides and amphotericin, which may enhance the nephrotoxicity of ciclosporin.

2 Drugs that alter the pharmacokinetics of ciclosporin.

Cytochrome P-450 inhibitors such as erythromycin and ketoconazole lead to increased ciclosporin blood levels. Conversely, drugs that induce cytochrome P-450 such as carbamazepine, phenytoin and rifampicin reduce ciclosporin blood levels.

Clinical use and dose

The introduction of ciclosporin revolutionised organ transplantation, allowing greater than 80% 1-year graft survival for kidney, heart and liver transplantation. Nearly all immunosuppressive protocols for organ transplantation include ciclosporin, although treatment regimens vary widely between centres (Table 16.1).

The daily oral dose in the immediate post-transplant period is usually 10–15 mg/kg and this is gradually reduced to a maintenance dose of 3–5 mg/kg, guided by ciclosporin blood levels and clinical assessment. Ciclosporin is used in the prophylaxis and treatment of graft versus host disease after bone marrow transplantation and increasingly in some types of autoimmune disease. It has been used either alone or in combination with methotrexate to treat severe rheumatoid arthritis.

Tacrolimus

This fungal macrolide acts in a very similar way to ciclosporin, although it has a different structure. It is increasingly used in organ transplantation as an alternative to ciclosporin and is also used in autoimmune disease such as polymyositis

Table 16.1 Immunosuppressive drugs used to prevent graft rejection.

Induction/maintenance of immunosuppression	Treatment of rejection
Ciclosporin (cyclosporin) monotherapy	High-dose prednisolone
or	*or*
Ciclosporin + prednisolone	Polyclonal/monoclonal antibody
or	
Ciclosporin + prednisolone + azathioprine (triple therapy)	
or	
Polyclonal/monoclonal antibody + ciclosporin + prednisolone + azathioprine (quadruple therapy)	

and dermatomyositis. Drug-specific side effects are broadly similar to those of ciclosporin. Gingival hypertrophy and hypertrichosis are not seen but neurological side effects may occur.

Sirolimus

This new drug is similar in structure to tacrolimus but acts at a different site within the lymphocyte. It may synergise with ciclosporin and has the potential advantage of reduced nephrotoxicity.

Leflunomide

Leflunomide inhibits the mitochondrial enzyme, dihydroorotate dehydrogenase (DHODH), involved in synthesis of pyrimidines. It thereby inhibits lymphocyte activation and growth. This drug has been shown to exhibit efficacy and disease-modifying activity in rheumatoid arthritis and may also be beneficial in psoriatic skin and joint disease.

Glucocorticoids

Prednisolone and other glucocorticoids have both anti-inflammatory and immunosuppressive properties (see 'Glucocorticoids', Chapter 17). They have many different effects on the immune system and interfere with the following:

1 Lymphocyte recirculation
2 T-cell activation
3 Generation of cytotoxic lymphocytes
4 Cytokine release
5 Macrophage and monocyte function.

Steroids are widely used as immunosuppressives but long-term use in high dose is associated with an unacceptable incidence of adverse effects, and it is therefore preferable to use low-dose steroids combined with other immunosuppressive agents.

Combination of drugs in treatment of immune-mediated disorders

The treatment of chronic inflammatory diseases, such as rheumatoid arthritis, and connective tissue diseases now often entails use of combinations of immune modulatory drugs. In rheumatoid arthritis, combination of methotrexate, sulfasalazine and hydroxycholorquine has proven superior to single therapy. Additional combinations shown to be beneficial include methotrexate/ciclosporin and methotrexate/sulfasalazine. Low-dose corticosteroids are often added to these combinations. It is unclear yet whether autoimmune diseases and chronic inflammatory disease should be treated with several drugs from outset with agents removed as disease improves (*step down therapy*) or whether disease should be treated by sequential addition of drugs until disease is in remission (*step up therapy*).

Other drugs that act by their effect on the immune system

Antihistamines

These block classical histamine (H_1) receptors and interfere with the actions of histamine released in type I immune reactions. They are used in hay fever, allergic rhinitis, urticaria and other acute allergic reactions. The vascular effects of histamine including flare, wheal and itch are prevented. They are of no use in asthma. Older antihistamines like promethazine and diphenhydramine have sedative and anticholinergic side effects. These are less prominent with cyclizine and chlorphenamine (chlorpheniramine). New agents like cetirizine cause little or no sedation, have non-reversible antagonist properties and can be given once daily. Antihistamines are also used to treat motion sickness and vestibular disease. Combination with type II histamine receptor antagonists may be beneficial in some forms of urticaria.

Drugs that block mediator release

Drugs that increase intracellular cyclic adenosine monophosphate (cAMP) stabilise the mast cell and prevent degranulation and mediator release. This reduces or attenuates the symptoms of IgE-mediated hypersensitivity reactions.

β$_2$-Adrenoceptor agonists

Drugs like adrenaline, terbutaline or salbutamol (Chapter 6) increase intracellular cAMP, reduce mediator release and improve symptoms.

Theophylline derivatives

These block phosphodiesterase, prevent cAMP breakdown, increase local levels and thus reduce mediator release.

Disodium cromoglicate and ketotifen

These agents stabilise the mast cell membrane and reduce mediator release. The precise mechanism is unknown but it may be related to inhibition of phosphodiesterase.

Biological therapies

Biological therapies consist of antibodies or receptors that can specifically bind soluble or cell-bound

molecules of demonstrable importance in pathological immune responses. They are usually developed following elucidation of pathophysiologically important pathways that appear amenable to immunomodulation. Broadly they can target cells mediating immune responses, or their soluble products, usually cytokines. They should be avoided in patients with a past history of serious infections such as Tuberculosis or a history of recent\break malignancy. All patients should be screened for TB prior to commencing therapy with these agents

Targeting cells, cell receptors and co-stimulatory molecules

Polyclonal anti-T-cell antibodies are raised by injecting animals (e.g. goats or rabbits) with human lymphocyte or thymocyte preparations. OKT3 is a mouse monoclonal antibody to the CD3 complex on T-lymphocytes. These antibody preparations are given intravenously and cause profound immunosuppression by depleting T-cells from the circulation. They are used in transplantation either as prophylaxis or to treat steroid-resistant acute graft rejection. Polyclonal antibody preparations often cause fever and thrombocytopenia and rarely serum sickness or anaphylaxis. OKT3 may result in the cytokine release syndrome (pyrexia, rigors, nausea, wheeze, diarrhoea and rash).

Several other monoclonal antibodies are currently being assessed for treatment of graft rejection and autoimmune disease. Monoclonal antibodies directed against the α chain of the IL-2 receptor such as basiliximab and dclizumab are now used in organ transplantation. Genetic engineering technology is being used to 'humanise' relevant mouse monoclonal antibodies to render them less immunogenic and therefore more effective. Several cell-targeted therapies are close to or already in clinical use.

Rituximab

This is a chimeric (part mouse/part human protein) monoclonal antibody directed against CD20 which is a receptor expressed on B-cells. Rituximab is effective in treatment of lymphoma but has beneficial effects also in rheumatoid arthritis and probably also in SLE and immune thrombocytopenic purpura. It is given by intravenous infusion together with methotrexate and corticosteroid to achieve maximal benefit. Clinical improvement in rheumatoid arthritis can last at least 6 months after a single therapeutic course.

Abatacept

This is a protein therapy that blocks co-stimulatory function. T-cells are activated upon receipt of two signals from a dendritic cell (*signal* 1 is mediated via the antigen receptor/MHC/peptide interaction and *signal* 2 comes from a co-stimulatory molecule such as CD28). CTLA-4 regulates the capacity of CD28 to mediated signal 2. If only one signal is received then the T-cell becomes anergic (unable to respond). Abatacept is a CTLA-4, immunoglobulin Fc fusion protein that can interfere with T-cell dendritic cell interactions. It has been shown to be effective in rheumatoid arthritis and psoriasis. It is given by subcutaneous injection. Benefit is noted within 3 months of starting therapy. Best effects may require co-prescription with methotrexate.

Alefacept

A further essential co-stimulatory pathway for T-cells is that mediated via CD2 and LFA3. Alefacept is a fusion protein containing LFA3 together with an Fc protein segment. It interferes with interactions between T-cells and adjacent dendritic cells and macrophages. It has been shown to be beneficial in psoriasis.

Efalizumab

Blocking adhesion between leukocytes as they migrate into an inflammatory lesion and receive activatory signals represents an attractive approach to therapy exemplified in this antibody that blocks the adhesion molecule LFA-1. Efalizumab has been introduced for the treatment of psoriasis thus far.

Targeting cytokines

Biologic agents that target cytokines have proven highly effective in the treatment of a variety of inflammatory diseases. A chimeric antibody (part mouse/part human immunoglobulin) against tumour necrosis factor (TNF) (infliximab) and a fully human antibody against TNF (adalimumab) have been successfully used to treat rheumatoid arthritis and Crohn's disease. Similarly, a soluble TNF receptor fused to the Fc portion of human immunoglobulin (etanercept) has similar efficacy in rheumatoid arthritis. All three agents also appear effective in psoriasis, psoriatic arthritis and ankylosing spondylitis and induce significant clinical responses in approximately 70% of patients. These agents carry with them the risk of potential side effects including infection and the theoretical risk of developing lymphoproliferative diseases or solid tumours. The risk:benefit ratio appears favourable, however, and is being monitored prospectively by national registries such as the British Society of Rheumatology Biologics Registry. In addition anti-TNF therapy appears to reduce the risk of cardiovascular and cerebrovascular events, particularly in patients who respond well to treatment. Effects in other autoimmune diseases are variable with some benefits reported in ulcerative colitis, vasculitis and uveitis.

Anakinra (IL-1 receptor antagonist) is also licensed for the treatment of rheumatoid arthritis although it is used rarely in comparison to TNF antagonists. Tocilizumab, a humanised monoclonal antibody to IL-6 receptor has been demonstrated to be effective in the treatment of rheumatoid arthritis and will shortly be licensed for this indication. Numerous other biological agents (monoclonal antibodies and soluble receptors) targeting cytokines, chemokines and pro-angiogenic factors implicated in autoimmune responses are in development.

Infliximab

This is an anti-TNF antibody given by i.v. infusion every 8 weeks. Beneficial effects on disease activity are usually observed within 4 weeks. It must be used in combination with methotrexate in rheumatoid arthritis with which it has synergistic benefit.

Etanercept

This is a TNF receptor Fc fusion protein given by s.c. injection once or twice weekly. It has synergistic benefit when used with methotrexate in rheumatoid arthritis.

Adalimumab

This is a fully human anti-TNF antibody given by s.c. injection every 2 weeks. It has synergistic benefit when used with methotrexate in rheumatoid arthritis.

Regardless of disease indication, before starting TNF blocking therapies, all patients should be screened for prior or current tuberculosis (usually CXR and skin testing), history of severe infection, malignancy or multiple sclerosis. Live vaccines are contraindicated. No information is yet available about safety during pregnancy. Monitoring is not required but is advisable since patients are often on complex drug regimes and exhibit co-morbidities together with the underlying inflammatory disorder.

Immunostimulatory and immunomodulatory agents

Effective strategies for stimulation of the immune system have proved elusive, although there has been some recent progress.

Cytokines

Cytokines are soluble proteins produced by a wide variety of cells and act primarily in an autocrine or paracrine manner. They have many important and complex actions and play a particularly im-portant role in the regulation of immune and inflammatory responses. Recombinant DNA tech-nology has allowed the large-scale production of many cytokines and these are being used increas-ingly to modify the biological response to malig-nancy and infection. Interferon-α is an effective therapy for hairy cell leukaemia (a rare form of chronic leukaemia) and is useful for Kaposi's sar-coma in patients with acquired immunodeficiency syndrome (AIDS). Selected patients with chronic hepatitis B or C infection may also respond to interferon-α therapy. Interferon-α and IL-2 have been used in the treatment of metastatic renal carcinoma and malignant melanoma but response rates are disappointing and, in view of the cost of therapy and side effects, this is a controversial area. Interferon-β has been employed successfully in multiple sclerosis. G-CSF and GM-CSF are be-ing used to shorten the duration of neutropenia after cytotoxic therapy for non-myeloid malig-nancies, and also in bone marrow transplanta-tion. The use of cytokines as biological response modifiers is at an early stage of development and holds much promise for the future. This may be of particular relevance in immune stimulation in patients with human immunodeficiency virus (HIV)/AIDS.

Other immunostimulatory agents

Bacille Calmette–Guérin (BCG) and other agents, e.g. levamisole and *Corynebacterium parvum*, have been tried as immunostimulants in a wide variety of malignancies because of their potential ability to enhance cell-mediated immunity. Results have been disappointing and they are not in widespread use with the notable exception of intravesical BCG which is used in the treatment of bladder carci-noma. Recently, adaptive transfer of live dendritic cells to recipients has been used to stimulate im-mune responses against tumours. These exciting studies remain at an early stage.

Chapter 17

Corticosteroids

Clinical scenario

A patient presents with a 3-month history of painful shoulders. The doctor who sees her thinks that there is tenderness and perhaps some weakness in the proximal muscles of the upper limb. The ESR has come back at 123 mm/hour. The provisional diagnosis of polymyalgia rheumatica is made. A decision has been made to put the patient on steroids. How should this be done, what are the potential side effects and how are steroids weaned in due course?

Introduction

Corticosteroids are usually given for one of the following three reasons:
1 Suppression of inflammation
2 Suppression of immune responses
3 Replacement therapy
  Corticosteroids are hormones synthesised from cholesterol by the adrenal cortex and have a wide range of physiological functions. Pharmacologically, they are divided according to the relative potencies of their physiological effects into:
1 Glucocorticoids that principally affect carbohydrate and protein metabolism (type II receptor)
2 Mineralocorticoids that principally affect sodium balance (type I receptor)

Lecture Notes: Clinical Pharmacology and Therapeutics, 8th edition. By Gerard McKay, John Reid and Matthew Walters. Published 2010 by Blackwell Publishing Ltd.

Production of the naturally occurring glucocorticoid, cortisol (hydrocortisone), is stimulated by the release of adrenocorticotropic hormone (ACTH) from the anterior pituitary. Production of the major naturally occurring mineralocorticoid, aldosterone, is controlled by other factors in addition to ACTH, including the activity of the renin–angiotensin system and plasma potassium. Synthetic steroids have largely replaced the natural compounds in therapeutic use as they are usually more potent, may be more specific with regard to mineralocorticoid and glucocorticoid activity and can be given orally. Prednisolone, betamethasone and dexamethasone are widely used as anti-inflammatory and immunosuppressant drugs.

Glucocorticoids

Cortisol and its derivatives

Glucocorticoids act primarily via binding to a cytosolic glucocorticoid receptor that in complex with glucocorticoid enters the nucleus and binds to glucocorticoid–response elements situated in the promoters of genes coding for proteins that regulate inflammation and immune responses (*transactivation*). The glucocorticoid receptor complex can also interfere directly with other transcription factor complexes and thereby further suppress inflammatory gene expression (*transrepression*).

Pharmacological effects

1 Inflammatory response. Irrespective of the injury or the insult, corticosteroids interfere non-specifically with all components of the inflammatory responses. This includes reduced capillary dilatation and exudation, inhibition of leucocyte migration and phagocytic activity and reduced fibrin deposition with diminution of subsequent scar formation (see 'Disease-controlling antirheumatic therapies', Chapter 19).

2 Immunological response. In high doses, lymphocyte mass and immunoglobulin production are reduced as are monocyte and macrophage function. This results in impaired immunological competence (see 'Immunopharmacology', Chapter 16).

3 Carbohydrate and protein metabolism. Steroids promote glycogen deposition in the liver and gluconeogenesis, an increase in glucose output by the liver and a decrease in glucose utilisation by peripheral tissues. There is a concomitant increase in protein catabolism with mobilisation of amino acids from peripheral tissues.

4 Fluid and electrolyte balance. Even glucocorticoids have some mineralocorticoid activity and can act on type I receptors. The principal effect is of enhanced sodium reabsorption from the distal tubule of the kidney, with an associated increase in the urinary excretion of potassium and hydrogen ions. Oedema is rare but moderate hypertension is not uncommon.

5 Lipid metabolism. Corticosteroids facilitate fat mobilisation by adrenaline and redistribution of body fat to 'centripetal' areas: face, neck and shoulders.

6 Mood and behaviour changes. Mild euphoria is quite common with higher doses.

7 Increase in the number of red cells, platelets and polymorphs, but a decrease in the number of eosinophils and lymphocytes. These effects may in part arise from altered cell migration.

8 Increased production of gastric acid and pepsin.

9 Reduction in bone formation: A decrease in calcium absorption from the intestine and an increase in calcium loss from the kidney. There is also reduced secretion of growth hormone and antagonism of its peripheral effects, and so there may be growth retardation in children.

Adverse effects

The adverse effects of corticosteroids are largely predictable from the wide range of known physiological and pharmacological effects.

1 Metabolic effects. Patients on high-dosage steroid therapy quickly develop a characteristic appearance: a rounded, plethoric face (moon face), deposits of fat over the supraclavicular and cervical areas (buffalo hump), obesity of the trunk with relatively thin limbs, purple striae typically on the thighs and lower abdomen and a tendency to bruising. Disturbed carbohydrate metabolism leads to hyperglycaemia and glycosuria and rarely proceeds to overt diabetes mellitus.

In addition to the loss of protein from skeletal muscle, patients also develop muscular weakness, which particularly affects the thighs and upper arms (proximal myopathy).

2 Fluid retention may be associated with hypokalaemic alkalosis and hypertension.

3 Increased susceptibility to infection.

4 Osteoporosis. It may cause compression fractures of the vertebral bodies and avascular necrosis of the head of the femur. UK national guidelines now dictate that osteoporotic prophylaxis be introduced in a proportion of patients destined to receive steroid treatment for prolonged periods; all patients starting steroids should be entered into prophylaxis algorithms and a bisphosphonate commenced if indicated.

5 Psychosis. A sense of euphoria frequently accompanies high-dosage steroid therapy and this may rarely proceed to overt manic psychosis. The increased sense of well-being leads to an improved appetite and contributes to weight gain.

Steroids may precipitate a depressive illness.

6 Cataract. This is a rare complication, usually in children, reflecting prolonged high-dosage therapy.

7 Gastrointestinal symptoms. Dyspepsia frequently accompanies high-dosage oral steroid therapy. Signs of peritonitis, which would

complicate a perforated peptic ulcer, may be masked by the anti-inflammatory effect of steroids.

These predictable and serious adverse effects should lead to particular caution in the use of steroid therapy in patients who have pre-existing peptic ulceration, severe hypertension, congestive cardiac failure and osteoporosis.

Adrenal suppression

The administration of exogenous corticosteroids results in negative feedback to the anterior pituitary, with inhibition of ACTH release and the consequent withdrawal of trophic stimulation to the adrenal cortex. In time, the adrenal cortex atrophies and when long-term steroid therapy is finally stopped it may be 6–12 months before normal pituitary–adrenal function recovers. An alternate-day steroid regimen may cause less adrenal suppression than daily treatment. Adrenal suppression has two consequences:

1 Impairment of patient's response to 'stress' (illness, injury, surgery) and susceptibility to infection. Chickenpox may be particularly severe: passive immunisation with varicella zoster immunoglobin should be given to non-immune patients.

2 The withdrawal of corticosteroid therapy must be slow and supervised. Short-term therapy (4–6 weeks) can be reduced quickly and stopped abruptly without difficulty. Long-term therapy, particularly with more than 7.5 mg prednisolone daily, or equivalent, carries the risk of adrenal and hypothalamic–pituitary suppression. Withdrawal must be undertaken cautiously and gradually. Assuming that there is no flare-up of the systemic disease for which the steroid therapy was originally prescribed, the daily dose should be reduced by 5 mg of prednisolone, or equivalent, every 1–2 weeks until the total daily dose is at the physiological replacement level of 5 mg daily. This dosage should be converted to a single morning administration, and at intervals of 2 weeks, decrements of 1 mg should be made. The safety of this gradual withdrawal can be monitored by the endogenous plasma cortisol level; full recovery can be verified by a Synacthen (ACTH) test. All these patients require supervision and advice for 6 months after steroid withdrawal.

Patients on long-term steroid therapy, and particularly those undergoing steroid withdrawal, require a temporary increase in the dose of steroid during periods of stress because of the inability of the hypothalamic–pituitary–adrenal axis to respond normally with an increased production of endogenous corticosteroid, e.g. in times of intercurrent illness. Similarly, patients on steroid therapy who undergo surgery require an increased steroid dosage to enable them to withstand the stress of the operation. Such patients need to carry a steroid card (or bracelet/necklace) so that they can be identified as steroid dependent in the event of an accident/emergency. They should understand the need for uninterrupted treatment and report any problem (vomiting/diarrhoea) immediately. Patients on steroids are now specifically advised to avoid contact with people who have chickenpox or shingles and to see their doctor if such contact occurs. If travelling to remote areas, they should be instructed in the self-administration of intramuscular hydrocortisone and given the appropriate equipment and drugs.

Topical therapy

Topically applied steroids are absorbed through the skin and in the case of very potent drugs, such as clobetasol or betamethasone, adrenal suppression and the toxic effects described above can occur. This usually happens only if recommended doses are exceeded, extensive areas of skin are covered or very prolonged administration is used.

Other effects seen with topical application are:
1 Worsening of local infections. This is particularly important in the eye, where ulcers caused by herpes simplex (dendritic ulcers) spread dramatically and dangerously following application of steroids.
2 Local thinning of the skin. This slowly resolves on stopping steroids, but some permanent damage may remain.
3 Atrophic striae. These are irreversible.
4 Increased hair growth.

5 The use of high doses of beclomethasone by aerosol inhalation can result in hoarseness or candidiasis of the mouth.

Clinical use and doses of commonly used steroids

Hydrocortisone

Hydrocortisone is used in three different situations:
1 Replacement therapy – when it is given orally in a dose of 20 mg in the morning and 10 mg in the afternoon. Body size needs to be taken into consideration (12–15 mg/m^2 surface area).
2 Shock and status asthmaticus – when it is given intravenously up to 200 mg 6-hourly.
3 Topical application – for example 1% cream or ointment in eczema; 100-mg dose as enema or foam in treating ulcerative colitis.

Prednisolone

Prednisolone is used orally in three types of condition:
1 Inflammatory diseases, e.g. rheumatoid arthritis, ulcerative colitis, chronic active hepatitis
2 Allergic diseases, e.g. severe asthma
3 Acute lymphoblastic leukaemia and non-Hodgkin lymphoma.

A single dose of up to 60 mg daily is given, depending on disease severity, reducing to a maintenance dose in the range 2.5–15 mg daily. It is used topically in ulcerative colitis as a 20-mg enema.

Beclometasone

Beclometasone is a fluorinated, and therefore polar, steroid that passes poorly across membranes. It is used topically in:
1 Asthma – when it is given by metered aerosol doses. About 20% reaches the lungs, and the rest is swallowed and destroyed by first-pass metabolism (Chapter 8).

2 Severe eczema – when it is used as 0.025% cream.

Betamethasone

Betamethasone is used for:
1 Cerebral oedema caused by tumours and trauma; given either orally or intramuscularly in doses up to 4 mg 6-hourly. It is ineffective in cerebral oedema resulting from hypoxia.
2 Severe eczema; given topically as 0.1% cream.

Dexamethasone

Dexamethasone is used in cerebral oedema.

Triamcinolone

Triamcinolone is used for:
1 Local inflammation of joints or soft tissue; given by intra-articular injection in doses up to 40 mg depending on joint size.
2 Severe eczema; given topically as 0.1% cream.

Mineralocorticoids

Pharmacological effects

These drugs produce retention of salt and water by the same mechanism as aldosterone on the distal renal tubule. Their main adverse effect is excessive fluid retention and hypertension.

Clinical use and dose

Fludrocortisone is a fluorinated hydrocortisone with powerful mineralocorticoid activity and very little anti-inflammatory action. It is used in:
1 Replacement therapy in doses of 50–200 μg/day.
2 Congenital adrenal hyperplasia in doses up to 50–200 mcg in adults (adjusted in infants depending on body surface area).
3 Idiopathic postural hypotension in doses of 100–200 μg/day.

Chapter 18

Drugs and the blood including anticoagulants and thrombolytic drugs

Clinical scenario

A 26-year-old woman presents with a swollen left leg. She has no past medical history of note, but is on the combined oral contraceptive pill. She smokes 20 cigarettes per day. On examination she is obese (BMI>30) with a red, swollen, painful left leg. Her D-dimers are raised and Doppler ultrasound confirms a deep venous throbosis (DVT). How should she be treated?

Key points

- There are different indications for and ways of anti-coagulating patients
- Anti-coagulation is always a balance between the benefit and risk
- Oral anti-coagulant therapy requires regular blood monitoring

Introduction

Vascular injury results firstly in vasoconstriction and formation of a platelet plug at the site of injury (primary haemostasis). The platelet plug is then stabilised by the formation of a fibrin meshwork, resulting from activation of the coagulation cascade. Eventually fibrin is cleared through digestion by fibrinolytic enzymes.

Lecture Notes: Clinical Pharmacology and Therapeutics, 8th edition. By Gerard McKay, John Reid and Matthew Walters. Published 2010 by Blackwell Publishing Ltd.

Primary haemostasis

When endothelial integrity is breached, platelets adhere to exposed subendothelial collagen. The adherent platelets become activated resulting in:

1 Exposure of fibrinogen receptors, allowing fibrinogen to bind and cross-link adjacent platelets. This process is known as platelet aggregation. The platelet fibrinogen receptor consists of a complex of glycoproteins IIb and IIIa on the platelet membrane.

2 Release of contents of secretory granules including substances such as adenosine diphosphate (ADP) which promote further platelet activation.

3 Synthesis of thromboxane A_2 which also acts to promote further platelet activation and vasoconstriction.

Activation of the coagulation cascade

As shown in Fig. 18.1, the coagulation cascade consists of a series of steps in which precursor proteins in plasma are converted to active enzymes in a sequential series of reactions. For convenience the coagulation cascade can be divided into three parts.

1 The *common* pathway consists of those reactions subsequent to the generation of factor X_a, culminating in the cleavage of fibrinogen by thrombin, with subsequent polymerisation of fibrin

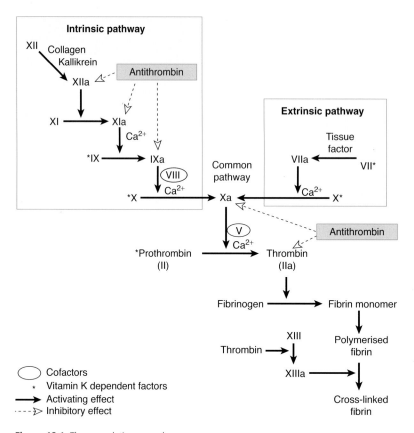

Figure 18.1 The coagulation cascade.

monomers into fibrin strands. Factor X_a may be generated either by the extrinsic pathway or by the intrinsic pathway.

2 In the *extrinsic* pathway, tissue factor is expressed by cells or released following tissue injury. Binding of tissue factor to factor VII greatly accelerates the activation of factor VII and also the action of factor VII$_a$ in the activation of factor X.

3 The *intrinsic* pathway is initiated by the activation of factor XII by contact of blood with a 'foreign' surface. *In vivo*, this is usually the subendothelial tissues. A sequence of reactions as illustrated in Fig. 18.1 then result in the activation of factor X. Most coagulation factors are synthesised in the liver, and the synthesis of the procoagulant forms of factors II, VII, IX and X is dependent on the availability of vitamin K.

Fibrinolysis

The fibrinolytic system, like the coagulation cascade, also consists of a series of enzymatic steps (see Fig. 18.2), this time resulting in the breakdown of polymerised fibrin by plasmin into small fibrin degradation products (FDP). Plasmin is generated from the plasma protein plasminogen by the action of tissue plasminogen activator (tPA), which is most efficient in activation of plasminogen, when it is bound to fibrin. Furthermore, such localisation of fibrinolytic reactions protects plasmin from potent inhibitors present in plasma.

Pathophysiology

Thrombosis is 'haemostasis in the wrong place'. When haemostasis proceeds unchecked within a

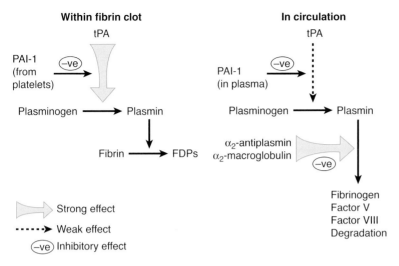

Figure 18.2 The fibrinolytic system. Exogenous thrombolytic agents are plasminogen activators. FDPs, fibrin degradation products.

large vessel, thrombosis occurs and vascular occlusion may result. Thrombi may also break up into small pieces and lodge at distant points within the circulatory system (embolism). The process of thrombosis in a blood vessel is promoted by one or more of three underlying pathological events: (i) abnormalities of the vessel wall; (ii) abnormalities of flow within a vessel; or (iii) abnormalities of blood constituents.

Thrombosis in arteries usually results from rupture of an atheromatous plaque, and arterial thrombi consist initially of platelets and subsequently of fibrin. Venous thrombosis often occurs in the context of stasis of blood flow, for example during periods of immobility or during pregnancy when pressure from the gravid uterus may impede venous return, and thrombi in veins are rich in fibrin enmeshing all the cellular constituents of blood.

Anticoagulant drugs

Parenteral anticoagulants

Anticoagulation can be achieved rapidly with heparins, and pentascharides such as fordaparinux.

They are the anticoagulants of choice in many acute thrombotic states such as treatment of deep vein thrombosis (DVT) or pulmonary embolism, and in the acute coronary syndromes in which they have an additive effect to aspirin.

Heparins

Chemistry and pharmacology

Unfractionated heparin (the original parenteral anticoagulant) is a mixture of naturally occurring glycosaminoglycans with polysaccharide chains of varying length, and molecular weights ranging from 5000 to 30,000. Low molecular weight heparins have several advantages over unfractionated herparin, and are progressively replacing it in clinical practice. They are manufactured from unfractionated heparin to produce material with an average molecular weight of 4000–6500.

All heparins exert their anticoagulant activity by binding to and greatly accelerating the action of antithrombin as an inhibitor of thrombin (factor IIa), factor X_a and other serine protease coagulation factors. Binding to antithrombin requires the presence of a specific pentasaccharide sequence on the heparin polysaccharide chain. A further requirement for heparin to enhance the anti-II$_a$ activity of antithrombin is the presence of a minimum chain length of 18 saccharides. As the proportion of chains of this length in low molecular weight heparins is less than in unfractionated heparin, it follows that low molecular weight heparins have a higher ratio of anti-X$_a$ to anti-II$_a$ activity.

All heparins must be administered parenterally, either by the intravenous or by the subcutaneous route. For treatment of thrombosis, unfractionated heparin has traditionally been given by continuous intravenous infusion. The half-life of standard heparin following intravenous administration is 45–60 minutes, but heparins have complex kinetics, depending on dose, molecular weight and route of administration. Unfractionated heparin can also be given twice daily subcutaneously for treatment of DVT or (in lower doses) for prevention of DVT. Low molecular weight heparins demonstrate less binding to cells and to heparin-neutralising proteins than unfractionated heparin. This leads to improved bioavailability and to a longer half-life. These properties allow a more predictable anticoagulant response and once-daily subcutaneous administration, and there is usually no need to monitor therapeutic doses with coagulation time assays.

Clinical use of unfractionated heparin

Heparin is used in the initial treatment of DVT and pulmonary embolism. Standard practice has been to administer 5000 IU unfractionated heparin intravenously as a loading dose, followed by a continuous infusion of 30,000–40,000 IU over 24 hours, and to monitor the anticoagulant effect. Heparin is also used in acute coronary syndromes (unstable angina and myocardial infarction) to reduce progression of coronary artery thrombosis, prevent coronary reocclusion following clot extraction or thrombolysis, and in the treatment and prevention of mural thrombus. It has a place as an adjunctive treatment to surgery or thrombolysis in the management of acute peripheral arterial occlusion. It is also used to prevent clotting in extracorporeal circulations such as renal dialysis circuits and cardiopulmonary bypass, and at low doses to flush indwelling vascular catheters (although sodium chloride 0.9% is as effective).

Perioperative subcutaneous administration of low-dose unfractionated heparin (usually 5000 IU b.d.) is effective in reducing the incidence of DVT and pulmonary embolism following general or orthopaedic surgery, and is also used for this purpose in acutely ill, immobile medical patients.

Clinical use of low molecular weight heparin

Low molecular weight heparins have effectively replaced unfractionated heparin in the prevention of venous thrombosis in patients at risk, including those undergoing general or orthopaedic surgery and high-risk medical patients. They have been shown to be of similar efficacy to unfractionated heparin in all of these situations, and the convenience of once-daily administration makes their use attractive. They also cause less bleeding in medical patients. In orthopaedic surgery, some orthopaedic surgeons prefer use of mechanical methods and aspirin as prophylaxis, to reduce the risk of bleeding.

Low molecular weight heparins administered once or twice daily subcutaneously (with dose adjusted for body weight) are as effective as unfractionated heparin administered intravenously in the treatment of DVT and pulmonary embolism. Once-daily administration allows outpatient treatment of DVT and minor pulmonary embolism in many patients, with savings on hospitalisation costs.

Monitoring of heparin

Administration of therapeutic doses of unfractionated heparin must be monitored in the laboratory. A prolongation of the activated partial thromboplastin time (APTT) and the thrombin time is observed. The APTT, which tests the intrinsic and common pathways of coagulation, is the test usually chosen for therapeutic heparin monitoring. For the treatment of thrombosis, one should aim for an APTT 1.5–2.5 times the mid-point of the normal range, and it is important to achieve this in the first 24 hours of treatment. An alternative is to measure plasma heparin levels that are based upon plasma anti-X_a activity. It is not usually necessary to monitor heparin given in low doses for prophylaxis, and such regimens do not lead to prolongation of the APTT.

The APTT is insensitive to the effects of low molecular weight heparins. These may be measured by anti-X_a assays (e.g. in renal failure, to prevent bleeding due to accumulation of heparins which are excreted by the kidneys) but monitoring is usually unnecessary because of the predictability of responses.

Adverse effects

Bleeding is a hazard, especially with full-dose heparin treatment. Bleeding complications are not entirely predictable by APTT monitoring of unfractionated heparin, and patient-related factors are also important. Hopes that low molecular weight heparins would have a substantially better safety profile compared with unfractionated heparin with respect to bleeding have not been confirmed for treatment, nor for prophylaxis in surgical patients.

Heparin induced thrombocytopenia occurs in approximately 3% of patients given full-dose unfractionated heparin. Mild early transient thrombocytopenia may be more common and is of no clinical significance. Thrombocytopenia occurring 4–14 days following heparin exposure is of greater significance, as potentially life-threatening thrombosis occurs in a small proportion of such patients. The thrombocytopenia is induced by a heparin-dependent antibody that causes platelet aggregation. Heparin-induced thrombocytopenia can occur with any dose or preparation of heparin (including heparin flushes of intravenous cannulae), and although it appears to be much less common with low molecular weight heparin, antibody cross-reactivity has been documented. It is therefore mandatory to monitor platelet counts during heparin therapy and prophylaxis from day 5 onwards: a baseline platelet count should be performed. If heparin-induced thrombocytopenia is suspected, heparin should be withdrawn and haematological advice sought imme-

diately. The haematologist may recommend substitution of heparin anticoagulation with alternative parenteral anticoagulants) e.g. heparinoids or hirudins? (see below).

Osteoporosis (Reduction in bone density) and bone fractures have been described following prolonged administration (usually greater than 20 weeks) and therefore have generally occurred in pregnant women. The mechanism is poorly understood. There appears to be a relationship with dose and duration of treatment, but individual susceptibility is also likely to be important. Monitoring of bone density may be considered in high-risk patients.

Hypersensitivity including local reactions at injection sites have been reported and, much more rarely, anaphylactoid reactions.

Reversal of anticoagulation with heparin

Because of the short half-life of heparin, in the absence of clinical bleeding, it is reasonable simply to withhold therapy temporarily if over-anticoagulation has occurred. In the presence of haemorrhage, protamine should be administered intravenously. Protamine 1 mg neutralises the effects of 100 IU of unfractionated heparin. Protamine should never be given in doses of greater than 50 mg and should always be administered slowly to avoid hypotension and bradycardia.

Contraindications to heparin

Active bleeding is an obvious contraindication. Others, including relative contraindications, are given below.

Contraindications to heparin

1 Uncorrected major bleeding
2 Uncorrected major bleeding disorder, e.g. thrombocytopenia, haemophilias
3 Active peptic ulcer, oesophageal varices, aneurysm, proliferative retinopathy or organ biopsy
4 Recent surgery, particularly neurosurgery or ophthalmic surgery
5 Severe renal or hepatic impairment (not including use for renal dialysis)

---

6 Recent stroke, intracranial or intraspinal bleed
7 Severe hypertension
8 Previous heparin-induced thrombocytopenia or thrombosis
9 Documented hypersensitivity

Heparinoids and hirudins

These do not cross-react with heparin-dependent antibodies; hence, they can be used in heparin-induced thrombocytopenia. Danaparoid is a heparinoid; desirudin and lepirudin are recombinant hirudins, developed from hirudin, the natural anticoagulant of the medicinal leech.

Fondaparinux

This is a pentasaccharide which selectively inhibits factor X_a. It is effective in prevention and treatment of DVT, and in treatment of acute coronary syndromes. Recent UK guidelines (SIGN and NICE) recommend its use in preference to heparins, due to increased ratio of efficacy to bleeding risk, in some of these indications.

Oral anticoagulants

Vitamin K antagonists

In current practice, warfarin, a derivative of 4-hydroxycoumarin, is by far the most extensively used oral anticoagulant and is the drug of choice. Acenocoumarol (nicoumalone) and phenindione are also available but are rarely used. All of these drugs act as vitamin K antagonists. The remainder of this section on vitamin K antagonists will refer only to warfarin, but similar principles apply to use of the other agents.

Pharmacology

The coagulation factors II, VII, IX and X require gamma carboxylation on glutamic acid residues in order to bind calcium during coagulation reactions. Vitamin K is required for this carboxylation reaction, which is essential for procoagulant activity. Whilst acting as a cofactor, vitamin K is converted to vitamin K epoxide. The epoxide is then recycled via reductase reactions to active forms of vitamin K. Warfarin inhibits the reductase enzymes involved in the recycling of vitamin K, thus leading to a deficiency of procoagulant forms of factors II, VII, IX and X. Because some of these factors have prolonged half-lives, anticoagulation is not achieved for several days after initiating warfarin therapy, and loading doses are usually given in acute thrombosis. In acute situations, it is necessary to overlap heparin and warfarin therapy.

Warfarin is rapidly absorbed from the gut and is extensively bound to plasma albumin. Elimination of warfarin is by oxidative metabolism in the liver, with a half-life of 15–50 hours.

Monitoring of warfarin therapy

Warfarin therapy is monitored by the prothrombin time, which assesses the extrinsic and common pathways of coagulation. Standardisation is achieved by calibrating laboratory reagents used for measuring the prothrombin time against an international standard, and assigning an international sensitivity index (ISI) to each reagent. This allows the prothrombin time for the patient on treatment to be converted to an international normalised ratio (INR). The INR is the ratio of the patient's prothrombin time over the mean value in a normal reference population determined using the same batch of reagent and corrected for the ISI of the reagent. The development of the INR system of monitoring oral anticoagulation has allowed comparability of results between laboratories.

Clinical use of oral anticoagulants

- Venous thromboembolism—prophylaxis and treatment
- Atrial fibrillation (high-risk patients)
- Valvular heart disease and prosthetic valve replacements, cardiomyopathy
- Mural thrombus

Warfarin is also used long-term if there is considered to be a significant risk of recurrent venous thrombosis. Table 18.1 shows recommended target INR ranges for some common indications for warfarin.

Table 18.1 Target INR ranges for oral anticoagulation.

INR	Clinical condition
2.0–2.5	Prophylaxis of DVT and pulmonary embolism in high-risk patients (e.g. previous DVT, pulmonary embolism or thrombophilias) (for hip surgery 2.0–3.0)
2.0–3.0	Treatment of DVT and pulmonary embolism
	Prevention of systemic embolism in atrial fibrillation, mitral valve disease and other cardiac sources of embolism in the presence of previous systemic embolism
	Bioprosthetic heart valves with embolic risk factors
	Prevention of cardiac thromboembolism in high-risk patients following myocardial infarction
3.0–4.5	Mechanical prosthetic cardiac valves Recurrent thrombosis in patients with antiphospholipid syndrome

Pregnancy

Warfarin crosses the placenta and is contraindicated in the first trimester of pregnancy because of teratogenicity, and in the last few weeks of pregnancy because of fetal bleeding at delivery. Placental passage of warfarin leads to fetal anticoagulation at any stage in pregnancy, and so warfarin is not generally recommended in the management and prevention of venous thromboembolism during pregnancy. However, because there is a high risk of embolisation, warfarin is still used in some patients as the anticoagulant of choice from 12 to 36 weeks of pregnancy in patients with mechanical prosthetic heart valves. An alternative approach now is to use low molecular weight heparin with dose adjustment depending on anti-Factor Xa activity. These patients are complicated and the decision on how their anti-coagulation managed through pregnancy should be made on a balance of risk and benefit with the input from the patient's obstetrician and cardiologist.

How to initiate anticoagulation with warfarin

As a result of the kinetic considerations described above, anticoagulation with warfarin is not achieved for several days after initiating therapy, and in acute thrombosis loading doses are given at the start of treatment. A baseline coagulation screen should be checked prior to initiating treatment. Common practice for loading would be to administer 5–10 mg warfarin on two consecutive days and to check the INR on the third day. The use of treatment algorithms such as the Fenerty chart will help in predicting final dose. Lower doses are usually required in congestive cardiac failure, in the presence of abnormalities of liver function or a prolongation of baseline prothrombin time, and in the elderly. It is also necessary to avoid loading doses in patients known to be suffering from familial protein C or protein S deficiency (see below).

Maintenance doses usually lie between 3 and 9 mg warfarin. Daily or alternate-day monitoring of the INR should be carried out until stable values are achieved within the target range. In many instances, patients being induced with warfarin will also be receiving heparin for treatment or prevention of thrombosis. It is important to continue heparin until a therapeutic INR is achieved with warfarin.

Once stabilised, all patients, before discharge from hospital, should be enrolled in their local anticoagulant service and should receive education (e.g. by a pharmacist), using a national anticoagulant book where warfarin dosage and INR results are documented. The book should also contain important information for the patient (or carers) regarding therapy, including side effects and information about drug interactions. The following information should always be supplied to the supervising anticoagulant clinic: full personal patient details, indication for anticoagulation, proposed duration of treatment, desired target INR, and full details of all of the patient's medication. The patient should be advised to show the book to all doctors whom they attend, as well as the dentist.

Drug interactions

Drug interactions are the most common reason for loss of anticoagulant control, bleeding and thrombosis in patients previously stabilised on warfarin. Great care should be taken in prescribing any additional medication to patients on oral anticoagulants. Drugs may potentiate the effects of warfarin by inhibiting liver enzymes involved in warfarin metabolism, by competing for protein binding, by reducing vitamin K availability or by affecting other aspects of haemostasis. Note that alcohol dose-dependently potentiates the effects of warfarin, and patients on oral anticoagulants should keep their alcohol consumption stable and less than 2 units/day. Drugs usually antagonise the effects of warfarin by inducing liver enzymes but in one case (colestyramine) the underlying mechanism is interference with warfarin absorption. Common drug interactions are illustrated in Table 18.2, but this list is by no means exhaustive: consult the resources such as the *British National Formulary* before any change of drugs.

Adverse effects

Bleeding is the most common adverse event encountered in patients on oral anticoagulants. Bleeding is usually related to prolongation of the INR above the therapeutic range, and underlying causes should be sought if bleeding occurs at therapeutic levels (e.g. endoscopy for gastrointestinal bleeding or haematuria).

Other adverse effects are rare and include alopecia and skin rashes. There was a high incidence of hypersensitivity reactions with phenindione, and so it is now rarely used.

Patients with protein C or protein S deficiency are susceptible to skin necrosis during induction phases of oral anticoagulation. This is a result of the suppression of these vitamin K dependent coagulation inhibitors by warfarin, which occurs quickly compared with the suppression of the procoagulant factors. Adequate heparinisation and the avoidance of loading doses of warfarin should help to prevent this complication in patients at risk. Such patients should be managed by haematologists.

Table 18.2 Important drug interactions with warfarin.

Potentiation	Antagonism
Analgesics	
NSAIDs—azapropazone, phenylbutazone	
Aspirin	
Co-proxamol	
Ketorolac (postoperative)	
Antibiotics	
Co-trimoxazole	Rifampicin
Metronidazole	Griseofulvin
Ampicillin	
Cephalosporins	
Erythromycin	
Aminoglycosides	
Tetracycline	
Miconazole	
Cardiovascular drugs	
Amiodarone	Spironolactone
Fibrates	Colestryramine (cholestyramine)
Endocrine agents	
Corticosteroids	
Thyroxine	
Tamoxifen	
Anabolic steroids	
Glucagon	
Gastrointestinal drugs	
Cimetidine	
Omeprazole	
Others	
Allopurinol	Vitamin K
Alcohol	Phenytoin
Chlorpromazine	Carbamazepine
Tricyclic antidepressants	Barbiturates
	Antihistamines

Treatment of haemorrhage and reversal of oral anticoagulation

For elective situations such as surgery including tooth extractions, warfarin should be stopped at least 48 hours in advance of the procedure and the INR monitored, with the option of substituting heparin for a few days (bridging) if there is high risk of thrombosis (e.g. mechanical heart valves).

When haemorrhage occurs in patients on oral anticoagulants, there are well-defined guidelines

Table 18.3 Reversal of oral anticoagulation.

Condition	Action
Major bleeding	Stop warfarin; give phytomenadione (vitamin K_1) 5 mg by slow intravenous injection; give prothrombin complex concentrate (factors II, VII, IX and X) 30–50 units/kg or (if no concentrate available) fresh frozen plasma 15 ml/kg
INR > 8.0, no bleeding or minor bleeding	Stop warfarin, restart when INR < 5.0; if there are other risk factors for bleeding give phytomenadione (vitamin K_1) 500 μg by slow intravenous injection or 5 mg by mouth (for partial reversal of anticoagulation give smaller oral doses of phytomenadione e.g. 0.5–2.5 mg using the intravenous preparation orally); repeat dose of phytomenadione if INR still too high after 24 hours
INR 6.0–8.0, no bleeding or minor bleeding	Stop warfarin, restart when INR < 5.0
INR < 6.0 but more than 0.5 units above target value	Reduce dose or stop warfarin, restart when INR < 5.0
Unexpected bleeding at therapeutic levels	Always investigate possibility of underlying cause, e.g. unsuspected renal or gastrointestinal tract pathology

for management. These are shown in Table 18.3. The advice of a haematologist should always be sought. Several general points are important regarding the use of vitamin K. Note that vitamin K takes 6 hours to have any effect, and in an emergency fresh frozen plasma or coagulation factor concentrates must be administered to provide an immediate source of vitamin K dependent factors. Small doses of vitamin K (0.5–2 mg) are sufficient for reversal of warfarin effects in all but the most extreme cases. Furthermore, caution should be exerted in the administration of vitamin K to patients with prosthetic cardiac valves. The administration of large doses of vitamin K, e.g. 10 mg, makes further use of oral anticoagulants impossible for several weeks.

Contraindications to oral anticoagulants

These are similar to the previously listed contraindications to heparin, except for the following:
1 Lack of patient co-operation for any reason (e.g. mental impairment, alcoholism) or continued intravenous drug use constitutes a contraindication to oral anticoagulants.
2 Oral anticoagulants are teratogenic and are contraindicated in the first trimester of pregnancy except in certain rare circumstances.

3 Heparin-induced thrombocytopenia is *not* a contraindication to oral anticoagulants, which may be used as antithrombotic agents when the platelet count has normalised.

New oral anticoagulant

Two new oral anticoagulants, which are not vitamin K antagonists, have recently been introduced. Rivaroxatin is a selective inhibitor of factor Xa, and dabigatran is a direct thrombin inhibitor. They do not require monitoring of coagulation times, and are given in fixed daily doses. They are currently licensed for prophylaxis of venous thromboembolism after major orthopaedic surgery. Ongoing randomised trials are assessing their efficacy and safety in treatment of venous thromboembolism, and in prophylaxis of thromboembolism in high-risk patients with atrial fibrillation.

Thrombolytic agents

Clinical use of thrombolytic agents

Thrombolytic agents have gained an established role in the treatment of acute myocardial infarction with ST segment elevation (STEMI) or left bundle branch block. Their early administration leads to angiographically demonstrable coronary artery patency, limitation of infarct size, improved left ventricular function and, most importantly, reduced mortality (for streptokinase and alteplase). However, current clinical guidelines recommend primary angioplasty for such patients when practicable, because this strategy is associated with lower mortality and lower risk of bleeding than thrombolytic therapy.

Thrombolysis is also used in selected cases of acute peripheral arterial occlusion (usually by local arterial infusion) and in massive ileofemoral vein thrombosis or massive pulmonary embolism. The role of thrombolysis in peripheral arterial or venous thromboembolism is less widely accepted.

The role of thrombolysis with alteplase (less than 3 hours after onset of symptoms although some evidence now exists that treatment is effective up to 4.5 hours) in acute ischaemic stroke has been established, under strictly controlled circumstances in acute stroke units. In particular, haemorrhage or established infarction must be excluded by brain imaging with computerised tomography (CT) or magnetic resonance (MR).

General aspects of thrombolysis

All thrombolytic agents act by activating plasminogen to plasmin, leading to degradation of fibrin, not only in thrombi but also in haemostatic fibrin plugs, which frequently causes major bleeding (there is a 1% risk of intracranial bleeding which is often fatal or disabling).

Streptokinase

This is a protein produced by group A β-haemolytic streptococci. Streptokinase requires a complex to be formed with plasminogen before it can cleave other plasminogen molecules to form plasmin. As it is a foreign protein, streptokinase may cause allergic reactions. Many patients already have antibodies to streptokinase because of previous streptococcal infection, but streptokinase administration also frequently leads to antibody formation. Use of an alternative agent such as tPA is recommended if a patient who has previously received streptokinase requires thrombolysis (such patients should carry a card indicating this).

Alteplase (tPA)

Recombinant tPA (alteplase) is developed from an endogenous fibrinolytic enzyme, release of which initiates physiological fibrinolysis. It lyses thrombi more rapidly, but carries a higher risk of intracranial haemorrhage than streptokinase and is more expensive. It is the thrombolytic agent of choice in selected cases of acute ischaemic stroke.

Other thrombolytic agents

Reteplase and tenecteplase are also licensed for treatment of acute myocardial infarction. They are given by intravenous injection (tenecteplase by a bolus injection).

Anaemia and haematinics

Aims

1 To relieve symptoms
2 To correct the underlying disorder
3 To replace any deficiencies: iron, vitamin B_{12}, folic acid.

Relevant pathophysiology

The cellular constituents of the blood—the red cells, white cells and platelets—exist as a result of the balance between production and destruction. Anaemia occurs when the concentration of haemoglobin in the blood falls below normal for the age and sex of the patient. The lower limits of normal are:
1 For adult males: 13.0 g/dL
2 For adult females: 11.5 g/dL.

The balance between production and destruction may be disturbed by:
1 Blood loss
2 Impaired red cell formation: haematinic deficiency or bone marrow depression
3 Increased red cell destruction: haemolysis.

Iron, vitamin B_{12} and folic acid are essential for normal marrow function. Deficiency of any or all of these results in defective red cell synthesis and eventual anaemia. As each of the agents plays a different part in cellular production in the marrow, individual deficiencies are manifested in different ways. Accurate diagnosis is therefore essential before any specific agent is given. Lack of iron causes a hypochromic, microcytic anaemia with low serum ferritin. Lack of vitamin B_{12} or folic acid causes a macrocytic anaemia with a megaloblastic bone marrow. If the marrow is deprived of either or both vitamin B_{12} and folic acid, the blood picture and the marrow look the same, but it is essential to determine which substance is missing. If folic acid is given to a patient who has vitamin B_{12} deficiency, neurological damage (subacute combined degeneration of the cord) may be provoked or aggravated.

Iron deficiency anaemia

As iron is usually absorbed from the gut, a satisfactory response is achieved in most patients when iron salts are given orally. Several ferrous salts are available. There is little to choose between them although they vary greatly in cost. The cheaper salts such as ferrous sulphate should be used unless gastrointestinal adverse effects are severe. Slow-release preparations should be avoided because of unreliable absorption. The duration of treatment, and its success, depends on the underlying cause of the anaemia. Haemoglobin should rise by approximately 1 g/dL/week. The achievement of normal haemoglobin levels should then be followed by further treatment for 6 months in an attempt to replenish iron stores throughout the body.

Adverse effects

Some people cannot tolerate oral iron preparations. The main complaints are nausea, epigastric discomfort, constipation and diarrhoea. A change in the ferrous salt form may help but improvement may be related to a lower content of iron in the alternative preparation.

Dose

Ferrous sulphate is given at a dose of 200 mg three times daily until anaemia is corrected and iron stores are replenished.

Parenteral iron

Oral iron therapy occasionally fails to achieve its objective because of lack of patient cooperation, severe adverse effects or gastrointestinal malabsorption. The total dose of parenteral iron required is calculated for each patient on the basis of body weight and haemoglobin level. Iron sucrose is given by slow intravenous injection of infusion only. Iron dextran is given either by deep intramuscular injection into the gluteal muscle or by slow intravenous injection or infusion. Anaphylactic reactions can occur with parenteral iron, and patients should be given a test dose initially, and carefully monitored.

Megaloblastic anaemia

Vitamin B_{12} deficiency requires vitamin B_{12} to be injected in adequate doses for life. Usually the underlying disease, such as pernicious anaemia, cannot be corrected and a route that bypasses the defective absorption mechanism in the gut therefore must supply the vitamin. Treatment should correct the anaemia and then maintain a normal blood picture. It should arrest, reverse or prevent lesions of the nervous system and replenish depleted stores.

A dramatic response often follows within 2–3 days of the start of vitamin B_{12} therapy. Symptoms improve and the haemoglobin concentration rises progressively to normal. An early index of success is a rise in the reticulocyte count, which reaches a peak after about 1 week and then gradually declines to normal in the next 2 weeks. Marrow changes reverse rapidly.

Adverse effects

These are rare and probably related to contamination or impurities in the injected solution.

Dose

Hydroxocobalamin is given at a dose of 1 mg on alternate days by intramuscular injection for 1 week, then at 2- to 3-monthly intervals for life.

Folic acid

Folic acid deficiency in Western countries is frequently the result of low dietary intake. Less commonly it is the consequence of malabsorption. Pregnancy makes such demands on iron and folic acid stores in the mother that it has been routine for iron and folic acid to be prescribed throughout pregnancy. Recent evidence that periconceptional maternal folic acid deficiency is associated with the birth of infants with neural tube defects has led to the recommendation of the use of supplements of small doses of folic acid by women who are planning pregnancy until at least 12 weeks gestation. Folic acid should never be given alone for vitamin B_{12} deficiency, as it may precipitate subacute combined deficiency of the spinal cord.

Dose

An oral dose of 5 mg daily is given for 4 months. When combined with iron for prophylactic use in pregnancy, 200–500 μg is given daily. A dose of 400 μg daily is recommended for routine periconceptional prophylaxis, but 5 mg daily (until week 12 of pregnancy) is recommended for women who have already given birth to an infant with a neural tube defect.

Haemopoietic growth factors

These naturally occurring glycoproteins have a physiological role in the regulation of haemopoiesis. Most are synthesised by bone marrow stromal cells. Some act on pluripotent stem cells, whilst others are lineage-specific and act only on committed progenitors. Molecular biological techniques have made possible the production of recombinant forms of some of the haemopoietic growth factors, and these are now in clinical use for a number of specialised indications. All these agents are given parenterally, usually by subcutaneous or sometimes by intravenous injection.

Recombinant erythropoietin (epoetin, darbepoetin alfa)

Physiologically, erythropoietin is synthesised in the kidney, and its synthesis is regulated by the oxygen tension in renal tissues. It acts on committed erythroid precursors to increase erythropoiesis. In severe renal failure erythropoietin production is defective and this contributes to the anaemia of renal disease. Recombinant human erythropoietin was the first of the growth factors to come into therapeutic use and is indicated for the treatment of anaemia associated with severe renal failure. Patients on dialysis and those not yet being dialysed are suitable. Haematinic deficiency, infections and aluminium accumulation should be ruled out as major contributory causes of anaemia before prescribing erythropoietin to renal patients. Potential adverse effects of erythropoietin include hypertension, clotting of vascular access sites, flu-like symptoms and seizures. It follows that erythropoietin is contraindicated in patients with uncontrolled hypertension.

Recombinant human granulocyte-colony stimulating factor (filgrastim, lenogastim, perfilgrastim)

Granulocyte-colony stimulating factor (G-CSF) is a growth factor that acts at relatively late stages of myelopoiesis in a lineage-specific manner to enhance the production and function of neutrophils. Recombinant human G-CSF (rhG-CSF) has been available for therapeutic use in recent years. It is effective in shortening the duration of neutropenias, e.g., following myelosuppressive chemotherapy, including bone marrow transplantation. Its use should be confined to specialised haematology or oncology units.

240

Drug-induced blood conditions

Drug-induced blood loss

Drugs used to relieve pain and inflammation in rheumatoid and osteoarthritis are often associated with chronic, occult blood loss from the gastrointestinal tract. Aspirin ingestion is a well-recognised cause of this type of anaemia and all other non-steroidal anti-inflammatory drugs, e.g. indomethacin, ibuprofen and COX-2 inhibitors, carry this risk (see Chapter 19). Oral anticoagulants carry a similar risk.

Drug-induced megaloblastic anaemia

Two important mechanisms result in drug-induced megaloblastic anaemia:
1 Interference with cellular DNA synthesis by cytotoxic drugs such as cytosine arabinoside, 5-fluorouracil or 6-mercaptopurine
2 Interference with folate absorption or use of anticonvulsants such as phenytoin and phenobarbital or the cytotoxic drug methotrexate, which inhibits dihydrofolate reductase.

Drug-induced sideroblastic anaemia

Some drugs and chemicals are involved in the aetiology of sideroblastic anaemia (a type of refractory anaemia) in a small proportion of patients. This can occur following administration of the anti-tuberculous drug isoniazid, or following excessive alcohol consumption or exposure to lead.

Drug-induced marrow depression: aplastic anaemia

This occurs when cellular activity in the bone marrow is suppressed and is usually associated with the suppression of white cell and platelet formation (pancytopenia). Rarely, pure red cell aplasia may occur. Cytotoxic drugs are the commonest cause.

Drugs causing aplastic anaemia usually incorporate a benzene ring with closely attached amino groups. The outcome depends on the dose and the length of exposure, and to less well-defined factors such as the degree of susceptibility, idiosyncracy or hypersensitivity exhibited by an individual.

Certain drugs have a high risk of causing aplastic anaemia. These include gold salts. In other cases this is a rare idiosyncratic adverse effect, e.g. with antimicrobials such as chloramphenicol and the sulphonylureas.

Some drugs have a tendency to suppress white cells, e.g. phenylbutazone, meprobamate and chlorpromazine, while others inhibit platelet production, e.g. gold salts.

Unless the risk is acceptable, as in the treatment of some forms of malignant diseases, aplastic anaemia should be prevented at all costs. The risks can be minimised by avoiding known marrow depressants, especially in patients with a history of allergy or idiosyncracy. If the risk is accepted, then every effort should be made to detect early signs and symptoms of bone marrow depression. The patient should be advised that sore throat, fever, malaise and bruising may be an indication. Regular peripheral blood examination should be performed. In many circumstances, where the degree of exposure to the causative agent has not been excessive, withdrawal of the agent leads to recovery within 2–3 weeks. Otherwise, intensive therapy is required, including reverse barrier nursing antibiotics, transfusion of blood products, administration of androgens or rhG-CSF and, in extreme cases, bone marrow transplantation.

Drug-induced haemolytic anaemia

A haemolytic anaemia occurs when the rate of red cell destruction is increased and red cells survive for a shorter time than the normal 100–200 days. Many drugs can reduce red cell survival:
1 Those that inevitably cause haemolytic anaemia (direct toxins)
2 Those that cause haemolysis because of hereditary defects in red cell metabolism
3 Drugs that cause haemolysis because of the development of abnormal immune mechanisms.

Direct toxins

Drugs and chemicals that have powerful oxidant properties are likely to cause haemolysis. Damage by these agents results in fragmentation and irregular contraction of red cells, spherocytosis, basophilic stippling, Heinz bodies, methaemoglobinaemia and sulphaemoglobinaemia. In addition to many domestic and industrial agents, haemolytic anaemia may follow the use of sulphones in the treatment of leprosy and sulphonamides, including sulphasalazine and dapsone.

Interaction with hereditary defects in red cells

Glucose-6-phosphate dehydrogenase deficiency in Negroid and Mediterranean races may give some protection against falciparum malaria, but the red cells in these individuals are abnormally sensitive to oxidising agents, resulting in haemolysis.

A large number of compounds may cause this haemolytic reaction, notably:

1 Antimalarial drugs, e.g. primaquine and pamaquin
2 The sulphones used in leprosy, e.g. dapsone
3 Some sulphonamides including co-trimoxazole
4 Quinolone antibiotics including ciprofloxacin and nalidixic acid
5 Water-soluble vitamin K analogues.

Immune mechanisms

Drugs can be associated with two immune haemolytic mechanisms.

Immune haemolytic anaemia

Antibodies may be formed against the drug or its metabolites. Antibodies can only be demonstrated *in vitro* in the presence of the drug. They may be stimulated by the drug binding directly to red cells forming a drug–red cell complex (the hapten cell mechanism, e.g. penicillin and cephalothin) or by the drug itself with subsequent adsorption on to the red cell surface. Activation of complement then causes lysis (immune complex mechanism, e.g. quinidine, *p*-aminosalicylic acid and rifampicin).

Autoimmune haemolytic anaemia

Antibodies are formed against the red cells. They can be demonstrated *in vitro* in the absence of the drug. This not uncommon form of haemolytic anaemia has been associated most often with the antihypertensive drug methyldopa. While at least 15% of patients on methyldopa develop a positive direct antiglobulin test, less than 0.1% develop overt haemolytic anaemia. If the drug is withdrawn, the haemoglobin level recovers but it may take many months for the antiglobulin test to become negative. Other drugs occasionally causing this kind of haemolytic anaemia are levodopa and mefenamic acid.

Neutropenia

Drugs and neutropenia

1 Antibiotics: chloramphenicol, co-trimoxazole
2 Anti-inflammatory drugs: phenylbutazone
3 Oral hypoglycaemics
4 Psychotropic drugs including phenothiazines and the antipsychotic agent clozapine which may cause agranulocytosis in 1 in 300 patients and which requires patient registration for use
5 Anticonvulsants: carbamazepine
6 Antithyroid drugs

The most common adverse effect of drugs on the white cell system is a reduction in the number of neutrophils below the lower limit of normal (neutropenia). Drugs causing this do so either as part of aplastic anaemia (pancytopenia) or as a selective neutropenia that does not involve the red cells or platelets. Drugs causing pancytopenia have been discussed in relation to aplastic anaemia. Drugs may also cause selective neutropenia. This may occur either because of selective myeloid suppression, or because of an immune mechanism that may affect mature neutrophils only, or may also involve late myeloid precursors in the bone marrow (agranulocytosis). A large number of agents have been documented as causes of neutropenia, and a careful drug history should be taken in patients presenting with neutropenia. In most cases individual patient susceptibility to a particular drug underlies the problem. The following have a particular association with neutropenia:

Treatment of drug-induced neutropenia calls for:

1 Withdrawal of the drug

2 Haematological advice and bone marrow examination

3 In severe cases expert supportive care for the prevention and treatment of infection

4 In selected cases treatment with myeloid growth factors, e.g. rhG-CSF.

Drug-induced thrombocytopenia

Platelets may be reduced in number (thrombocytopenia) or function by drugs and chemicals. This may be part of aplastic anaemia or selective thrombocytopenia. The latter is a rare effect of various drugs, including heparins, thiazides, sulphonamides and sulphonylureas, and sodium valproate. Drug-induced thrombocytopenia may occur as a result of suppression of platelet production or may involve an immune mechanism, akin to drug-induced immune haemolysis. A further mechanism is drug-induced platelet aggregation, for example, heparin-induced thrombocytopenia which is a consequence of antibody-dependent platelet aggregation. Rarely, drugs may be involved in the aetiology of microangiopathic syndromes associated with thrombocytopenia (thrombotic thrombocytopenic purpura and haemolytic uraemic syndrome). Oral contraceptive agents and ciclosporin have occasionally been implicated in such cases.

Drug-induced thrombocytopenia should be treated according to haematological advice. The offending agent should be withdrawn and a bone marrow examination is usually indicated. If an immune mechanism is implicated, intravenous immunoglobulin treatment may be helpful. In others, particularly if platelet production is suppressed and the thrombocytopenia is severe or the patient is haemorrhagic, platelet transfusion may be indicated. Platelet transfusion should *not* be given in suspected cases of heparin-induced thrombocytopenia. Heparin should be stopped and advice regarding alternative anticoagulation sought from a haematologist. Platelet transfusions are also contraindicated in microangiopathic syndromes.

Comment

Whenever a disorder of blood cell formation is observed and an adverse drug effect suspected, take a careful drug history and consult reference books describing adverse effects.

Chapter 19

Drugs and inflammatory joint disease

Clinical scenario

A 58-year-old lady with a 3-year history of rheumatoid arthritis is referred by her GP with a flare up of her arthritis. She has a high ESR and CRP and is rheumatoid factor positive. In the last year she has been taking various NSAIDs and 3 months ago was found to have iron deficient anaemia. An upper GI endoscopy showed a gastric ulcer, NSAIDS were stopped and she was prescribed a proton pump inhibitor. Since then she has been taking co-codamol for pain relief but this has resulted in constipation. Her other medical problem is hypertension treated with atenolol. How would you treat this lady's rheumatoid arthritis?

Introduction

In inflammatory joint disease, the aims are as follows:

1 To reduce pain.
2 To reduce stiffness and improve function.
3 To prevent chronic deformity by arresting the inflammation that results in synovial membrane proliferation and bone erosions.

Relevant pathophysiology

Anti-inflammatory analgesic drugs are used to relieve the painful symptoms of joint diseases, including those listed below.

Key points

- Drugs used in inflammatory joint disease are aimed at symptom relief and preventing joint damage
- Many of the drugs used, whether for symptom relief or to prevent joint damage, have considerable side effects and need careful clinical and laboratory monitoring
- DCARTs (disease controlling antirheumatic therapies) and immune modifying therapies are increasingly used early in the course of the disease to prevent joint damage

Joint diseases	
Rheumatoid arthritis	Gout
Osteoarthritis	Reactive arthritis (including Reiter's syndrome)
Psoriatic arthritis	Arthritis associated with systemic lupus erythematosus (SLE)
Ankylosing spondylitis	

Lecture Notes: Clinical Pharmacology and Therapeutics, 8th edition. By Gerard McKay, John Reid and Matthew Walters. Published 2010 by Blackwell Publishing Ltd.

The aetiology of these diseases is varied and in most cases not entirely clear. There is a disturbance in immune response which may also be a feature in gout and even osteoarthritis. In rheumatoid arthritis (RA), for example, activated T-cells and cytokine release from macrophages result in a cascade of events that result in proteolytic enzyme release which damages cartilage, while prostaglandins promote synovial vasodilatation and exacerbate pain. Thus, there are a number of areas where an anti-inflammatory drug might be effective:

1 Immunosuppression
2 Inhibition of cell migration
3 Inhibition of enzyme release
4 Inhibition of prostaglandin synthesis
5 Inhibition of pro-inflammatory cytokines.

Principles of drug treatment

The chronicity of inflammatory joint disease such as RA necessitates long-term follow-up and management within a multi-dimensional framework aimed at preserving the patient's quality of life. This is achieved by attempting to improve functional ability, mental and social health and vocational status, and reduce disease activity. While drugs are an important part of the treatment of patients with inflammatory joint disease, other non-pharmacological aspects demand careful consideration. These include rest, exercise and psychological management.

Rest

Inflammatory arthritis is typically a disease of exacerbation and remission. During an acute attack it may be necessary to recommend bedrest and splinting of the affected joints.

Exercise

After an acute attack, carefully graded exercises in the form of physiotherapy and hydrotherapy are required to ensure an early return to normal activities. Exercise also has psychological goals. It can enhance a feeling of well-being and provide active recreation. Excessive exercise, however, can be harmful. Assessing activities of daily life is an important role for occupational therapists.

Psychological management

Psychological factors are implicated in pain perception. The intensity of pain is in part related to patients' beliefs in their ability to cope with or control the effect of their disease. Counselling about employment is also important, as the patient's self-esteem often depends on useful and purposeful work. The development of support groups for various inflammatory arthritides has an important role in improving patients' education, and these 'group therapies' encourage self-management behaviour and better adaptation to a chronic, incurable disease, often leading to psychological, social and perhaps financial well-being.

Various physical aids are available to allow those with disabilities to maintain independence while protecting the affected joints.

The previous treatment of inflammatory arthritis was represented by a pyramid starting with non-steroidal anti-inflammatory drugs (NSAIDs) and progressing to disease-controlling antirheumatic therapies (DCARTs) such as antimalarials, sulphasalazine (sulfasalazine), gold, D-penicillamine, methotrexate, leflunomide, azathioprine and other immunosuppressive agents. Over the past decade, there has been an increasing use of DCARTs, and monoclonal antibody therapy especially in the early course of the disease, together with an NSAID because the majority of patients who develop joint damage do so in the first 2 years.

Symptom modifying antirheumatic therapies

Simple analgesics

Simple analgesics such as paracetamol may be used to supplement other therapy, but they are relatively ineffective when used alone in RA. They do not retard the progress of the disease and cannot provide adequate pain relief. They may be adequate in the management of some patients with OA.

Non-steroidal anti-inflammatory drugs

NSAIDs act in a variety of ways but their prime mode of action is via the inhibition of cyclooxygenase (Cox), which exists in two isoforms – Cox-1 and Cox-2. It is now known that Cox-1 is the constitutive form and Cox-2 is the inducible form of the enzyme. Most currently available NSAIDs primarily inhibit Cox-1 but there are now several highly selective Cox-2 inhibitors available. Although lysosome-stabilising effects and inhibition of cellular migration have also been demonstrated, the clinical significance of this observation is unclear. The available NSAIDs come in a variety of chemical classes (Table 19.1). Differences in physicochemical characteristics may influence their pharmacokinetics and give rise to differences in their efficacy and adverse effects.

Aspirin and related salicylates

Aspirin is the longest established and most traditional of the anti-inflammatory drugs and is relatively cheap. However, in the United Kingdom, its role has been supplanted by other NSAIDs. Benorilate (benorylate) is a compound in which aspirin is linked with paracetamol, and diflunisal is a difluorophenyl salicylic acid derivative however these drugs are used relatively infrequently.

Pharmacokinetics

The pharmacokinetics of aspirin are complex and when used in relatively high doses for long periods of time, plasma levels should be monitored. Aspirin is readily absorbed from the gastrointestinal tract and is given orally. Elimination normally follows first-order kinetics, but after very large doses the enzymes that metabolise aspirin become saturated.

Adverse effects

1 Gastrointestinal effects. Nausea and vomiting follow high doses of aspirin. Dyspepsia, gastric irritation and occult or frank blood loss are common

Table 19.1 Examples of the principal groups of NSAIDs.

Drug	Dose* (mg)	Dosage interval (hour)
Salicylates		
Aspirin	900	4[†]
Diflunisal	500	12
Benorilate (benorylate)	4000	12
Pyrazolones		
Phenylbutazone	100	8
Azapropazone	300	8
Indoles		
Indometacin (indomethacin)	50	8
Sulindac	200	12
Etodolac	400	8
Fenamates		
Mefenamic acid	500	8
Flufenamic acid	200	8
Propionates		
Ibuprofen	400	8
Naproxen	250	8
Ketoprofen	50	6
Phenylacetates		
Diclofenac	50	8
Oxicams		
Piroxicam	20	Daily
Tenoxicam	20	Daily
Meloxicam	7.5–15	Daily
Other		
Nabumetone	1000	Daily
Cox-2 inhibitors		
Celecoxib	200	Daily
Etoricoxib	60–120 mg	Daily
Valdecoxib	10–20	Daily

*These doses are near the upper limit and therapy should be commenced with approximately half doses.
[†]Adjust according to serum concentration.

adverse effects, particularly when aspirin is associated with alcohol ingestion. Blood loss results from superficial gastric erosions or peptic ulceration. Inhibition of prostaglandin synthesis is probably responsible because some prostaglandins increase gastric mucosal blood flow and have other protective effects. Gastrointestinal blood loss occurs even with parenteral aspirin or aspirin by suppository.

However, fewer erosions and ulcers are found with these and more recent enteric-coated formulations. Newer NSAIDs have been claimed to cause less gastric irritation. These comparisons have not usually been made with enteric-coated aspirin. At present, there appears to be a dose-dependent relationship between anti-inflammatory analgesic effect, prostaglandin synthetase inhibition and the frequency of gastric irritation. Less active analgesics cause less gastric irritation.

2 Prolonged bleeding time may result from the inhibition of thromboxane synthesis and impaired platelet aggregation (Chapter 18) or reduced hepatic clotting factor synthesis.

3 Bronchospasm, urticaria or hay fever may rarely occur in sensitive individuals and appear to result from release of immune mediators secondary to prostaglandin synthesis inhibition.

4 Tinnitus, dizziness and deafness are dose and plasma level related adverse effects. Vomiting and tachypnoea may also occur.

5 In overdose, confusion, convulsions and hyperpyrexia are seen. Refer to Toxbase for management. (see Chapter 26).

Dose

Aspirin tablets of 300–900 mg are given 4- to 6-hourly. In RA, up to 4.5 g/day may be required in divided doses.

Phenylbutazone

This belongs to the pyrazolone class and has analgesic, antipyretic and potent anti-inflammatory actions. However, unfortunately, it can cause serious and sometimes fatal marrow depression. Its use is now limited to the treatment of ankylosing spondylitis and even for this indication is rarely used. It is available on hospital prescription only.

Azapropazone

Azapropazone is chemically related to phenylbutazone but it does not apparently give rise to the marrow depression that led to the severe restrictions on the use of phenylbutazone. In addition to

acting as a non-steroidal anti-inflammatory agent, it has a uricosuric effect and is used in the treatment of gout. In the treatment of OA, RA and ankylosing spondylitis, dosage in elderly patients with a creatinine clearance of less than 60 mL/minute should not exceed 300 mg twice daily. If creatinine clearance in these patients is greater than 60 mL/minute, dosage may be increased to 900 mg daily. In younger patients who have normal renal function, the standard dose is 1200 mg daily.

Drug interactions

Azapropazone increases plasma concentrations of phenytoin and combined use should be avoided. It also potentiates the action of warfarin and should not be used with this anticoagulant. It should be used with great caution, if at all, with any other oral anticoagulants. Combination with oral hypoglycaemics may result in excessively low blood sugars, and again, its concurrent use should be avoided if possible.

Adverse effects

Skin rashes, fluid retention, angioneurotic oedema, dyspepsia and gastrointestinal bleeding have been reported.

Indometacin and related drugs

Indometacin has been widely used in inflammatory and non-inflammatory joint diseases for years. It is given by mouth or by suppository, and is generally very effective. Gastric adverse effects are a predictable problem, but headache, mental confusion and dizziness may also present problems. Salt and water retention with oedema may aggravate cardiac failure or hypertension and reduce the efficacy of antihypertensive drugs. Rectal administration may be associated with pruritus, discomfort and bleeding. Sulindac is chemically related to indometacin and is a prodrug, reversibly metabolised by the liver into its active metabolite. This might explain its relatively lower incidence of gastric side effects. Etodolac, another member of this group, is extensively metabolised and excreted in both urine and bile. The kinetics of etodolac are unchanged in the elderly and in renal impairment.

Dose

Indometacin: Oral, 25–50 mg two to three times daily. The 75-mg sustained release capsule is designed to deliver 25 mg of the drug immediately and the remaining 50 mg over the next 8–12 hours. Rectal suppository, 100 mg at night; this may be repeated in the morning.

The recommended dose for sulindac is 200 mg twice daily and that of etodolac, 600 mg slow release once a day.

Propionic acid derivatives

A large number of agents from this group of drugs have been marketed. They are well absorbed orally and have fewer gastric adverse effects than plain aspirin. This has led some rheumatologists to favour their use. This group consists of the drugs listed below.

Propionic acid derivatives	
Ibuprofen	Flurbiprofen
Fenoprofen	Fenbufen
Ketoprofen	Tiaprofenic acid
Naproxen	

Note that fenbufen is a prodrug with no direct effect on the stomach. None of these propionic acid derivatives has been shown to interact significantly with oral anticoagulants, and if a patient must also receive warfarin, this group of drugs may be preferable.

Phenylacetic acid derivatives

Diclofenac is very similar to the propionic acid derivatives. It may sometimes cause hepatitis.

Fenamates

The long-established mefenamic acid and flufenamic acid are mildly effective in inflammatory joint disease, but they share the problems of salicylates to which they are chemically related. Thus, they share the gastric adverse effects but, in addition, they cause diarrhoea, a dose-related phenomenon for which the basis is not clear.

Piroxicam and related oxicams

Piroxicam is an anti-inflammatory agent that is chemically unrelated to other drugs. It does, however, share their propensity to cause gastrointestinal adverse effects, and potentiates the effect of oral anticoagulants. It is contraindicated in asthmatic patients who cannot tolerate aspirin. It may cause fluid retention, a particular hazard in the elderly. Tenoxicam is reported to have less gastric toxicity and meloxicam has some Cox-2 selectivity.

Nabumetone

This is a non-acidic compound and a poor inhibitor of prostaglandin synthesis. After absorption, it is metabolised rapidly by the liver into an acidic metabolite that has effective anti-inflammatory actions. In comparison to other NSAIDs, nabumetone is less gastrotoxic. The recommended dose is 1000 mg daily.

Cox-2 inhibitors

There are now several Cox-2 inhibitors available for the treatment of RA and OA. They have been shown to reduce gastrotoxicity with a decrease in perforations, ulcers and bleeds, but some such as rofecoxib, celecoxib and valdecoxib may also increase the incidence of cardiovascular events such as stroke and myocardial infarction. Rofecoxib has been withdrawn from the market and the others should only be used in patients with no cardiovascular risk factors. Etoricoxib is a long-acting Cox-2 inhibitor that has not been implicated to date in patients with an increased cardiovascular risk, although the possibility of a class effect has not been ruled out. Recent studies also implicate non-selective NSAIDs (with the exceptions of naproxen and aspirin) in increased vascular risk. NSAIDs and Cox inhibitors should therefore be used with caution in patients with vascular risk factors or history, and should be used at the lowest dose necessary and for limited periods if possible.

Key points

- NSAIDS form the mainstay of symptom modification in inflammatory joint disease
- There is a wide selection of agents but no drug has been clearly shown to be superior in terms of efficacy and safety
- It is important that a constant vigilance is maintained for side effects and drug interactions especially in the elderly
- Individual response to a particular drug may vary

Disease-controlling antirheumatic therapies

Disease-controlling antirheumatic therapies (DCARTs) are used in the management of inflammatory arthritis to achieve disease remission and slow down the progression of joint erosions. These antirheumatic agents comprise a group of widely different chemical entities, including hydroxychloroquine, sulphasalazine, gold, D-penicillamine, immunosuppressant drugs (methotrexate, leflunomide, azathioprine, cyclophosphamide, chlorambucil and ciclosporin) and corticosteroids. Mechanisms of action of these drugs are not clear. There is a lag between starting therapy and observing an effect. They are indicated in the earlier years of the disease. It is usual to continue with conventional anti-inflammatory drugs. Unlike NSAIDs, DCARTs may influence the underlying disease process. For example, in RA, decreasing erythrocyte sedimentation rate and rheumatoid factor titre will be associated with an increase in haemoglobin in patients who respond and a slowing down of the rate of radiological progression. There is evidence that combination therapy with several DCARTs, e.g. methotrexate, sulphasalazine and hydroxychloroquine, is more effective than using single agents alone.

Chloroquine and hydroxychloroquine

These drugs, originally developed as antimalarials, have been used to treat RA and SLE since the 1950s, and responses in RA are similar but somewhat less than those observed with other DCARTs except for auronofin (oral gold). However, they have a major advantage in their lack of life-threatening toxicity compared to other DCARTs and are being increasingly used early in the course of disease and in combination regimens with other DCARTs. The mechanisms of action of these preparations may be by lysosome stabilisation and inhibition of phagocytic functions.

They are well absorbed orally, taken up by many tissues and then very slowly excreted in the urine. The most disturbing toxic effect (although rare) is a retinopathy as a result of gradual accumulation of the drug in the retina and is dose-dependent. Irreversible retinal damage with permanent blindness has been reported in patients taking high doses of chloroquine. Rashes and marrow toxicity are rarely seen. Neuropathies and myopathies have been reported.

Clinical use

Hydroxychloroquine employed in the usual doses is less likely to be associated with adverse effects and has largely superseded chloroquine in clinical practice. Initially, 400 mg is given daily and this dose can be reduced after 6–12 months depending on response. Careful ophthalmological screening at baseline and after 2 years should be done to identify any potential retinal damage, which is reversible if diagnosed early, although this complication is rare provided dosage is kept below 6.5 mg/kg. Patients with renal failure are more at risk from retinal toxicity.

Sulphasalazine

Sulphasalazine is an effective and relatively safe antirheumatic drug in RA and also in ankylosing spondylitis and HLA-B27 related arthropathies such as reactive arthritis and psoriatic arthritis. It consists of 5-aminosalicylic acid joined to sulphapyridine (sulfapyridine) by an azo bond. In the gut, these two moieties are liberated following bacterial reduction of the azo bond. Sulphapyridine is thought to be the principal antirheumatic agent, while 5-aminosalicylic acid is the active anti-inflammatory moiety when sulphasalazine is used in the treatment of inflammatory bowel disease.

Adverse effects

These include skin rashes, nausea, headache and occasional leucopenia, neutropenia and thrombocytopenia. The blood abnormalities usually occur early on in the course of treatment (within 6 months) and reverse if the drug is stopped.

Clinical use and dose

Sulphasalazine ranks with antimalarials and auronofin as the best tolerated of the DCARTs. The oral dose is initially 500 mg daily, usually increased by 500 mg at 1-week intervals to a maximum of 2–3 g daily. or 40 mg/kg. Blood counts are performed fortnightly in the first 12 weeks, and 3-monthly thereafter.

Gold salts

These have been used for over 40 years in the management of RA. Previously, gold salts were thought to act by reducing macrophage activity. A potentially important new finding is that gold salts affect the immune system by regulating gene expression and consequent protein synthesis. One-third of patients derive considerable benefit, one-third have only a modest response and one-third have adverse effects that require interruption of treatment.

Adverse effects

1 Pruritic rashes are common and present in many forms, including mouth ulcers.
2 Proteinuria secondary to a membranous glomerulonephritis occurs in 10% of patients but it resolves on stopping gold treatment.

3 Vasodilatation with orthostatic hypotension may acutely follow drug dosing and is more likely to occur in patients on ACE inhibitors.
4 Neutropenia and thrombocytopenia may occur suddenly or develop slowly.
Recovery is usually assured provided no more gold is given. Aplastic anaemia is extremely rare now if it occurs; it has a high fatality rate.

Gold treatment is closely supervised with haematological checks before each dose.

Clinical use and dose

An intramuscular injection of sodium aurothiomalate is given initially as a 10-mg test dose followed by 50 mg weekly for up to 6 months or until a response or toxic effects are observed. Dose frequency may be reduced to monthly and continued for years. An oral preparation (auronofin) is also available. It is safer and less toxic than injectable gold, but is commonly associated with diarrhoea and lower abdominal discomfort. It is also much less effective than other DCARTs. Gold therapy is no longer as commonly used as in the past.

D-Penicillamine

First introduced as a copper-chelating agent in Wilson's disease, D-penicillamine modifies the formation of immunoglobulin. It has a similar action to gold salts but relapse may occur with continuing therapy.

Adverse effects

These are similar to those with gold. Cross-toxicity with gold has been reported but is disputed.
1 Skin rashes are common.
2 Taste disturbance is usually transient.
3 Proteinuria, as with gold.
4 Marrow toxicity is similar to gold, consisting of thrombocytopenia and neutropenia. As these changes develop gradually, routine fortnightly haematological monitoring is essential during the initial stages of therapy.

5 Immunological effects. Up to 50% of patients develop positive antinuclear antibodies. Rarely, SLE or myasthenia gravis may be precipitated.

Clinical use and dose

D-Penicillamine is given as a 125-mg dose initially followed by monthly increments of 125 mg until response is satisfactory or a maximum dose of 1000 mg is achieved. It is now rarely used as a first-line DCART.

Cytotoxic drugs

Methotrexate, azathioprine, leflunamide, cyclophosphamide and chlorambucil are used in inflammatory arthritis because of their immuno-suppressant effects. They are discussed in Chapter 15. In rheumatic diseases, these drugs are indicated in resistant inflammatory joint disease, and commonly used together with corticosteroids in the presence of potentially serious extra-articular disease involvement, systemic vasculitis and connective tissue diseases such as SLE and dermato-myositis. Methotrexate is currently considered as the DCART of choice, especially in early aggressive inflammatory joint disease. It works quickly and significant improvement in the disease is observed within the first 4–6 weeks. It shares similar side effects with other cytotoxic agents.

Immunotherapy

Ciclosporin, mycophenolate, corticosteroids and anti-cytokine therapy are used in the treatment of inflammatory joint disease and other inflammatory conditions. They are discussed elsewhere (see Chapter 16)

Combination therapy

Rheumatologists are now using selected DCARTs in combination with clinical evidence of a synergistic effect. Two combinations have been shown to be efficacious: (i) ciclosporin with methotrex-ate, and (ii) methotrexate with sulphasalazine and hydroxychloroquine. The incidence of side effects is not increased when these drugs are used in combination.

Key points

- Inflammatory joint disease remains an important and difficult therapeutic challenge
- The chronicity of disease, variable expression, with remissions and exacerbations, and its implications for the patient's life must all be considered when deciding on treatment
- Rheumatologists are now treating inflammatory joint disease early and aggressively with DCARTS and im-munotherapy
- In most cases the approach in using a DCART or immunotherapy is to work through the drugs available, continuously weighing the risk of serious toxicity against the benefits of pain relief and minimising joint destruction

Drugs used in gout

Clinical scenario

A 45-year-old obese man presents with an acutely swollen first metatarsal phalangeal joint. He is on ben-droflumethiazide for his blood pressure and drinks 30 units of alcohol per week. He has a clinical di-agnosis of acute gout. How should this patient be managed?

Key points

- Acute gout should be managed symptomatically with high doses of NSAIDs
- Chronic management of gout aims to reduce uric acid formation prophylactically by xanthine oxidase inhibition using allopurinol, thus preventing arthritis and renal damage
- Uricosuric drugs are now used less commonly and are only indicated in patients who are intolerant of allopurinol
- Management should also include lifestyle advice and avoiding, if possible the use of diuretics which may precipitate an acute episode

Introduction

It managing gout it is important to distinguish the following:

1 Management of the acute attack
2 Long-term management

Management of the acute attack

An acute attack of gout is extremely painful and effective anti-inflammatory drugs should be given at once. The drugs used are:

1 NSAIDs such as indometacin, naproxen, diclofenac, piroxicam and etoricoxib in large doses for 24–48 hours.
2 Colchicine: This drug can still be used in acute gout (orally or intravenously) or in the early months of treatment with allopurinol. Adverse effects – nausea, vomiting, abdominal pain and diarrhoea – can be less common with low-dose regimens.

Long-term management

As the underlying mechanism in gout involves excess production of uric acid and/or reduced renal excretion of urate, long-term management aims at reducing uric acid in the body in two ways:

1 Inhibition of uric acid formation from purines by xanthine oxidase inhibition
2 Promotion of urate excretion in the urine.

Xanthine oxidase inhibition

Allopurinol

Pharmacokinetics
Allopurinol is well absorbed from the gastrointestinal tract and is rapidly cleared from the plasma with a half-life of 2–3 hours. It is converted to alloxanthine and this metabolite in turn inhibits the metabolism of the parent drug. Alloxanthine is also a xanthine oxidase inhibitor.

Adverse effects
These are not common. Hypersensitivity reactions, which subside on withdrawing the drug, consist of a skin rash accompanied by fever, malaise and muscle pain. Rarely, leukopenia or leukocytosis with eosinophilia occur.

Drug interactions
Drugs depending on xanthine oxidase for their metabolic conversion should be given with caution in association with allopurinol. This applies to 6-mercaptopurine and azathioprine. Inhibition of warfarin metabolism may also occur; anticoagulant control should be monitored closely in circumstances such as these.

Clinical use and dose
Allopurinol must not be used in an acute attack of gout because this will be prolonged. Initially, 100 mg allopurinol is given daily as a single dose, increasing to about 300 mg daily depending on serum uric acid levels. The aim is to keep serum uric acid levels in the bottom half of the normal range. Colchicine or indometacin may be given concurrently over the first 2 months to prevent acute gout.

Allopurinol should be considered in:

1 Urate overproduction, primary or secondary
2 Acute uric acid nephropathy (tumour lysis syndrome)
3 Nephrolithiasis of any type
4 Renal impairment (dose 100 mg/day per 30 mL/minute glomerular filtration rate)
5 24 hours urinary uric acid >0.42 g
6 Intolerance or allergy to uricosuric agents
7 Chronic tophaceous gout.

Uricosuric drugs

Probenecid

Probenecid inhibits the transport of organic acids across lipid membranes, including the renal tubule. Whereas this leads to an increase in the plasma concentration of a number of acidic drugs, the uric acid concentration falls because its reabsorption from tubular fluid is inhibited.

Pharmacokinetics
Probenecid is well absorbed from the gastrointestinal tract and peak concentrations are achieved in 2–4 hours. Metabolism and renal excretion result

in a half-life of about 9 hours; a large proportion of the parent drug is actively secreted by the proximal tubules.

Adverse effects

About 25% of patients experience dyspepsia and this limits its use in peptic ulceration. Hypersensitivity reactions occur occasionally as skin rashes. Drug-induced nephrotic syndrome has been reported.

Drug interactions

The uricosuric effect of probenecid may be inhibited by large doses of salicylates. Aspirin should therefore be avoided in patients receiving probenecid.

Dose

A 250-mg dose of probenecid is given twice daily initially, increasing to a maximum of 2 g daily over 2–3 weeks, depending on serum uric acid concentrations.

Sulphinpyrazone (sulfinpyrazone)

Sulphinpyrazone inhibits the tubular reabsorption of uric acid when given in sufficient dose. Like probenecid, it reduces the renal tubular secretion of many other organic acids.

Pharmacokinetics

Sulphinpyrazone is well absorbed from the gastrointestinal tract. It is strongly bound (98–99%) to plasma albumin; 90% is excreted unchanged in the urine; 10% is metabolised to the N-p-hydroxyphenyl metabolite, itself a potent uricosuric.

Adverse effects

Ten to fifteen per cent of patients receiving sulphinpyrazone develop gastrointestinal symptoms; as a rule it should be avoided in patients with a history of peptic ulceration. Rarely, it causes skin rashes and fever.

Drug interactions

As with probenecid, salicylates inhibit the uricosuric effect of sulphinpyrazone and more than occasional doses of aspirin should be avoided. Decreased excretion of oral hypoglycaemic agents may lead to hypoglycaemia and sulphinpyrazone may enhance the effect of warfarin.

Dose

A 100- to 200-mg dose of sulphinpyrazone is given daily, increasing over 2–3 weeks to about 600–800 mg daily, depending on serum uric acid concentrations.

Azapropazone

Azapropazone has a uricosuric effect and is used in acute attacks of gout and in long-term prophylaxis.

Dose

During the first 24 hours of an acute attack, 2400 mg azapropazone is given in divided doses and then 1300 mg daily until acute symptoms subside, followed by 1200 mg daily until symptoms have disappeared. In chronic gout, 600 mg twice daily is given unless the patient is elderly (over 65 years of age; see above).

Chapter 20

Anaesthesia and the relief of pain

Introduction

Modern anaesthetic practice involves a wide variety of pharmacological strategies to minimise pain, control physiological parameters and facilitate surgery. This chapter provides an overview of drugs used by anaesthetists, including analgesics, drugs which induce local and general anaesthesia, and neuromuscular blocking agents.

Relevant pathophysiology

Sensory receptors for pain are found in all tissues of the body. A variety of noxious stimuli (thermal, chemical, mechanical or electrical) cause them to respond and lead to the subjective experience of pain.

1 The first-order afferent neurones transmitting pain impulses are of two types:
- The rapidly conducting (12–30 m/second) small-diameter myelinated fibres of the A group (delta)
- The slow (0.5–2 m/second) non-myelinated C fibres.

Both the rapidly and slow-conducting fibres terminate in the dorsal horns of the spinal cord.

Lecture Notes: Clinical Pharmacology and Therapeutics, 8th edition. By Gerard McKay, John Reid and Matthew Walters. Published 2010 by Blackwell Publishing Ltd.

2 Second-order neurones carry the pain stimuli to the thalamus in the lateral spinothalamic tracts. Branches from both A and C fibres form synapses with cells in the dorsal horns of the spinal cord. A network of cells in this area, which includes the substantia gelatinosa, regulates transmission between the nociceptive neurones and those in the spinothalamic tract. Descending fibres from higher centres act to inhibit transmission.

3 From the thalamus, third-order neurones convey pain impulses to the post-central gyri of the cerebral cortex. The thalamus is the main region responsible for the integration of pain input but the cortical area is concerned with the exact and meaningful subjective interpretation of pain.

The transducing qualities of free nerve endings are affected by chemical changes in the immediate vicinity, e.g. changes in the concentrations of hydrogen ions, substance P, 5-hydroxytryptamine (5-HT), histamine, bradykinin and eicosanoids. Bradykinin and related substances are formed in extracellular fluid whenever there is tissue damage and account for the vascular and exudative changes of inflammation. Bradykinin sensitises and stimulates nerve endings and causes pain. The analgesic effects of aspirin and other non-steroidal anti-inflammatory drugs result from the impaired release of mediator by mechanisms including inhibition of prostaglandin synthesis.

Within the central nervous system (CNS), opioid receptors are localised in the spinal cord dorsal horn, and in the brain stem, thalamus and cortex, in what constitutes the ascending pain transmission system, as well as structures that comprise a descending inhibitory system that modulates pain at the level of the spinal cord. There are four distinct opioid receptor types and each of these has an endogenous ligand. Mu and kappa receptors, stimulated naturally by β-endorphins and dynorphins respectively, are responsible not only for analgesia but also for many of the adverse effects of morphine including respiratory depression and miosis. The consequences of stimulating the delta receptor, whose endogenous ligand is the enkephalins, with morphine in humans are unclear. The opioid receptor-like (ORL1) receptor is stimulated naturally by nociceptin/orphanin FQ (N/OFQ). Although the ORL1-N/OFQ system clearly belongs to the opioid receptor family and has a role in a variety of processes such as pain modulation and anxiety, it does not bind classical opiates and has distinct pharmacological actions. It is no longer believed that there is a sigma opioid receptor.

In addition to the endogenous ligands of the opioid receptor family, many other substances influence the pain pathways of the CNS including nitric oxide, cholecystokinin, substance P, biogenic amines like 5-HT and excitatory amino acids such as glutamate.

Principles of drug treatment

From a practical point of view, there are two types of pain:

1 Visceral pain, which is a dull, poorly localised pain, e.g. peritoneal pain

2 Somatic pain, which is sharply defined, e.g. pain of a fractured femur.

Pain is a valuable symptom of underlying pathology and may be vital in the diagnosis of disease, e.g. in management of the acute abdomen. However, inadequate administration of relief to a patient in distress while steps are taken to confirm the diagnosis should be avoided.

There is a pronounced placebo effect in the treatment of pain. Thirty per cent of patients in pain experience some relief from a doctor taking an interest in their pain and prescribing any drug.

Key points

- Use analgesics in adequate doses
- Titrate doses for individual patients
- Consider administration of analgesia 'by the clock' to prevent pain, rather than 'as required' when pain occurs
- Develop a management plan for breakthrough pain
- Use the oral route whenever possible
- Review and reassess requirement for analgesia on a regular basis
- Keep the treatment regimen as simple as possible

Opioid analgesics

Opiates are drugs derived from opium, a term for the juice of the poppy plant. Opioid is a more inclusive term, applying to all agonists or antagonists with morphine-like activity. The term narcotic is no longer used pharmacologically because of its pejorative legal meaning.

Morphine

Mechanism of action

Morphine produces a range of depressant effects by a central action on mu opioid receptors within the CNS and in peripheral tissues.

The CNS effects include analgesia, euphoria and sedation; depression of respiration; depression of the vasomotor centre resulting in hypotension; cough suppression; release of antidiuretic hormone; miosis; and nausea and vomiting. Peripheral effects include smooth muscle contraction with reduced motility of the gastrointestinal tract; reduced secretion of gastrointestinal tract; biliary spasm; urinary retention; constriction of bronchi partly as a result of histamine release; vasodilatation; and itching.

Pharmacokinetics

Morphine is unreliably absorbed after oral administration and subject to high first-pass metabolism in the gut wall and the liver; the oral bioavailability of morphine is typically 20%. However, there is a slow-release oral preparation that results in delayed but sustained therapeutic plasma morphine concentrations. The drug can be given intravenously, intramuscularly or subcutaneously. After intramuscular injection, peak brain concentrations occur between 30 and 45 minutes but relatively little of the administered drug crosses the blood–brain barrier. Morphine can also be injected into the subarachnoid and epidural spaces although its high water solubility makes it a less attractive drug for this purpose than diamorphine or fentanyl (because of the risk of secondary respiratory depression) and its side-effect profile is relatively poor when administered via these routes.

The major route of elimination is conjugation with glucuronic acid to form morphine-3-monoglucuronide, which is excreted in the urine. Only a very small amount of free morphine appears in the urine, bile or faeces. About 90% of the administered dose is eliminated within the first 24 hours.

Adverse effects

Many of the adverse effects of morphine represent an extension of its pharmacological effects as a result of relative overdosage (see below).

Adverse effects of morphine

1 Respiratory depression, periodic breathing or apnoea
2 Hypotension
3 Nausea and vomiting
4 Constipation
5 Tremor
6 Urticaria and itching
7 Tolerance and addiction to the drug. These are rare when morphine is given during anaesthesia or for the relief of pain after surgery

---

Drug interactions

Morphine delays the absorption of other drugs when they are given orally. In addition, other drugs such as phenothiazines and tricyclic antidepressants potentiate its depressant effects. Morphine will, in turn, potentiate the effect of most hypnotics and all volatile anaesthetic agents.

Clinical use and dose

1 The relief of visceral and somatic pain
2 The relief of anxiety and pain after myocardial infarction
3 In acute left ventricular failure (pulmonary oedema) to reduce preload by venodilation
4 Before, during and after anaesthesia, as part of a balanced anaesthetic technique

The usual intramuscular or subcutaneous dose for relief of severe pain is 0.1–0.2 mg/kg but this dose may need to be adjusted to take into account factors such as age and co-morbidity that may alter an individual's response. For post-operative pain, morphine is often given intravenously using syringe drivers activated by the patient (patient-controlled analgesia)
5 Opioids, particularly codeine derivatives, are used as antidiarrhoeal agents (Chapter 3).

Other opioid analgesics

Many opioid drugs are available and the properties of some are summarised in Table 20.1. Others such as papaveretum, pentazocine, butorphanol, dextromoramide, levorphanol and dipipanone have very limited use.

Diamorphine or heroin

This is more potent and more lipid-soluble than morphine. It is metabolised to monoacetylmorphine and then morphine. It is claimed to be less emetic than morphine but there is little evidence for this. When patients receiving palliative care require large doses of morphine for pain relief, diamorphine can be administered by continuous subcutaneous infusion in a smaller volume of solution than the equivalent dose of morphine. This is an important consideration in patients with cachexia.

Table 20.1 Comparison of opioid analgesic drugs.

	Dose	Route	Duration of action	Notes
Natural opiates				
Morphine	10–15	i.m., s.c.	4	
	10–30	Oral as sustained release	8	Slow onset, needs regular dosage
			8	To be useful
Semi-synthetic				
Diamorphine	5	i.m., s.c.	4	
Oxycodone	10	i.m.	4–6	Used in chronic pain
	30	Rectal	4–8	
Dihydrocodeine	50	i.m., s.c.	4	
	30–60	Oral	4	
Synthetic				
Pethidine	100–150	i.m., s.c.	2–3	
Buprenorphine	0.3	i.m., s.c.	8	Partial agonist
	0.3	Sublingual	8	Slow onset
Methadone	5–10	Oral/i.m.	5–6	Used in chronic pain
Tramadol	50–100	Oral	5–6	Used in chronic pain
	100	i.m.	5–6	Used in post-operative pain

Codeine or methylmorphine

The actions of codeine are similar to those of morphine but codeine is a less potent analgesic. A number of fixed dose preparations containing paracetamol, ibuprofen or aspirin in combination with codeine phosphate are available for the treatment of pain of mild to moderate severity. Codeine is also used as a cough suppressant and to control diarrhoea. Ten per cent of the dose is demethylated in the liver to form morphine.

Pethidine

This is a synthetic analgesic that has a more rapid onset than morphine and a shorter duration of action. Smooth muscle contraction is less prominent and therefore pethidine is used in biliary and ureteric colic. Constipation does not occur to the same extent. One of its metabolites, norpethidine, is active and may accumulate and cause convulsions in patients with hepatic or renal impairment. The risk of toxicity may be increased in patients taking other drugs that induce hep-atic enzymes. Pethidine effectively inhibits post-anaesthetic shivering.

Fentanyl

This is the most potent analgesic used in the United Kingdom. When given in small intra-venous doses, it has a rapid onset and a short duration of action (about 30 minutes), whereas large doses may be effective for several hours. Cardiovascular stability is present even when the drug is administered in large doses and the role of fentanyl in cardiovascular anaesthesia is well established. Because fentanyl is highly lipid-soluble, it may be absorbed transdermally and this property is exploited in palliative care.

Alfentanil

This is given solely by the intravenous route. When compared to fentanyl, alfentanil has a slightly faster onset of action but, following a bolus dose, its effects last only 5–10 minutes. The pharmacokinetics of alfentanil is consistent with administration by a continuous intravenous infusion and it can be included in the sedation regimes of intensive care units. The clearance of alfentanil is unaffected by renal disease.

Remifentanil

This is given solely by the intravenous route. It has a rapid onset of action (similar to alfentanil) and an ultra-short duration of action. The context-sensitive half-time of a drug is a pharmacokinetic measure of the time required for the drug's plasma concentration to decrease by 50% after cessation of an infusion; the 'context' is the duration of the infusion. By virtue of its relatively small volume of distribution and widespread metabolism by non-specific esterases, the context-sensitive half-time of remifentanil remains consistently short (3.2 minutes) even following an infusion of long duration (>8 hours). This clinically important feature distinguishes remifentanil from other opioids, the context-sensitive half-times of which are highly dependent upon the duration of the infusion, and is largely independent of the degree of hepatic and renal function.

Tramadol

Tramadol is a non-selective agonist at mu, kappa and delta opioid receptors. It also inhibits neuronal reuptake of 5-HT and noradrenaline, and enhances 5-HT release. It is used in the management of moderate to severe acute pain, in chronic pain and in palliative care. Advantages include a low incidence of respiratory depression and a low potential for abuse. The main disadvantages are nausea, sedation and diaphoresis.

Partial agonists and opiate antagonists

Buprenorphine

This is a partial agonist at mu opiate receptors. It is a potent long-lasting analgesic drug that can be absorbed sublingually. Dependence or addiction potential is claimed to be low. Respiratory depression is not reversed by the opiate antagonist naloxone except in very high doses (15 mg or more). Hallucinations can occur. Note that it is not advisable to give buprenorphine to augment inadequate analgesia from morphine and more potent agents.

Nalbuphine and meptazinol

These are synthetic opioids used parenterally in the treatment of surgical and chronic pain.

Naloxone

This is a specific opioid antagonist without agonist activity. It is used to antagonise all of the actions of opioid analgesic drugs. It precipitates withdrawal symptoms if given to addicts or the neonate born to a mother addicted to opioids. Naloxone may be given intravenously or intramuscularly in a dose of 0.4–1.2 mg. When given intravenously, the onset of action occurs within 1–2 minutes and it lasts 20–30 minutes. Thus, if it is used to reverse an opioid that has a longer duration of action it may have to be given repeatedly, preferably by intravenous infusion.

Local (regional) anaesthesia

Transmission of impulses in peripheral nerves is associated with depolarisation of the nerve cell membrane, which is the result of increased membrane permeability to sodium ions. Local anaesthetic agents produce a localised, reversible block to nerve conduction by reducing the permeability of the membrane to sodium. Most of the clinically useful local anaesthetic agents act by reversibly blocking the sodium channel through a direct interaction between the anaesthetic molecule and a few amino acids of the receptor protein. These agents may exist in the charged and uncharged form in solution. The uncharged form diffuses more readily through the neural sheath while the charged form attaches to the receptor. The relative proportion of the charged and uncharged form depends upon the pK_a of the drug, the pH of the solution and the pH at the injection site.

The smaller the nerve fibre, the more sensitive it is to local anaesthetic block. Thus it is possible, but practically difficult, to block pain and autonomic fibres and leave proprioception, i.e. touch and movement, intact.

Local anaesthetics are administered locally and do not rely on the circulation to take them to their site of action. However, uptake into the systemic circulation terminates their effects. The rate of systemic absorption is determined by the factors listed below.

Systemic absorption of local anaesthetics

1 Pharmacokinetic properties of the drug
2 Vascularity of the injection site
3 Concentration of the solution used
4 Rate of injection

A vasoconstrictor, such as adrenaline, may be used in solution with the local anaesthetic to delay systemic absorption, prolong the local block and limit toxicity.

Local anaesthetics are weak bases with pK_a values between 7.5 (mepivacaine) and 8.9 (procaine). Marked changes in the ratio of ionised to non-ionised drug occur with changes in acid–base balance. They are extensively bound to plasma proteins. Differences in binding between agents may influence the intensity and duration of effect and placental transfer.

Local anaesthetic drugs are of two types:
1 *Esters*, e.g. procaine, which are metabolised in the plasma by esterases
2 *Amides*, e.g. lidocaine (lignocaine), which are extensively metabolised in the liver, the clearance being dependent on liver blood flow. In the liver, N-dealkylation of the tertiary amine produces a more soluble secondary amine that may be active and is in turn dealkylated. Very little of an injected dose of local anaesthetic is excreted unchanged in the urine.

The physicochemical and pharmacokinetic properties of several local anaesthetics are shown in Table 20.2.

Lidocaine

Lidocaine (lignocaine) has both local and systemic effects. Local effects include loss of pain and other sensations, vasodilatation and loss of motor power. Various preparations of lidocaine are used for topical, infiltration, conduction and epidural anaesthesia. One or two per cent solutions, containing 10 or 20 mg/mL of lidocaine respectively, are popular and the first effects are noted 5–10 minutes after administration with the duration of action being around 2–3 hours. Systemic effects follow absorption from the site of local administration or systemic administration and result from generalised membrane stabilisation.

Table 20.2 Comparison of local anaesthetic drugs.

Agent	Relative dosage	pKa	$t_{1/2}$ (hour)	Onset	Duration
Amides					
Lidocaine	1.0	7.9	1.6	Rapid	Medium
Bupivacaine	0.25	8.1	2.7	Slow	Long
Prilocaine	1.0	7.9	—	Slow	Medium
Ropivacaine	0.33	8.1	3.3	Slow	Long
Esters					
Cocaine	1.0	—	*	Slow	Medium
Procaine	2.0	8.9	*	Slow	Short
Tetracaine (Amethocaine)	0.25	8.5	*	Slow	Long
Chloroprocaine	3.0	8.7	*	—	—

*$t_{1/2}$ is very short owing to hydrolysis in plasma.

Myocardial excitability is depressed and lidocaine may be used in the treatment of ventricular tachyarrhythmias (Chapter 4) because it possesses class I anti-arrhythmic activity.

Adverse effects include anxiety and excitement progressing to sedation, disorientation, lingular and circumoral anaesthesia, restlessness, twitching, tremors, convulsions and unconsciousness. Coma may be accompanied by apnoea and cardiovascular collapse. The maximum 'safe' dose of lidocaine is 3 mg/kg without adrenaline and 7 mg/kg with adrenaline. However, factors that influence toxicity include peak plasma level and rate of rise of plasma level. Adverse effects can therefore occur not only after an overdose, but also following a rapid injection into a highly vascular area; recommended maximum doses are a guide only.

Other local anaesthetics

Bupivacaine

This is an amide that is four times as potent as lidocaine. It is available in 0.25, 0.5 or 0.75% solutions, containing 2.5, 5 or 7.5 mg/mL of bupivacaine respectively, and these are used for infiltration, conduction, spinal and epidural anaesthesia. The maximum 'safe' dose is 2 mg/kg (with or without adrenaline) and, in comparison with lidocaine, its action has a slower onset but a longer duration.

Levobupivacaine

Bupivacaine exists as a racemic mixture of two enantiomers – levobupivacaine and dextrobupivacaine. Levobupivacaine has a similar efficacy but an enhanced safety profile when compared to bupivacaine and, as a result of progress in chiral synthetic technology, is now available in 0.25, 0.5 or 0.75% solutions.

Prilocaine

This is equipotent with lidocaine and can be used for all types of local analgesia. It is less toxic than lidocaine because of its greater degree of tissue uptake. Large doses may produce methaemoglobinaemia, which is caused by a metabolite, O-toluidine. The maximum dose is 6 mg/kg (8 mg/kg with felypressin). The drug is widely used for intravenous regional anaesthesia. Reformulated in a mixture of prilocaine and lidocaine crystals (eutectic mixture of local anaesthetic – EMLA), it is absorbed transdermally and gives good surface analgesia for procedures such as venepuncture in children.

Ropivacaine

Although structurally similar to bupivacaine, ropivacaine may cause less motor block and cardiotoxicity. However, this may simply relate to reduced potency.

Cocaine

This is an ester and is unique in that, in addition to its local anaesthetic properties, it may act as a CNS stimulant. It has been used clinically for topical anaesthesia and for its central euphoriant effects in the management of terminal malignant disease.

General anaesthesia

General anaesthesia is characterised by a balanced technique in which drugs are used specifically to produce loss of consciousness, analgesia and muscle relaxation. Nowadays, a single drug is rarely used to produce all the components of general anaesthesia.

Intravenous anaesthetic agents

These drugs are used to produce a rapid and pleasant induction of sleep. In most cases, other agents will maintain anaesthesia and thus it is rapidity of onset and not brevity of action that is the most desirable property. The mechanism of action of these agents remains unclear. They are all highly lipid-soluble agents and cross the blood–brain barrier rapidly. Their rapid onset of action is a result of this rapid transfer into the brain and high cerebral blood flow. Action is terminated by distribution of the drugs away from the brain to less well-perfused tissues.

Non-barbiturate anaesthetics

Propofol

Propofol is the most widely used intravenous anaesthetic. It is a phenol derivative that is available as a white oil-in-water emulsion containing 1 or 2% propofol in soybean oil, glycerol and purified egg phosphatide. After administration of 1.5–2.5 mg/kg, sleep occurs in one arm–brain circulation time (10–20 seconds) but this may be delayed in patients with cardiac disease or shock. Loss of consciousness is pleasant and lasts for 2–5 minutes. Recovery is rapid following redistribution of propofol from the brain to other tissues. Elimination is faster than with other intravenous anaesthetics because of glucuronide conjugation in the liver. There is thus no pronounced after-effect. Similarly, infusion of the drug does not produce significant cumulation, making it suitable for total intravenous anaesthesia. Advantages include depression of upper airway reflexes and an anti-emetic effect; disadvantages are hypotension, respiratory depression and pain on injection.

Etomidate

This is an imidazole derivative with a very short duration of action owing to rapid redistribution. It has minimal effect on the cardiovascular system and traditionally it has been the induction agent of choice in very sick patients. It is metabolised in the liver and has a half-life of 4.6 hours. Injection may be painful and causes muscle twitching with involuntary movements. Post-operative nausea and vomiting are also associated with etomidate. The drug blocks 11-β-hydroxylation in the adrenal cortex, inhibiting cortisol synthesis for up to 24 hours after a bolus dose. The clinical implications of this finding are unclear but the use of etomidate infusions for sedation in the intensive care unit is associated with an increased mortality.

Ketamine

This is a derivative of phencyclidine. It may be administered intravenously, intramuscularly or into the epidural space. It is now used infrequently in the United Kingdom but is given extensively in developing countries. It is almost devoid of hypnotic properties and produces a state of dissociative anaesthesia characterised by anterograde amnesia and profound analgesia. In contrast to other intravenous anaesthetic agents, ketamine stimulates respiration and increases blood pressure. Adverse effects include emergence delirium, unpleasant dreams and hallucinations. Post-operative nausea and vomiting are common.

Barbiturates

Thiopental (thiopentone)

Thiopental, the sulphur analogue of pentobarbitone, was once the most widely used intravenous anaesthetic. After administration, the initial decay of plasma concentration is very rapid and the half-life of the initial distribution phase is 2.5 minutes. Elimination is by hepatic metabolism and the terminal half-life is 6.2 hours (Table 20.3).

The adverse effects of thiopental include respiratory depression, myocardial depression and vasodilatation. Laryngeal reflexes are not depressed and laryngospasm may occur. The drug has no analgesic properties. Thiopental, like all barbiturates, may exacerbate porphyria.

Table 20.3 Comparison of intravenous anaesthetic induction agents.

Drug	Distribution volume (L/kg)	Clearance (mL/minute)	Plasma half-life $t_{1/2}$ (hour)
Propofol	5.0	1500	2.0
Etomidate	4.5	740	4.6
Ketamine	3.3	1296	3.4
Thiopental	1.6	144	6.2

Inhalation anaesthetic agents

These agents, usually with others, such as intravenous analgesics, are used to maintain a state of general anaesthesia after induction. The depth of anaesthesia produced is related to the tension of the agent in the blood. Because the alveolar epithelium of the lung presents virtually no barrier to diffusion, the partial pressure of the agent in the alveoli determines the depth of anaesthesia. This alveolar partial pressure is influenced by several factors including inspired concentration, pulmonary ventilation and cardiac output. However, the rate of onset of anaesthetic action is mainly determined by the agent's solubility in blood; as a general rule, drugs with low blood–gas solubility, such as sevoflurane, act rapidly and drugs with high blood–gas solubility, such as ether, act slowly.

Factors affecting alveolar concentration of anaesthetics

1 The concentration of the drug in the inspired gas
2 Alveolar ventilation
3 Cardiac output
4 The solubility of the drug in the blood

The potency of these agents is related to, but is not dependent on, fat solubility. The minimum alveolar concentration (MAC) is the alveolar concentration that produces a state of surgical anaesthesia in 50% of patients. Put another way, it is the dose that abolishes movement in response to incision in 50% of patients. MAC is a population median that varies with age and other factors.

In practice, clinical signs are used to monitor depth of anaesthesia. Inspired and end-tidal concentrations of inhalational agent are routinely measured but depth of anaesthesia monitors have not gained widespread acceptance in the United Kingdom.

Nitrous oxide

This is a vapour at room temperature. Although it cannot produce surgical anaesthesia when administered alone (i.e. its MAC is over 100%), a concentration of 70% in oxygen is conventionally used as an adjunct to more potent inhalational agents. An equal mixture of nitrous oxide and oxygen is used to produce analgesia during labour and other painful procedures. Adverse effects include postoperative nausea and vomiting, and prolonged exposure to nitrous oxide may result in bone marrow depression.

Isoflurane

This is a halogenated ether that is a liquid at room temperature and must be vaporised before use. Over 99% of an administered dose is excreted unchanged by the lungs and the remainder is metabolised in the liver. In common with other volatile anaesthetics, it depresses the respiratory and cardiovascular systems but causes less myocardial depression and arrhythmias than other agents.

Desflurane

This differs from isoflurane by the substitution of a fluorine for a chlorine atom. It boils at around room temperature and requires a heated, pressurised vaporiser. Its solubility in blood is similar to that of nitrous oxide allowing rapid uptake and, more importantly, rapid elimination of the drug. Its properties are otherwise similar to those of isoflurane.

Sevoflurane

Like desflurane this is an ether halogenated solely with fluorine atoms. Its low solubility in blood allows rapid emergence from anaesthesia and its low level of airway irritation makes it suited for inhalational induction of anaesthesia.

Halothane

This is a halogenated hydrocarbon. The liver metabolises 20%; hepatic damage very rarely occurs 7–10 days after halothane anaesthesia, especially following repeated exposures, because of an immunological response to one of its metabolites. This has virtually abolished the use of halothane in adults. Arrhythmias, bradycardia and myocardial depression are more troublesome than with other volatile agents.

Enflurane

A halogenated ether, its properties are similar to those of halothane. As the liver metabolises much less enflurane than halothane, the risk of hepatitis is reduced.

Neuromuscular blocking drugs

When an electrical impulse in a motor nerve reaches the nerve ending it releases acetylcholine at the neuromuscular junction. Acetylcholine acts on nicotinic cholinergic receptors on the muscle membrane, resulting in a wave of depolarisation. The acetylcholine is then destroyed rapidly by a specific cholinesterase.

Neuromuscular blocking drugs may interfere with neurotransmission in one of two ways:

1 Prolongation of the normal depolarisation, e.g. suxamethonium

2 Competitive inhibition of acetylcholine at the receptors, e.g. vecuronium, atracurium.

These drugs are used during general anaesthesia to:

1 Facilitate tracheal intubation and controlled ventilation

2 Facilitate surgery, e.g. abdominal surgery, if muscle relaxation is deemed advantageous.

After administration, the anaesthetist must always ventilate the patient's lungs because paralysis includes all voluntary muscles, notably the respiratory muscles. The use of these drugs is an integral part of a balanced anaesthetic technique, but great care must be taken to ensure that the patient is unconscious.

Factors that influence the action of neuromuscular blocking drugs are listed below.

Factors affecting neuromuscular blockade

1 Muscle blood flow (the most important factor). Muscles with high blood flow have the earliest onset and shortest duration of action

2 Changes in temperature

3 pH

4 Potassium concentrations influence the degree of paralysis

5 Aminoglycoside antibiotics prolong competitive blockade by reducing acetylcholine release

6 Drugs that produce central muscle relaxation, e.g. benzodiazepines or isoflurane, prolong the muscle paralysis

7 Renal disease, as most competitive blockers are excreted unchanged in the kidney to a greater or lesser extent. Atracurium is, however, metabolised in the blood

8 Hereditary atypical cholinesterase markedly prolongs the effect of suxamethonium

---

Suxamethonium

This is a very short-acting depolarising neuromuscular blocking drug. A dose of 1 mg/kg produces muscle fasciculations within 30 seconds followed by complete paralysis for 3–5 minutes.

Respiration must be maintained artificially. The drug is broken down very rapidly by plasma cholinesterase. In patients with a genetically determined abnormality in this enzyme's activity, paralysis is prolonged. Adverse effects of suxamethonium include bradycardia, muscle pains and raised intraocular pressure.

Non-depolarising muscle relaxants

Vecuronium

This is an aminosteroid that produces competitive neuromuscular paralysis. It has replaced the traditional relaxants tubocurarine, a benzylisoquinolinium compound, and pancuronium, also an aminosteroid. Its advantages are its lack of effects on the heart and an intermediate duration of action (20–40 minutes). Rocuronium is structurally similar. Duration of action is similar to that of vecuronium but its onset is more rapid.

Neuromuscular blockade may be reversed at the end of surgery by administering an anticholinesterase such as neostigmine. This drug is always given with atropine or glycopyrrolate, which prevent the muscarinic effects of acetylcholine and allow the nicotinic effects to be manifest.

Atracurium

This is a benzylisoquinolinium compound with few cardiovascular side effects. It has an intermediate duration of action because of rapid non-enzymatic degradation in plasma and is particularly favoured in patients with renal or hepatic disease. The principal disadvantage is histamine release. This can be avoided by using cisatracurium, an isomer of atracurium, which does not provoke histamine release.

Mivacurium

Mivacurium is also a benzylisoquinolinium compound. It is hydrolysed rapidly by plasma cholinesterase and has a shorter duration of action than atracurium or vecuronium, making it suitable for shorter procedures.

Part 3

Practical Aspects of Prescribing

Chapter 21

Clinical pharmacokinetics: dosage individualisation

Clinical scenario

A 76-year-old man has been referred with sepsis probably secondary to a urinary tract infection. He is unwell and the hospital guidelines suggest giving him gentamicin. He has a past history of renal impairment which has been stable for some time. What information do you need to know and what dose of gentamicin would you give?

Key points

- There a number of factors that contribute to a lack of therapeutic effect of a dosed drug in an individual
- Blood monitoring of drug levels is a useful way of ensuring maximum benefit whilst minimising the risk of complications of a particular drug
- Therapeutic drug monitoring is most useful for drugs such as digoxin, phenytoin and gentamicin which have a narrow therapeutic index

Introduction

There are a various reasons why a prescribed dose of drug leads to a different plasma drug concentration and therefore clinical effect. These include:

- Individual differences in absorption, first pass metabolism, volume of distribution and clearance
- Altered pharmacokinetics because of gastrointestinal, hepatic or renal disease

- Drug interactions
- Poor adherence to therapy

For most drugs there is an accepted 'target' range, i.e. a range of concentrations below which the drug is usually ineffective and above which it is usually toxic. In order to maintain drug concentrations within this range, knowledge about factors that influence the relationships between drug dose and blood concentration is used to design dosage regimens. Dosage adjustments based on age, renal function, hepatic function or other drug therapies are often recommended, especially for drugs with a narrow therapeutic index. For example, the initial dose of gentamicin, a renally cleared antibiotic, is based on the patient's renal function. As a consequence of an interaction that increases digoxin concentrations, the dose of digoxin is usually halved when amiodarone is added to a patient's therapy.

Therapeutic drug monitoring

In many cases it is relatively easy to evaluate the pharmacological effects of a drug by clinical observation, and initial dosage regimens can be modified to increase the therapeutic effect or to eliminate unwanted effects. Measurement of drug concentrations in blood can be performed to help with diagnosis or to optimise therapy for those drugs where response (therapeutic or toxic effects) cannot be readily evaluated from clinical

Lecture Notes: Clinical Pharmacology and Therapeutics, 8th edition. By Gerard McKay, John Reid and Matthew Walters. Published 2010 by Blackwell Publishing Ltd.

Table 21.1 Examples of target ranges.

Drug	Target range	
	Mass units	**Molar units**
Digoxin	0.8–2 μg/L	1–2.6 nmol/L
Carbamazepine	4–12 mg/L	20–50 μmol/L
Phenytoin	10–20 mg/L	40–80 μmol/L
Gentamicin	5–12 mg/L	
	(1 hour post-dose)	
Vancomycin	5–10 mg/L	
	(trough)	
Theophylline	5–20 mg/L	28–110 μmol/L

In some hospitals, high aminoglycoside doses (e.g. gentamicin doses of 5–7 mg/kg) are given at intervals of 24–48 hours and the normal target peak and trough ranges do not apply. Samples are usually taken 6–14 hours after the dose and the dose is adjusted (if necessary) according to a nomogram.

observation alone. Examples of drugs where monitoring can usefully aid clinical judgement, together with target ranges, are shown in Table 21.1.

As a result of pharmacokinetic and pharmacodynamic variability, the following factors should be considered when interpreting drug concentration measurements:

1 Is the patient responding to therapy or showing symptoms of toxicity?
2 Was the sample taken at steady state?
3 Was the sampling time appropriate for the drug?
4 Where is the concentration relative to the 'target' range?
5 If the patient is not responding or has toxicity, how should the dose be modified? Unexpectedly low concentrations may indicate poor adherence or an absorption problem (e.g. secondary to vomiting).

Clearance estimates

The clinical significance of clearance is that it determines an individual patient's maintenance

Table 21.2 Factors influencing theophylline clearance and therefore dose requirements.

Factor	Adjustments required
Smoking	×1.6
Congestive cardiac failure	×0.4
Hepatic cirrhosis	×0.5
Acute pulmonary oedema	×0.5
Severe chronic obstructive airways disease	×0.8

dose requirements. Clearance varies between individuals and within an individual in response to changes in his or her clinical condition.

The physiological and pathological factors that affect the clearance of a drug depend mainly on which organ is primarily responsible for its elimination. For example, clearance of the bronchodilator theophylline, a drug that is eliminated by hepatic metabolism, is influenced by age, weight, alcohol consumption, cigarette smoking, other drugs, congestive cardiac failure, hepatic cirrhosis, acute pulmonary oedema and severe chronic obstructive airways disease.

Clearance in any individual is most accurately determined from concentration measurements. However, in many cases, relationships between clearance and clinical factors have previously been established. For example, the average value for theophylline clearance is 0.04 L/hour per kg and this is modified according to the patient's clinical characteristics by multiplying by the factors shown in Table 21.2. This means that on average, smokers require 1.6 times the theophylline dose of non-smokers and patients with cirrhosis require half the dose of patients without cirrhosis.

For drugs primarily excreted by the kidney, e.g. digoxin and gentamicin, creatinine clearance closely reflects drug clearance. Thus, digoxin clearance can be estimated from the equation:

$$\text{Digoxin clearance} = \text{Creatinine clearance} + 0.33$$
$$\text{(mL/min/kg)} \qquad \text{(Eqn. 21.1)}$$

The value 0.33 in this equation represents the elimination by routes other than the kidney, such as metabolism and clearance by the hepatobiliary system.

An estimate of clearance can then be used to calculate the required dose to achieve a target concentration:

$$\text{Maintenance dose rate} = \text{Clearance}$$
$$\times \text{Target } Cs_{\text{average}} \qquad \text{(Eqn. 21.2)}$$

$$\text{Maintenance dose} = \text{Clearance} \times \text{Target } Cs_{\text{average}}$$
$$\times \frac{\text{Dosage interval}}{F} \qquad \text{(Eqn. 21.3)}$$

where F represents oral bioavailability. Factors that influence clearance are now routinely investigated for all new drugs so that dosage adjustments can be made for patients with a low clearance, who might be at risk from toxicity.

Interpretation of serum concentrations

Serum concentrations can be measured for a number of reasons and it is important to interpret the measured concentration in the light of the clinical situation. If the aim is to assess the patient's maintenance dose requirements, samples should ideally be taken at steady state. However, confirmation of steady state is not necessary if the aim is to confirm toxicity and adherence or to assess the need for a loading dose in a patient who is acutely unwell.

Steady state normally requires that 4–5 half-lives elapse since treatment started or since any change in dose. Doses should be given at regular intervals and it is important to confirm that no doses have been omitted. If these conditions can be satisfied and the pharmacokinetics of the drug are linear, clearance depends on the ratio of the dosing rate to the average steady-state concentration (Cs_{average}) as can be seen by rearranging Eqn. 21.2:

$$\text{Clearance} = \frac{\text{Maintenance dose rate}}{Cs_{\text{average}}} \qquad \text{(Eqn. 21.4)}$$

This means that doses can be adjusted by simple proportion, i.e.

$$= \frac{\text{Desired } Cs_{\text{average}}}{\text{Measured } Cs_{\text{average}} \times \text{Current dose}}$$
$$\text{(Eqn. 21.5)}$$

Concentrations that are not at steady state cannot be used in this way; although if accurate details of dosage history and sampling time are available, clearance may be estimated with the help of a pharmacokinetic computer package.

It is important to remember that drugs with non-linear kinetics (such as phenytoin) require special consideration, and different techniques are applied to the interpretation of their concentrations. Successful interpretation of a concentration measurement depends on accurate information. The minimum usually required is:

1 Time of sample collection with respect to the previous dose. Samples taken at inappropriate times may be misinterpreted. Usually, the simplest approach is to measure a trough concentration (i.e. at the end of the dosage interval).

2 An accurate and detailed dosage history – drug dose, times of administration and route(s) of administration. This information can be used to assess whether the sample represents steady state. Samples taken without knowledge of dosage history can result in an inappropriate clinical action or dosage adjustment.

3 Patient details such as age, sex, weight, serum creatinine (and estimated Glomerular Filtration Rate) and assessments of cardiac and hepatic function. This information helps to determine expected dose requirements and is necessary for all computerised interpretation methods. Knowledge about the stability of the patient can help to determine the frequency of monitoring, especially if the drug is cleared by the kidneys and renal function is changing.

4 Changes in other drug therapy that might influence the pharmacokinetics of the drug being measured.

5 The reason for requesting a drug analysis should be considered carefully. 'On admission' or

'routine' requests are usually of little value and are a waste of valuable resources.

Clinical examples of therapeutic drug monitoring

Digoxin

Clinical scenario

Mr AR, a 78-year-old man weighing 72 kg and with a creatinine clearance of 24 mL/min, has been taking 250 µg digoxin daily to control atrial fibrillation. He presents to his general practitioner with anorexia and nausea a month after starting therapy. A digoxin concentration of 3.6 mg/L (4.6 nmol/L) is measured.

Is this concentration expected?

His expected digoxin clearance can be calculated from Eqn. 21.1, i.e.

$$\text{Digoxin clearance} = \frac{24}{72} + 0.33 \ (\text{mL/min/kg})$$
$$= 0.663 \ \text{mL/min/kg}$$
$$= 2.91/h$$

His average steady-state concentration can be estimated from Eqn. 21.2, i.e.

$$\text{Predicted } Css_{average} = \frac{0.6 \times 250 \ \mu g}{2.9 \times 24 \ h}$$
$$= 2.2 \ \mu g/l(2.8 \ \text{nmol/L})$$

0.6 is an estimate of the bioavailability of digoxin tablets. The reason the measured concentration is higher than expected should be investigated. In this case, it was found that the sample had been withdrawn 2.5 hours after the dose. Digoxin is absorbed quickly but distributes slowly to the tissues. Samples taken before distribution is complete (i.e. less than 6 hours after the dose) cannot be interpreted. As concentrations fall only by about 20% from 6 to 24 hours after the dose, samples can be taken at any time during this period.

A further (trough) sample withdrawn 24 hours after the last dose measured 2.4 µg/L (3.1 nmol/L). This result is more consistent with the expected concentration but suggests that the dose

Table 21.3 Predicted steady-state digoxin concentrations for clinical scenario.

Dose (µg)	$Css_{average}$ (µg/L)	Css_{trough} (mg/L)
250	3.0	2.4
187.5	2.2	1.8
125	1.5	1.2
62.5	0.75	0.6

is too high and may be contributing to his symptoms.

What dose adjustment should be made?

Digoxin has linear pharmacokinetics therefore the new dose can be determined by simple proportion. Table 21.3 shows that there are three dosage options for Mr AR. A reduction to 125 µg daily is the most obvious first choice, but further adjustment (up or down) could be made if necessary on clinical grounds (e.g. poor control of atrial fibrillation or persistence of adverse effects).

Comment. This case illustrates the importance of sampling time for the correct interpretation of digoxin concentrations. Although digoxin is traditionally prescribed to be taken in the morning, changing to a night-time dose can reduce the chances of samples being withdrawn during the distribution phase. Digoxin has a long elimination half-life (50–100 hours) and elimination is slow beyond 6 hours after the dose. If samples are taken at steady state, dosage adjustment can be performed by simple proportion.

Gentamicin

Clinical scenario

Mr JL, a 64-year-old man who weighs 80 kg and has an estimated creatinine clearance of 35 mL/minute, requires gentamicin therapy for a suspected gram-negative infection. The aim is to achieve a peak concentration around 8 mg/L and a trough around 1 mg/L.

What dosage regimen should be prescribed?

Gentamicin is cleared by excretion through the kidneys and its clearance can be approximated by creatinine clearance. The volume of distribution of gentamicin is around 0.25 L/kg. A dosage interval of about 3 half-lives will allow the concentration to fall from 8 to 1 mg/L ($8 \rightarrow 4 \rightarrow 2 \rightarrow 1$). The elimination half-life can be calculated from Eqn. 21.3, i.e.

$$t_{1/2} = \frac{\ln 2}{k}$$

$$t_{1/2} = \frac{0.693 \times V}{Cl}$$

$$t_{1/2} = \frac{0.693 \times 0.25 \, l/kg \times 80 \, kg}{35 \, mL/min \times (60/1000)}$$

$$= \frac{0.693 \times 20 \, L}{2.1 \, L/h}$$

$$= 6.6 \, h$$

It will therefore take $3 \times 6.6 = 20$ hours for the concentration to fall from 8 to 1 mg/L. Because the 'peak' is measured 1 hours after the dose, the dosage interval should be 21 hours. A 'practical' dosage interval is therefore 24 hours. The dose administered should increase the concentration by 7 mg/L (i.e. from 1 to 8 mg/L). It can be calculated from the volume of distribution, i.e.

$$\text{Dose (mg)} = 7 \, mg/L \times 0.25 \, L/kg \times 80 \, kg$$

$$= 140 \, mg$$

Mr JL was started on a daily dose of 140 mg and after two days of therapy his peak concentration (1 hour post-dose) was 6 mg/L and his trough (24 hours post-dose) was 0.5 mg/L.

Has steady state been reached?

Mr JL's estimated elimination half-life is 6.6 hours; therefore, steady state should be reached in $5 \times 6.6 = 33$ hours. He will be at steady state after 2 days of therapy.

How should the dose be adjusted?

The peak is slightly lower than the target and the trough is satisfactory. As these represent steady-state concentrations and gentamicin has linear pharmacokinetics, the dose can be adjusted by proportion. Increasing the dose to 200 mg daily should achieve a peak of $(200/140) \times 6 = 8.6$ mg/L and a trough of $(200/140) \times 0.5 = 0.7$ mg/L.

Comment. Elimination half-life is a useful guide to dosage interval and is particularly important when the target concentration–time profile includes both peak and trough concentrations. In this case, because the peaks and troughs were both low, the dose can be adjusted by direct proportion. If the trough had been high, an increase in the dosage interval would also have been necessary.

Phenytoin

Clinical scenario

Mrs DL, a 38-year-old woman who weighs 55 kg, was prescribed phenytoin at a dose of 300 mg daily (5.5 mg/kg per day) after carbamazepine failed to control her epilepsy. She attended the outpatient clinic 3 weeks later and her 24-hours post-dose trough phenytoin concentration was 6 mg/L (24 μmol/L). As her seizures were not well controlled, her dose was increased to 350 mg daily (6.4 mg/kg per day). She presented to her general practitioner 2 weeks later complaining of fatigue and difficulty in walking properly. Her trough phenytoin concentration was 28 mg/L (112 mol/L).

Why was the first concentration so low?

There are two possibilities: the dose was too low, or she was not adhering with her prescribed dose. As patients generally require phenytoin maintenance doses in the range 4.5–5 mg/kg per day, both doses were higher than average. Phenytoin has non-linear pharmacokinetics at concentrations normally seen clinically, and standard pharmacokinetic equations cannot be used. The relationship between dose rate and average steady-state concentration is controlled by V_{max} (the maximum amount of drug that can be metabolised by the enzymes per day) and K_m (the concentration at half V_{max}). Using average values of V_{max} (7.2 mg/kg per day) and K_m (4.4 mg/L), Mrs DL's expected concentration can be calculated from the Michaelis–Menten equation;

$$\text{Dose rate} = \frac{V_{max} \times Css}{K_m + Css}$$

$$Css = \frac{\text{Dose rate} \times K_m}{V_{max} - \text{Dose rate}}$$

$$Css = \frac{300 \text{ mg/day} \times 4.4 \text{ mg/L}}{(7.2 \times 55) \text{ mg/day} - 300 \text{ mg day}}$$

$$= \frac{1320}{96}$$

$$= 14 \text{ mg/l } (55 \text{ μmol/L})$$

The measured concentration of 6 mg/L is much lower than expected and suggests poor adherence with therapy.

Why was the second concentration so high?

The predicted concentration on her increased dose can be calculated as before, i.e.

$$Css = \frac{350 \text{ mg/day} \times 4.4 \text{ mg/L}}{(7.2 \times 55) \text{ mg/day} - 350 \text{ mg/day}}$$

$$= \frac{1540}{46}$$

$$= 33 \text{ mg/l } (147 \text{ μmol/L})$$

In this case, the measured concentration was reasonably consistent with the predicted value and her actual V_{max} can therefore be estimated from the measured concentration, i.e.

$$V_{max}(\text{mg/day}) = \frac{\text{Dose rate} \times (K_m + Css)}{Css}$$

$$V_{max}(\text{mg/day}) = \frac{350 \text{ mg/day} \times (4.4 + 28) \text{ mg/L}}{28 \text{ mg/L}}$$

$$= 450 \text{ mg/day}$$

Using her actual V_{max} and a K_m of 4.4 mg/L, average steady-state concentrations can be pre-

Table 21.4 Predicted steady-state phenytoin concentrations for clinical scenario.

Dose	Steady-state concentration	
(mg/day)	(mg/L)	(μmol/L)
225	6	24
250	7	28
275	9	36
300	13	52.
325	18	72
350	28	112
375	55	220

dicted for various doses (Table 21.4). Note that a small change in the dose produces a disproportionately large increase in concentration, especially at higher concentrations.

It is known that a concentration of 6 mg/L does not control her seizures and she experiences toxicity with 28 mg/L. Her ideal dose is therefore likely to lie in the range 275–325 mg daily. It would be sensible to start with 300 mg daily and adjust the dose (if necessary) according to her response. It would also be useful to emphasise to the patient that she must comply with her prescribed dose in order to obtain the maximum benefit from her therapy.

Comment

This case illustrates the non-linearity of phenytoin dose–concentration relationships and the difficulty of interpreting phenytoin concentrations when dosage history is uncertain (as frequently occurs with outpatients). It also demonstrates the value of using serial measurements (the two results were clearly inconsistent with each other) and average dose requirements to assess adherence.

Chapter 22

Influence of renal and hepatic disease on pharmacokinetics and pharmacodynamics

Drugs are usually considered in terms of their effect on disease processes. However, several diseases can influence the pharmacokinetics of a drug or its pharmacological effect on target organs. Diseases of the liver and kidney are of particular importance due to the role of these organs in elimination of drugs. This chapter will discuss the important considerations which arise when prescribing for a patient with these comorbidities.

Clinical scenario

A 45-year-old woman is admitted to hospital with severe urosepsis. She gives a background history of recurrent urinary infections and chronic renal impairment secondary to structural abnormalities of the urinary tract. Blood and urine culture reveals growth of gram negative bacilli sensitive to gentamicin. How may this patient's renal function influence the treatment of her presenting complaint, and what precautions should be considered?

Lecture Notes: Clinical Pharmacology and Therapeutics, 8th edition. By Gerard McKay, John Reid and Matthew Walters. Published 2010 by Blackwell Publishing Ltd.

Influence of impaired renal function

Key points

Impaired renal function can influence drug therapy for the following reasons:
- Pharmacokinetics may be altered as result of:
  - Decreased elimination of drugs that are normally excreted entirely or mainly by the kidneys
  - Decreased protein binding
  - Decreased hepatic metabolism
- Drug effect may be the altered
- Existing clinical condition may be worsened
- Adverse effects may be enhanced

Altered pharmacokinetics

Elimination

Because the kidney represents one of the major routes of drug elimination, a decline in renal function can influence the clearance of many drugs. If a drug normally cleared by the kidney is given to someone with decreased renal function without altering the dose, the steady-state blood concentrations of that drug will be increased. This is of considerable importance in the case of drugs showing concentration-related effects, particularly those that have a narrow therapeutic range.

When such drugs are given to patients with renal dysfunction, the general aim is to achieve similar concentrations to those seen in patients with normal kidneys.

Therapeutic concentrations can be maintained by:

1 Determining renal function, usually by estimating creatinine clearance.

2 Modifying the dose using a nomogram, either by increasing the dosage interval, or by giving a lower dose at the same interval or by altering both the dose and the interval. The extent and precision of dose modification depend very much on the toxicity of the drug concerned. In the case of the aminoglycosides, even minor impairment of renal function requires some dosage alteration, while the dose of penicillins need only be reduced in severe renal failure (creatinine clearance <10 mL/minute). Guidance on dosage modification is readily available for most commonly used drugs. It should be noted that the loading dose is usually not changed by renal impairment because this depends more on the volume of distribution of the drug than its rate of elimination.

3 Monitoring drug concentrations. This is useful for drugs with concentration-related adverse effects, such as the aminoglycosides, digoxin, aminophylline, phenytoin and carbamazepine, and mandatory for lithium, ciclosporin and methotrexate. Nomograms are useful guides to the doses likely to be appropriate, but every patient is different. Concentrations of drugs in the blood can be used to assess clearance and to determine the most appropriate dose for individual patients.

Decreased protein binding

The following changes occur in patients with impaired renal function:

1 Acidic drugs are less bound to serum albumin and the decrease in binding correlates with the severity of renal impairment. The binding of basic drugs (to α_1-acid glycoprotein) undergoes little or no change.

2 The structure of albumin is changed in renal failure and endogenous compounds may compete with drugs for binding.

3 Haemodialysis does not return binding to normal, but renal transplantation does.

In most cases changes in protein binding have limited clinical relevance and do not require alterations in dose. However, protein binding is important for the interpretation of serum phenytoin concentrations.

Hepatic metabolism

The hepatic metabolism of some drugs (e.g. nicardipine, propranolol) may be decreased in patients with renal failure. The reasons for this are not clear, but may indicate the presence of a metabolic inhibitor in uraemic plasma because regular haemodialysis appears to normalise the clearance of these compounds.

Altered drug effect

There are several examples of increased drug sensitivity in patients with renal failure. Opiates, barbiturates, phenothiazines and benzodiazepines all show greater effects on the nervous system in patients with renal failure than in those with normal renal function. The reasons are not known, but increased meningeal permeability is one possible explanation.

Various antihypertensive drugs have a greater postural effect in renal failure. Again the reasons are not clear, but changes in fluid balance and autonomic dysfunction may be partly responsible.

Worsening of the existing clinical condition

Drug therapy can result in deterioration of the clinical condition in the following ways:

1 By further impairing renal function. In patients with renal failure it is clearly advisable to avoid drugs that are known to be nephrotoxic and for which alternatives are available. Examples include aminoglycosides, amphotericin, cisplatin, gold, mesalazine, non-steroidal anti-inflammatories, penicillamine and vancomycin.

2 By causing fluid retention. Fluid balance is a major problem in the more severe forms of renal

failure. Drugs that cause fluid retention should therefore be avoided, e.g. carbenoxolone and non-steroidal anti-inflammatory drugs (NSAIDs) such as indometacin (indomethacin).

3 By increasing the degree of uraemia. Tetracyclines, except doxycycline, have an anti-anabolic effect and should be avoided.

Enhancement of adverse drug effects

In addition to decreased elimination, digoxin is more likely to cause adverse effects in patients with severe renal failure if there are substantial electrolyte abnormalities, particularly hypercalcaemia and/or hypokalaemia.

Because potassium elimination is impaired in renal failure, diuretics that also conserve potassium (amiloride, spironolactone) are more likely to cause hyperkalaemia.

Influence of liver disease

Impaired liver function can influence the response to treatment

1 Altered pharmacokinetics:
 • Increased bioavailability resulting from reduced first-pass metabolism or, potentially, decreased first-pass activation of pro-drugs.
 • Decreased protein binding.
 • Worsening of metabolic state.
2 Altered drug effect.
3 Worsening of metabolic state.

Altered pharmacokinetics

The liver is the largest organ in the body, has a substantial blood supply (around 1.5 L/minute) and is interposed between the gastrointestinal tract and the systemic circulation. For these reasons it is uniquely suited for the purpose of influencing drug pharmacokinetics.

Decreased first-pass metabolism

A decrease in hepatocellular function decreases the capacity of the liver to perform metabolic processes, while portosystemic shunting directs drugs away from sites of metabolism. Both factors are usually present in patients with severe cirrhosis.

Knowledge of the drugs that undergo first-pass metabolism is important in situations where it is decreased as a result of disease. Considerably greater quantities of active drug then reach the site of action and any given dose of drug has unexpectedly intense effects.

Examples of changes in bioavailability found in some patients with severe cirrhosis are:
• Clomethiazole (chlormethiazole) (100% increase)
• Labetalol (91% increase)
• Metoprolol (65% increase)
• Nicardipine (500% increase)
• Paracetamol (50% increase)
• Propranolol (42% increase)
• Verapamil (140% increase)

Conversely, first-pass activation of pro-drugs such as many ACE inhibitors (e.g. enalapril, perindopril, quinapril) may potentially be slowed or reduced.

Decreased elimination by liver metabolism and decreased protein binding

High extraction drugs
These are drugs which the liver metabolises at a very high rate. Their bioavailability is low and their clearance is dependent mainly upon the rate of drug delivery to the enzyme systems. The clearance of these drugs is therefore relatively sensitive to factors that can influence hepatic blood flow, such as congestive cardiac failure, and relatively insensitive to small changes in enzyme activity or protein binding. Examples include labetalol, lidocaine, metoprolol, morphine, propranolol, pethidine, nortriptyline and verapamil.

Low extraction drugs
In low extraction drugs the rate of metabolism is so sufficiently low that hepatic clearance is relatively insensitive to changes in hepatic blood flow, and dependent mainly on the capacity of the liver enzymes. Examples include chloramphenicol, paracetamol and theophylline. The hepatic clearance of

drugs in this group that are also highly protein-bound, such as diazepam, tolbutamide, phenytoin and valproic acid, depends on both the capacity of the enzymes and the free fraction. It is thus difficult to predict the consequences of hepatic disease on total drug concentration. However, as with renal disease, care must be taken in the interpretation of concentrations of highly protein bound drugs such as phenytoin.

The influence of liver disease on drug elimination is complex; the type of liver disease is critical. In acute viral hepatitis the major change is in hepatocellular function, but drug-metabolising ability usually remains intact and hepatic blood flow can increase. Mild to moderate cirrhosis tends to result in decreased hepatic blood flow and portosystemic shunting, while severe cirrhosis usually shows reduction in both cellular function and blood flow. Cholestasis leads to impaired fat absorption with deficiencies of fat-soluble vitamins and impairment of absorption of lipophillic drugs. Alcoholic liver disease is common and chronic ethanol abuse is associated with increased activity of the microsomal ethanol-oxidising system. This effect is a result primarily of induction by ethanol of a specific cytochrome P-450 (CYP2E1) responsible for enhanced oxidation of ethanol and other P-450 substrates and, consequently, for metabolic tolerance to these substances. This may lead to enhanced clearance and, hence, decreased response to certain drugs such as benzodiazepine sedatives, anticonvulsants (phenytoin) and warfarin. By contrast, simultaneous alcohol ingestion may decrease clearance of drugs metabolised via the P-450 (CYP2E1) enzyme system.

Comment. Unlike the measurement of creatinine clearance in renal disease, there is no simple test that can predict the extent to which drug metabolism is decreased in liver disease. A low serum albumin, raised bilirubin and prolonged prothrombin time give a rough guide.

The fact that a drug is metabolised by the liver does not necessarily mean that its pharmacokinetics is altered by liver disease. It is not easy, therefore, to extrapolate the findings from one drug to another. This is because superficially similar metabolic pathways are mediated by different forms of cytochrome P-450.

The documentation of modestly altered pharmacokinetics does not necessarily imply clinical importance. Even normal subjects show quite wide variations in pharmacokinetic indices and therefore pharmacokinetics should not be viewed in isolation from alterations in drug effect, which are much more difficult to assess. However, if a drug is known to be subject to substantial pharmacokinetic changes, clinical significance is much more likely.

Table 22.1 Drugs that can cause liver damage.

Hepatitis
  Halothane (repeated exposure)
  Isoniazid
  Rifampicin
  Methyldopa
  Phenelzine
  Trimipramine
  Desipramine
  Carbimazepine
  Trasidone
  Propylthiouracil
  Augmentin
  Erythromycin
  Nitrofurantoin
  Chloroguanidee
  Tienilic acid
  Dihydralazine
  Azothiaprine
  Sulfasalazine (sulphasalazine)
  Naproxen
  Amiodarone
Cholestasis with mild hepatic component
  Phenothiazines
  Carbamazepine
  Tricyclic antidepressants
  Non-steroidal anti-inflammatory drugs
  (especially phenylbutazone)
  Rifampicin, ethambutol, pyrazinamide
  Sulphonylureas, trimethoprin
  Sulphonamides, ampicillin, nitrofurantoin,
  erythromycin estolate
  Oral contraceptives (stasis without hepatitis)
Cirrhosis
  Methotrexate

If it is clinically desirable to give a drug that is eliminated by liver metabolism to a patient with cirrhosis, it should be started at a low dose and the drug levels or effect monitored very closely.

Altered drug effect

Deranged brain function

The more severe forms of liver disease are accompanied by poorly understood derangements of brain function that ultimately result in the syndrome of hepatic encephalopathy. However, even before encephalopathy develops, the brain is extremely sensitive to the effects of centrally acting drugs and a state of coma can result from administering normal doses of opiates or benzodiazepines to such patients.

Decreased clotting factors

Patients with liver disease show increased sensitivity to oral anticoagulants. These drugs exert their effect by decreasing the vitamin K dependent synthesis of clotting factors II, VII, IX and X. When the production of these factors is already reduced by liver disease, a given dose of oral anticoagulant has a greater effect in these patients than in subjects with normal liver function.

Worsening of metabolic state

Drug-induced alkalosis

Excessive use of diuretics can precipitate encephalopathy. The mechanism involves hypokalaemic alkalosis, which results in conversion of NH^+_4 to NH_3, the un-ionised ammonia crossing easily into the central nervous system (CNS) to worsen or precipitate encephalopathy.

Fluid overload

Patients with advanced liver disease often have oedema and ascites secondary to hypoalbuminaemia and portal hypertension. This problem can be worsened by drugs that cause fluid retention, e.g. NSAIDs, and antacids that contain large amounts of sodium. NSAIDs should be avoided anyway, because of the increased risk of gastrointestinal bleeding.

Hepatotoxic drugs

Where an acceptable alternative exists, it is wise to avoid drugs that can cause liver damage (Table 22.1), e.g. sulphonamides or rifampicin, and repeated exposure to halothane anaesthesia.

Chapter 23

Prescribing at extremes of age

Influence of ageing

The elderly (65 years and over) constitute approximately 16% of the population, yet they consume 40% of the drug prescriptions in the United Kingdom. Two-thirds of those over the age of 65 receive regular medication. This high consumption of drugs is related to an increasing prevalence of acute and chronic disease, resulting in increasing numbers of prescriptions. Multiple drug prescribing can lead to problems with adherence and carries increased risk of side effects. The overall incidence of drug side effects in the elderly is up to three times that seen in the young. Adverse drug reactions in the elderly tend to be dose related rather than idiosyncratic and are related to changes in pharmacokinetics and pharmacodynamics. The drugs that have the highest incidence of side effects in the elderly are those that are most commonly prescribed (sedatives, diuretics and non-steroidal anti-inflammatory drugs). However, in one study, insulin and nitrofurantoin had the highest incidence of adverse effects when related to the total number of doses administered.

Drug absorption, distribution, metabolism, excretion and activity can all change as a result of ageing. However, the presence of multiple pathology in the old frequently has a greater effect than ageing alone.

Drug absorption

Ageing is associated with increased gastric pH, delayed gastric emptying, decreased intestinal motility and reduced splanchnic blood flow. Despite these changes, there is little evidence to suggest that intestinal drug absorption changes with age. For example, the rate of absorption of digoxin is slower in the elderly but the overall bioavailability remains the same.

Drug distribution

Age-related changes in body composition, in protein binding and in organ blood flow can all affect drug disposition.

Ageing is associated with a relative increase in body fat and corresponding reduction in body water. The volume of distribution of water-soluble drugs is smaller and this tends to cause an increase in initial drug concentration (e.g. digoxin and cimetidine). Lipid-soluble drugs tend to have an increased volume of distribution (e.g. nitrazepam and diazepam), which prolongs the elimination half-life and may prolong effect.

The extent of plasma protein–drug binding changes little with age but the plasma albumin may fall considerably with the onset of disease.

Lecture Notes: Clinical Pharmacology and Therapeutics, 8th edition. By Gerard McKay, John Reid and Matthew Walters. Published 2010 by Blackwell Publishing Ltd.

There is no strong evidence that protein-binding interactions are more common in the elderly than in the young.

Drug metabolism and age

There is evidence for age-related changes in the rates of metabolism of some drugs. In general, drugs that undergo microsomal oxidation (e.g. chlordiazepoxide) are likely to be metabolised more slowly in the elderly. Despite this, there is no evidence that the concentration or activity of hepatic microsomal oxidising enzymes is reduced in the elderly. The age-related reduction in oxidising capacity may be related to the reduction in hepatic volume and blood flow that occurs in the elderly. Conjugation pathways do not appear to be affected by age. Overall, the changes in metabolism with age alone are not of great clinical significance.

First-pass metabolism may be reduced considerably in the elderly (see below). This is probably the consequence of the age-associated reduction in liver mass and blood flow. As a result, drugs that undergo extensive first-pass metabolism (e.g. labetolol and propranolol) may show considerably increased bioavailability in the elderly.

This effect is amplified by the presence of chronic liver disease.

Renal excretion

In old age there is a fall in both renal blood flow and renal function. Glomerular filtration falls by approximately 30% by the age of 65 years, as compared to young adults. Digoxin and the aminoglycoside antibiotics are excreted mainly by glomerular filtration and these will tend to accumulate in the elderly if the dose is not reduced. Renal tubular function also declines and drugs such as penicillin and procainamide, which undergo active tubular secretion, have a marked reduction in clearance. In addition, the elderly are more likely to suffer a further reduction in renal function as a result of renal tract disease such as infection. Illness in the elderly is frequently accompanied by dehydration and this reduces renal function even further. The overall effect of physiological ageing and disease considerably diminishes the elderly kidney's capacity to excrete drugs.

Receptor sensitivity

In practice, it is very difficult to assess accurately drug receptor numbers or sensitivity. In most cases information is derived from drug effect related to drug plasma concentration. Using this approach it can be shown that the elderly are more sensitive to the effect of benzodiazepine drugs such as nitrazepam, temazepam and diazepam. Warfarin is more potent in the elderly because of a greater effect on coagulation factor synthesis and this is a reflection of the increased receptor affinity to warfarin that occurs in the elderly.

Perhaps most is known about the effects of ageing on the autonomic receptors. On the one hand there is a modest decline in the tachycardia produced by stimulation of β_1-adrenoceptors; on the other, there appears to be no age-related change in β_2-adrenoceptor-mediated vascular or bronchial relaxation. The effect of the vasconstrictor α_1-adrenoceptor is also unchanged with age.

Impairment of homeostasis

The effect of drugs in the elderly may be affected by a loss of homeostatic control that is often seen in the elderly patient.

Cardiovascular postural reflexes are commonly less effective in the aged. Elderly patients tend to fall more easily than the young and this is made worse by the use of drugs that cause postural hypotension. There are many such drugs, including diuretics, antihypertensive agents and sedatives.

The elderly have impaired thermoregulation. Many of the major tranquillisers may precipitate hypothermia. This is the result not only of a direct hypothermic effect, but also of a reduction in physical activity.

Adherence

There is no evidence that an elderly patient whose mental function is normal is more likely to make mistakes with their medication than a younger patient. However, one of the main contributory factors to poor drug adherence at all ages is polypharmacy – the rate of errors when three drugs are prescribed is approximately 20% but it is close to 100% when 10 drugs are prescribed – and the high consumption of drugs in the elderly results in a greater opportunity to make errors. This is often made worse by the prevalence of mental impairment, which is as high as 25% in those over the age of 85 years. Physical handicap can also contribute to poor adherence. Arthritic hands have great difficulty in opening 'child-proof' containers or 'bubble-packed' drugs.

Key points – prescribing for the elderly

- Make an accurate diagnosis. The presentation of disease in the elderly is often non-specific (e.g. confusion, dizziness and incontinence). It is important to make an accurate diagnosis to allow appropriate therapy.
- Treat only important disorders. Elderly patients frequently have multiple pathology. This can lead to polypharmacy with a resultant increase in side effects and poor adherence.
- Avoid ineffective drugs. Prescriptions for marginally effective or ineffective drugs can only lead to side effects and poor adherence.
- Review drugs regularly. It is important to review the need for each prescription. If a drug is considered necessary, make sure the minimum dose required is used.
- Understand the changes in pharmacology with age for each drug used, remembering that relative renal insufficiency is very common in the elderly.

Pharmacokinetics/pharmacodynamics in the elderly

Reduced first-pass metabolism
- propranolol (in sick elderly)

Reduced protein binding (in sick elderly)
- phenytoin
- diazepam

Increased volume of distribution (relative increased body fat)
- diazepam

Decreased hepatic oxidation
- chloridiazepoxide

Decreased renal excretion
- digoxin
- gentamicin
- cimetidine

Decreased drug-receptor sensitivity
- cardiac β_1-adrenoceptor drugs

Increased drug receptor sensitivity
- warfarin
- benzodiazepines

Considerations when prescribing for infants and children

When prescribing for children it is important to be mindful of the significant differences between children and adults in kinetics, dynamics and practical aspects of drug treatment. Children should not be regarded simply as small adults, and given the complexities inherent in prescribing for children; pharmacological treatment should not generally be initiated by inexperienced doctors.

Pharmacokinetics

A variety of factors influence pharmacokinetics in the very young. Drug absorption may be affected by relatively high gastric pH in infants, and topical preparations are better absorbed in this group because the skin is relatively thin. Low body fat content may reduce the volume of distribution of lipophilic drugs, and lower plasma albumin concentration reduces plasma protein binding. Immaturity of neonatal hepatic enzyme systems and renal excretion mechanisms may impair drug elimination, necessitating dosage reduction in the first months of life.

Pharmacodynamics

There is a paucity of research into altered receptor sensitivity in children. Despite this, the differential effects of some drugs in children compared to adults are well recognised. Perhaps the best-known example being the sedative effect of amphetamine derivatives in children, a paradoxical effect used in the management of hyperactive states.

Drug administration

Practical aspects of prescribing are of particular importance whenever a child is being treated. After appropriate dosage modification to compensate for the factors discussed above, medicines may still be ineffective if their unpleasant taste or bulky formulation prevent them from being swallowed by the child. Many proprietary children's medicines contain excipients to make them more palatable to children; however, less-widely-used medicines may not be available in more palatable formulations and this may make administration more difficult. Other practical considerations should be borne in mind whenever a child is being treated. For example, the management of common childhood complaints like asthma can be complicated by the need to acquire an effective inhaler technique which younger children often find difficult. In such circumstances the use of a 'spacer' device (see Chapter 6) should be considered.

Development and regulation of medicines for children

Pharmacological research in children is complicated by ethical issues such as inability of the very young to provide informed consent, and by concerns over potential long-term harm induced by exposure of developing tissues to drugs. The paucity of clinical information limits the number of drugs which obtain a regulatory licence for use in children. Valuable resources such at the BNF for children are validated against what evidence exists, and are helpful in the safe and appropriate management of diseases in childhood.

Chapter 24

Drugs in pregnant and breastfeeding women

Drugs in pregnancy

Clinical scenario

A 28-year-old woman attends her general practitioner (GP) for preconception advice. She has epilepsy and has been on carbamazepine 800 mg bd for several years. She has been seizure-free for over 12 months. She has recently got married and wishes to discuss the implications of her epilepsy on planning a pregnancy. She has no other medical or family history of note. What are the risks of the medication on a developing baby? Is there anything she can do to minimize this risk?

Key points

- The greatest risk of teratogenesis occurs at a stage when a women might not know that she is pregnant
- Only a few drugs are known definitely to be teratogenic, but many more could be under certain circumstances
- When prescribing for a woman of childbearing age, remember that she might be pregnant and ask yourself if the benefits of drug use outweigh the risks of teratogenesis

---

Introduction

Nearly 40% of women in the United Kingdom take at least one drug during pregnancy, exclud-

Lecture Notes: Clinical Pharmacology and Therapeutics, 8th edition. By Gerard McKay, John Reid and Matthew Walters. Published 2010 by Blackwell Publishing Ltd.

ing iron, vitamins and drugs used during delivery. Once in the maternal circulation, drugs are separated from the fetus by a lipid placental membrane, which any given drug crosses to a greater or lesser extent depending on the physicochemical properties of the molecule.

Drugs in pregnancy can be viewed from two perspectives:

1 Effect of drugs on the fetus
2 Effect of pregnancy on the drug

Effect of drugs on the fetus

Drugs can influence fetal development at three separate stages:

1 Fertilisation and implantation period: conception to about 17 days gestation
2 Organogenesis: 18–55 days
3 Growth and development: 56th day onwards

The possible consequences of drug exposure are different at each stage. In addition, drugs given at the end of pregnancy can influence structure or function in the neonate.

Fertilisation and implantation period

Interference by a drug with either of these processes leads to failure of the pregnancy at a very early and probably subclinical stage. Therefore, very little is known about drugs that influence this process in humans.

Organogenesis

It is during this period that the developing embryo shows great sensitivity to the teratogenic effects of drugs. A teratogen is any substance (virus, environmental toxin or drug) that produces deformity. Before discussing the teratogenic properties of certain drugs, the following points must be appreciated:

1 Teratogenesis in humans is very difficult to predict from animal studies because of considerable species variation. Thalidomide, the most notorious drug teratogen of recent times, showed no teratogenicity in mice and rats.

2 Serious congenital deformities are present in 1–2% of all babies; therefore, a drug is only readily identified as teratogenic if its effects are frequent, unusual and/or serious. A low-grade teratogen that infrequently causes minor deformities is likely to pass unnoticed.

Table 24.1 lists some drugs that are known to be teratogenic. It is important to emphasize that, even for known teratogens, first trimester use often results in a normal baby; for example, phenytoin is teratogenic in about 4% of exposures and warfarin in up to 5%. Also, there will be occasions, such as the use of warfarin in women with prosthetic heart valves, where the risks to the mother of not using the drug outweigh the risks of exposure in the fetus. The greatest risk of teratogenesis occurs at a time when a woman might not even be aware that she is pregnant.

Growth and development

During this stage, major body structures have been formed, and it is their subsequent development and function that can be affected:

1 Antithyroid drugs cross the placenta and can cause fetal and neonatal hypothyroidism.

2 Tetracyclines inhibit bone growth and discolour teeth.

3 Angiotensin-converting enzyme inhibitors can seriously damage fetal kidney function.

4 Warfarin can cause bleeding into the fetal brain.

5 Drugs with dependence potential, for example benzodiazepines and opiates, which are taken regularly during pregnancy, can result in withdrawal symptoms in the neonate.

Drugs given at the end of pregnancy

1 Aspirin in analgesic doses can cause haemorrhage in the neonate.

2 Indomethacin (and possibly other non-steroidal anti-inflammatory drugs (NSAIDs) causes premature closure of the ductus arteriosus with resulting pulmonary hypertension.

3 Central nervous system (CNS) depressant drugs (e.g. opiates, benzodiazepines) can cause hypotension, respiratory depression and hypothermia in the neonate.

Effect of pregnancy on drug absorption, distribution and elimination

The substantial physiological changes that occur in pregnancy can influence drug disposition, while pathological conditions in pregnancy can accentuate these changes.

Table 24.1 Drugs that are known to be teratogenic.

Drug	Deformity
Danazol	Virilisation of female fetus
Lithium	Cardiac (Ebstein's complex)
Phenytoin	Craniofacial; limb
Carbamazepine	Craniofacial; limb
Retinoids	Central nervous system
Valproate	Neural tube; neurodevelopment
Diethylstilbestrol (stilboestrol)	Adenocarcinoma of vagina in teenage years
Warfarin	Multiple defects; chondrodysplasia punctata

Drug distribution

Maternal plasma volume and extracellular fluid volume increase by about 50% by the last trimester, and this may decrease the steady-state concentration of drugs with a small volume of distribution. Considerable changes in protein concentration occur during the last trimester, with serum albumin falling by about 20% while α_1-acid glycoprotein increasing in concentration by about 40% in normal pregnancies. These changes are accentuated in pre-eclampsia, with albumin concentration falling by about 35% and glycoprotein rising by as much as 100%. This means that the free fraction of acidic drugs can increase substantially, while that of basic drugs can be decreased greatly, in the last trimester. Diazepam, phenytoin and sodium valproate have been shown to have significantly elevated free fractions in the last trimester.

Drug elimination

Effective renal plasma flow doubles by the end of pregnancy, but this has been shown to be important in only a few cases; for example the clearance of ampicillin doubles and the dose must also be doubled for systemic (but of course not for renal tract) infections. The hepatic microsomal mixed function oxidase system undergoes induction in pregnancy, probably as a result of high circulating levels of progesterone. This leads to an increased clearance of drugs that undergo metabolism by this pathway, and there is evidence that the steady-state concentrations of the anticonvulsants sodium valproate, phenytoin and carbamazepine may be decreased to a clinically significant extent during the second and third trimesters. Therefore, higher doses may be required as the pregnancy progresses.

Drug treatment of common medical problems during pregnancy

Infection

Urinary tract infections are common during pregnancy. Penicillins and cephalosporins are the pre-ferred treatment (subject to appropriate sensitivity testing), because these drugs have never been implicated in teratogenesis and are generally well tolerated. Nitrofurantoin is not harmful to the fetus but frequently causes nausea. Tetracyclines are contraindicated. Trimethoprim should be avoided in early pregnancy since it can possibly cause limb reduction and cleft palate.

Severe infections in pregnancy are rare. Aminoglycosides cause fetal eighth nerve damage, and the benefits of their use must be seen in this context. The risk is smallest with gentamicin, and if indicated, the levels should be monitored closely. In the case of viral infection, including primary herpes simplex and varicella-zoster, acyclovir is thought to be safe to administer in pregnancy. With regard to TB, present data suggests that the most commonly used agents including isoniazid, rifampicin, pyrazinamide and ethambutol are safe to use in pregnancy and the benefits of treatment of active TB outweigh any concerns of drug toxicity. Vitamin K should be given with isoniazid and rifampicin from 36th week to reduce the incidence of post-partum haemorrhage and hemorrhagic disease of the newborn. Because of concerns of hepatotoxicity in pregnancy with isoniazid, liver function should be monitored prior to treatment and at monthly intervals. Vitamin B6 should be given with isoniazid to reduce the risk of neuropathy. Streptomycin causes auditory damage in the fetus and is contraindicated in pregnancy.

Nausea and vomiting

Nausea affects about 90% of pregnant women, and nausea and vomiting around 50%. Non-drug treatments include dietary modification, hypnotherapy, acupressure and ginger. Antiemetics considered safe to use in pregnancy include antihistamines (e.g. cyclizine), phenothiazines (e.g. procholperazine), metoclopramide and the 5HT3 antagonist ondansetron (although as there is less evidence regarding fetal effects, this should be reserved as a second line agent). In severe cases, IV fluid and electrolyte replacement with thiamine supplementation may be required.

Diabetes

Diabetes in pregnancy is divided primarily into pre-existing diabetes (type 1 and type 2) and gestational diabetes (GDM). Diabetes is associated with increased risk for both the mother and the fetus and the most important goal of treatment is to achieve as near to normoglycaemia in the mother as possible to reduce these risks. For type 1 and type 2 diabetes, tight diabetic control is achieved ideally pre-pregnancy to reduce the risk of congenital malformations. For type 1 diabetes as standard, a four times daily basal bolus regimen, such as an intermediate acting insulin, to be taken at night and three pre-meal injections of fast acting insulin allow maximum flexibility. As pregnancy progresses, there will be increased insulin requirements which rapidly returns to pre-pregnancy levels post-delivery. The short-acting insulin analogues, insulin aspart and insulin lispro, are not known to be harmful, and may be used during pregnancy and lactation. The safety of long-acting insulin analogues in pregnancy has not been established; therefore, isophane insulin is recommended where longer-acting insulins are needed. Insulin is adjusted mainly on the basis of post-prandial blood glucose monitoring (1 hour < 7.8 mmol/L) and fasting levels (3.5–5.9 mmol/L).

Women with type 2 diabetes are usually converted to insulin either pre-pregnancy or in early pregnancy, with the aim of optimising glycaemic control. The sulphonylureas are generally avoided in pregnancy as they cross the placenta and theoretically cause neonatal hypoglycaemia. The thiazolidinediones are contraindicated due to teratogenesis in animal studies. Metformin can be used either alone or in combination with insulin in type 2 and gestational diabetics; however, at present the long-term effects of metformin on the fetus are not known.

Asthma

Poorly controlled asthma is associated with increased perinatal mortality. Maternal hypoxia and respiratory alkalosis are the major determinants of fetal distress in asthmatic pregnancies. Inhaled short acting B2 agonists, inhaled anticholinergics, theophyllines and steroids have good safety records at all stages of pregnancy. There has been limited human data with long acting beta 2 agonists but is still felt to be safe when administered by inhalation.

Pregnancy should not alter the general approach to asthma as described in Chapter 6. It is important to control bronchospasm and avoid prolonged abnormalities of blood gases or acid–base balance. Although asthma management is largely unchanged in pregnancy the leukotriene antagonists should be avoided, as there is extremely limited safety data in human pregnancy.

Epilepsy

Epilepsy is the commonest neurological disorder encountered in pregnancy affecting 0.5% of pregnant women. The main issues are possible teratogenicity associated with anticonvulsants and adjustment of doses of drug to control fits. The incidence of congenital malformations in children of mothers with epilepsy is about 3–5%, which is three times higher than in the general population. In part, this could reflect a genetic predisposition, but anticonvulsants seem largely to be responsible. Most evidence exists for the older drugs: carbamazepine, phenytoin and valproate, with cleft palate, neural tube defects and congenital heart disease being the most common findings, and there is increasing evidence of neurodevelopmental delay with valproate. There is much less evidence for the newer anticonvulsant drugs, but preliminary data suggests low rates of malformations (Table 24.2), particularly with lamotrigine and oxcarbazepine. There is a dose response relationship for valproate (>1 g/day) and lamotrigine (>400 mg/day). Co-administration of anticonvulsants produces a greater risk than when either drug is used alone (Table 24.3). To increase our knowledge on the effects of epilepsy and its drug treatment on pregnancy, all pregnant women with epilepsy should be added to the UK epilepsy and pregnancy register Table 24.4 summarises the key points to managing pregnant women with epilepsy.

Table 24.2 Data from UK Epilepsy and Pregnancy Register, 2005.

Anticonvulsant	Major malformation rate (%)
Carbamazepine	2.2
Sodium valproate	6.2
Lamotrigine	3.2
Phenytoin	3.7

Table 24.3 Influence of anti-epileptic drug treatment on rates of congenital malformations.

	Major congenital malformation rate
No AED	3.5%
Monotherapy	3.7%
Polytherapy	6.0%

AED, anti-epileptic drug.

The pharmacokinetic changes associated with pregnancy are clinically important in the treatment of epilepsy. There are several factors in pregnancy which influence drug levels including altered protein binding, changes in absorption, increased plasma volume, and increased metabolism and excretion. Non-compliance is also an issue in mothers concerned about the effects of the drugs. Therapy should be monitored by the clinical response and seizure activity and the lowest effective dose should be used. Generally dose increases are required in pregnancy particularly for drugs with little protein binding such as lamotrigine, which may need to be increased two- to threefold. After delivery, if drugs were increased during pregnancy they should be reduced to preconception levels by around 1 week post-partum. Breastfeeding should be encouraged as most anticonvulsants are secreted in very small amounts in breast milk. Neonates should be monitored for sedation. Higher doses of oestrogen in the combined oral contraceptive pill and progesterone in progesterone-only contraception are required in women on hepatic enzyme inducing drugs.

Hypertension

Methyldopa is widely used in the management of essential hypertension during pregnancy. This drug is now rarely used outside of pregnancy because of a wide range of side effects, notably

Table 24.4 Key points in the management of pregnant women with epilepsy.

1 Management should begin before conception
- Use the lowest effective dose of medication
- Consider replacing sodium valproate before conception
- Withdraw any unnecessary medication and use monotherapy wherever possible
- It may be possible to wean women who have been seizure-free for several years and require low doses of medication after careful counselling and discussion with a neurologist

Do not change if well controlled and already pregnant

2 Discuss increased incidence of congenital malformations using drug specific rates (Table 24.2). In general, the benefits of drug therapy on mother and fetus outweigh the risks.

3 All women require to take folic acid 5 mg preconceptually

4 Antenatal screening for neural tube defects by detailed anatomy scan should be performed at 12 weeks and again at 18–20 weeks

5 Vitamin K supplementation during the last month of pregnancy for enzyme inducing anticonvulsants

6 Monitor therapy by seizure frequency and adjust doses accordingly

7 Continue anticonvulsant medication during labour

8 Minimise triggers of seizures

9 Neonate should receive vitamin K and breastfeeding should be encouraged tiredness and dizziness. However, it has an unrivalled safety record in pregnancy. Therefore, it is the drug of choice when prescribing in pregnancy, particularly for chronic hypertension.

Beta-blockers successfully lower blood pressure in pregnancy, but have not been shown conclusively to improve fetal outcome. They are not teratogenic. Long-term use of beta-blockers in pregnancy has been associated with growth retardation of the fetus, although this is thought to be secondary to a reduction in blood pressure rather than associated with a particular class of drug. They !!!!!have minimal side effects in comparison with methyldopa and are often favoured by clinicians.

Nifedipine, a calcium channel blocker, is used as a second line agent for the treatment in hypertension in pregnancy. It has no major maternal or fetal side effects.

Hydralazine is used intravenously (IV) for acute or severe hypertension and also orally as a second line agent for chronic hypertension in pregnancy. It can cause tachycardia and headache if given IV. Its maternal and fetal effects compare unfavourably with nifedipiene and labetalol. There are also reported cases of maternal and fetal lupus-like syndromes associated with its use.

Angiotensin-converting enzyme (ACE) inhibitors and angiotensin II inhibitors are contraindicated in pregnancy. The use of ACE inhibitors is associated with an increased risk of major congenital malformations after first trimester exposure and causes oligohydramnios, renal dysplasia and pulmonary hypoplasia if administered in the second or third trimester of pregnancy. Ideally, they should be discontinued pre-pregnancy.

Statins are also contraindicated due to reported teratogenesis associated with their use, which may be secondary to interference with cholesterol biosynthesis in the fetus.

Hyperthyroidism

Propylthiouracil tends to be used more often than carbimazole during pregnancy. Propylthiouracil is less lipid-soluble and more protein-bound and crosses less well into the fetus and breast milk. The dose should be titrated against maternal thyroid function and adjusted to maintain free T4 in the upper non-pregnant range. Requirements tend to decrease in pregnancy. Propranolol may be used to treat symptoms and there are no know teratogenic effects. Radioactive iodine should not be given to any women who is or may be pregnant.

Thrombosis

Pregnancy is associated with a 10-fold increased risk of developing venous thromboembolic disease (VTE) than in non-pregnant and is the major direct cause of maternal mortality in the United Kingdom. Treatment and prophylaxis of VTE requires anticoagulants which have special considerations in pregnancy. Warfarin is teratogenic when given between sixth and twelfth week of pregnancy – a 5% risk of major abnormality and 0.6% risk of warfarin embryopathy. It is also associated with bleeding during pregnancy and at delivery, and is generally avoided except in very high risk cases. Low molecular weight heparins (LMWH) are usually the treatment of choice and have a much lower incidence of side effects such as heparin induced thrombocytopaenia, allergic reactions and osteoporosis than unfractionated heparin.

Depression

There are several factors to take into consideration when prescribing antidepressant medication in pregnancy. All antidepressants will cross freely across the placenta and the fetus and neonate are susceptible to side effects. A balance of the risk of treatment against the risk of serious mental illness should be made, and there should be consideration of efficacious non-pharmacological treatments. The older drugs such as tricylic antidepressants have been used for many years and there are no known teratogenic effects. Therefore, they are the drugs of choice in pregnancy. They can cause withdrawal symptoms or anticholinergic side effects in the neonate, and reducing the dose in the third trimester, wherever possible, may minimize this risk. They are safe in breastfeeding; the newer selective serotonin reuptake inhibitors

Table 24.5 Special considerations made when prescribing in pregnancy.

Drugs	Considerations in pregnancy
Paracetamol	First line analgesic – no known adverse effects
NSAIDs	Can be used in first and second trimester Avoid third trimester – can affect fetal kidneys and cause premature closure of ductus arteriosus
Corticosteroids	Prednisolone safe in pregnancy. Increased risk of GDM. If on long-term steroids, needs parental therapy to cover stress of labour
Antimalarials	Hydroxychloroquine drug of choice. No known teratogenic effects. Increased risk of flare of SLE if discontinued, steroid sparing agent in SLE
Azathioprine	Safe in pregnancy. No known fetal effects. Useful steroid sparing agent
Sulfazalazine	Safe in pregnancy. Should prescribe 5 mg folic acid in addition to reduce risk of neural tube defects
Pencillamine/Gold	Avoid in pregnancy
Cytotoxic agents	Methotrexate and cyclophosphamide are teratogenic and should be avoided 3 months prior to conception

(SSRI) are commonly used as first line agents out with pregnancy and will often be taken by women around the time of conception. It is not wise to abruptly stop these drugs as this may cause withdrawal in the mother. There appears to be a modest increased risk of congenital malformations and, in particular, cardiac defects with first trimester exposure. Paroxetine, in particular, is associated with an increased risk of fetal abnormalities and should either be discontinued or switched to another antidepressant in pregnancy. SSRIs are also associated with a neonatal withdrawal syndrome if taken in late pregnancy.

Connective tissue disease

This group of disorders includes conditions such as systemic lupus erythematosus (SLE) and rheumatoid arthritis. Special considerations are made when prescribing in pregnancy (Table 24.5).

Drug use in breastfeeding

Clinical scenario

A 40-year-old woman attends her doctor for advice. She was diagnosed with diabetes during pregnancy and treated with insulin. After pregnancy she continues on metformin alone. Her doctor is keen to start her on simvastatin for primary cardiac prevention. She is concerned that her baby might be exposed to the metformin and any other drugs the doctor is recommending, because she is breastfeeding and plans to continue to do so. Is her baby at risk, and how should her doctor deal with this enquiry?

Key points

- Most commonly used drugs can be safely used in women who are breastfeeding
- If prescribing a drug in a woman who is breastfeeding and you do not know whether it is safe, always seek further information

The factors that determine the transfer of drugs into breast milk are the same as that influencing

Table 24.6 Drugs safe for breastfeeding mothers.

Penicillins, cephalosporins
Theophylline, salbutamol by inhaler, prednisolone
Valproate, carbamazepine, phenytoin
Beta-blockers, methyldopa, hydralazine
Warfarin, heparin
Haloperidol, chlorpromazine
Tricyclic antidepressants

Table 24.7 Commonly used drugs that should be avoided in women who are breastfeeding.

Drug	Effect of drug
Amiodarone	Iodine content may cause neonatal hypothyroidism
Aspirin	Theoretical risk of Reye's syndrome
Barbiturates	Drowsiness
Benzodiazepines	Lethargy
Carbimazole	Hypothyroidism at higher doses
Contraceptives (combined oral)	May diminish milk supply and reduce nitrogen and protein content
Cytotoxic drugs	Potential problems include immune suppression and neutropenia
Ephedrine	Irritability
Tetracyclines	Theoretical risk of tooth discoloration

drug distribution in general (see Chapter 1). Most drugs enter breast milk to a greater or lesser extent but, because the concentration has been greatly reduced by distribution throughout the mother's body, the amount of drug actually received by the breast-fed baby is usually clinically insignificant.

Drugs that can safely be given to breastfeeding mothers are listed in Table 24.6. Certain drugs achieve sufficient concentration in breast milk, and they are sufficiently potent that their use in breastfeeding mothers should be avoided and are listed in Table 24.7.

Chapter 25

Pharmacoeconomics: the economic evaluation of new drugs

Clinical scenario

A 45-year-old man has recently been diagnosed with an advanced form of cancer. The patient presents at your clinic to discuss treatment options and has brought with him several printouts from the internet which he wants to ask you about. He has read that there is a new drug for his condition which has shown some promising early results in a phase III clinical trial. The drug showed some modest survival benefits compared to current standard therapy, alongside relatively manageable side effects, and your patient would therefore like to be prescribed the drug. However, you know that this new medicine is very expensive and that it has recently had a health economic evaluation. The result is that it is not recommended for use for patients you look after. What tools are used by health economists to decide whether a drug offers value for money?

Key points

- Resource scarcity in health care systems means that choices have to be made on how resources are spent.
- Economic evaluations are increasingly used in health-care decision making to provide an indicator of the cost-effectiveness of different treatment options and aid resource allocation decisions.

Lecture Notes: Clinical Pharmacology and Therapeutics, 8th edition. By Gerard McKay, John Reid and Matthew Walters. Published 2010 by Blackwell Publishing Ltd.

- Cost-utility analysis is a commonly used type of economic evaluation used by health technology assessment agencies.
- Quality adjusted life years (QALYs) are a standard outcome measure used to capture both the morbidity and mortality profile associated with a disease and its treatment.

Introduction – why do we need economic evaluations?

Over the last few decades, there has been an increased interest in applying economic analysis to health care interventions, as evidenced by the use of such evaluations by organisations such as the National Institute for Health and Clinical Excellence (NICE) and the Scottish Medicines Consortium (SMC) in the UK. The reason relates to a basic problem in economics, tackling the linked issues of scarcity and choice.

Scarcity of resources exists in health care systems worldwide, and means that there will never be sufficient funds to meet all the competing demands for health care. Difficult choices have to be made over how to spend resources in order to meet the many objectives of the healthcare system.

Pharmacoeconomics, defined as the economic evaluation of pharmaceutical interventions, is often used by healthcare decision makers in the NHS and elsewhere It is increasingly also used by pharmaceutical companies, who have to demonstrate the cost-effectiveness of new drugs in addition to achieving the traditional hurdles of safety and efficacy required for drug licensing.

Economic evaluation

Economic evaluation is defined as the *comparative analysis of alternative courses of action in terms of both their costs and consequences* (Drummond *et al.* 2005). Such evaluation can provide a systematic way of considering solutions to the problems of scarcity and choice that are faced in the healthcare system. The aim is to identify what is most *efficient*, defined as the greatest amount of health benefit that can be bought for a given level of resource.

Perspective

The specific costs and benefits that are included in any economic evaluation depend on the *perspective* that has been chosen for the analysis. The perspective is often that of the 'healthcare payer', who is generally only interested in the direct costs to the health care system and benefits to the patient treated. Alternatively, a 'societal' perspective may be adopted, which will aim to take into account a much wider range of costs and benefits by, for example, including costs that are borne by patients themselves, the income losses patients experience as a consequence of being ill or the wider benefits by reducing demands on social security resources. While the societal perspective may seem more logical and comprehensive, many of the costs and benefits are hard to quantify and/or realise.

Costs

Cost, in a health economic evaluation, comes in many forms and is more than the simple acquisition cost of the drug in question.

One of the key concepts in economic evaluation is that of *opportunity cost*. This is defined as the benefit foregone when selecting one course of action rather than another. When resources are limited, the decision to spend money in one way means that we cannot spend the money on something else, and therefore are foregoing the benefits associated with the thing we can no longer do. In a competitive market, opportunity costs should be reflected by market prices, but where they are not (as is usually the case in healthcare systems), opportunity costs have to be estimated by economists.

Economists also distinguish between *direct*, *indirect* and *intangible* costs. Direct costs are those that are consumed in the provision of a health intervention, e.g. staff costs, hospital operating costs, drug acquisition costs, etc. These are generally easy to measure. Indirect costs relate to costs from a societal perspective, for example, the loss of earnings or costs borne by patients and their carers as a consequence of illness. These costs are more difficult to measure and are not always included in economic evaluations. Intangible costs relate to things like pain, worry and distress caused by illness; these are very difficult to quantify in monetary terms and are often only described rather than quantified in economic evaluations.

The last distinction to note is the importance of *marginal* costs, rather than average costs, in economic evaluation. An example to explain this concept is to envisage a new treatment that results in a patient being able to be discharged from hospital a day earlier than the current treatment allows. It might seem that the average cost of this bed day saved should be incorporated into the analysis but from an economist's point of view, the average cost would overstate the savings that arise. This is because, unless the hospital ward can be closed, the fixed costs (such as staff costs, heat and light) will still be incurred. The marginal cost of the bed day is a better reflection of the resource change brought about by the new treatment as this will take into account only the costs that change, for example, the savings in the patient's meals, drugs and perhaps some small savings in staff time.

Linking costs to benefits

To aid decision-making, pharmacoeconomics aims to link the costs of a treatment to the benefits that it produces. There are four common types of economic evaluation, all of which use similar approaches to measuring the costs they include but which differ in the way that they treat the outcomes or consequences of treatment.

Cost-minimisation analysis

Cost-minimisation analysis (CMA) is the simplest form of economic evaluation. It is used where two or more treatments are known to have exactly the same outcomes, for example, in terms of proportion of patients successfully treated. The analysis is therefore simply reduced to a search for the least costly treatment. An example would be where a clinical trial had shown two antibiotic drugs to be equally effective in clearing an infection. The CMA would then simply compare the costs of the two treatments and the preferred treatment would be the lower cost alternative. The cost differences would include not only the drug acquisition costs but also any costs involved in drug administration, drug monitoring or management of adverse drug reactions.

Cost-effectiveness analysis

The term 'cost-effectiveness analysis' or CEA is often used loosely to refer to all types of pharmacoeconomic evaluation but does refer to a specific technique that compares alternative treatments in terms of a single *natural unit* which is common to both alternatives. It is of use where the alternative treatments achieve the outcome to different degrees i.e. one treatment is more effective than the other. Treatments are then compared in terms of the cost per additional unit of benefit, for example, cost per life year saved, cost per ulcer healed or cost per extra mmHg BP reduction. Cost-effectiveness analysis is frequently used to compare interventions within a single disease area. For many decision-makers it has a significant limitation as it does not allow comparisons to be made between different areas of clinical practice with different outcomes (e.g. ulcer-healing drug v blood-pressure lowering drug).

Cost-benefit analysis

In cost-benefit analysis (CBA) both the costs and the outcomes of alternative interventions are ex-

pressed in monetary units. This requires a financial value to be attached to the benefit of treatments, often by asking patients or the public to state how much they would be willing to pay for the effects of the intervention. In cost-benefit analysis, treatments are judged to offer value for money if the cost of the treatment is less than the value placed on the benefits of the treatment. CBA is a problematic form of analysis because of the difficulties in asking people to place a notional monetary value on health benefits, and is encountered less frequently in pharmacoeconomics literature.

Cost-utility analysis

Cost-utility analysis (CUA) is a special form of cost-effectiveness analysis where alternative interventions are compared in terms of their impact on a single measure which tries to capture all the benefits (and adverse effects) of the intervention in question. The cost per QALY, a measure that combines the impact of both the additional length of life and quality of life available from a treatment, is the most commonly used measure in CUA.

It is useful to have a working knowledge of CUA in today's health care environment, because it is the preferred method of economic evaluation of organisations such as NICE, SMC and other health technology assessment (HTA) agencies worldwide. CUA has been widely adopted, largely because it can be used to compare the cost-effectiveness of the many different types of interventions that HTA organisations must assess.

Why use CUA and QALYs?

It is helpful to use an example to explain why CUA is such a useful form of economic evaluation. In cardiovascular disease there are many different treatments available and each treatment will give rise to a specific pattern of costs and effects. For example, in seeking to manage a patient's weight, clinicians could use lifestyle interventions or drug therapy. If drug therapy provided greater benefits but at an increased cost compared to lifestyle modification, then economic evaluation can provide a marker to help the decision-maker judge

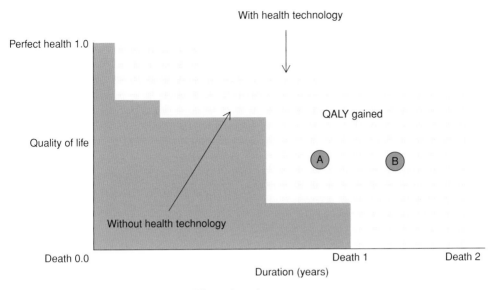

Figure 25.1 The concept of quality adjusted life year (QALY).

whether the additional costs are justified by the additional benefits. In comparing two (or more) treatment options in an economic evaluation, the convention is to calculate the additional benefit provided by the more effective treatment and then present the findings in terms of 'cost per additional unit of benefit', e.g. 'cost per additional life year gained'. Frequently, treatments offer a range of effects such as an improvement in symptoms and better survival. Cost-effectiveness analysis using an outcome measure such as a 'cost per additional life year gained' would struggle to take account of both dimensions of benefit.

QALYs have the advantage of being able to capture gains in quality of life and quantity of life (survival) in a single measure. The QALY adjusts length of life for quality of life by assigning a value (known as a *utility value*) between 0 and 1 (where 0 represents death or health states considered as bad as being dead and 1 represents perfect health) for each year of life. Negative utility values are also possible for some conditions that are considered to be worse than being dead, such as the end stage of a degenerative illness. Figure 25.1 illustrates the concept of a QALY. Without the new health technology the individual's quality of life, measured on

the *y*-axis, would deteriorate over time until they die ('Death 1'). However, with the new technology the individual's quality of life is maintained at a higher level until they die, a few years later than they would have done with the original treatment ('Death 2'). Area A represents the quality of life gain with the new treatment while area B corresponds to the survival gain with the treatment. Added together, they represent the total QALY gain associated with the new treatment.

How are the constituent parts of QALYs estimated?

Estimating the survival component of the QALY is often relatively straightforward as it can be taken directly from clinical trial data. Frequently, however, patient survival is not the primary end-point of the trial and, if an intermediate end-point shows significant benefit from the new intervention, the trial may be stopped early before mature survival data can be obtained. Under these circumstances, some mathematical modelling of the likely survival benefit may be required. Extrapolation always introduces an element of uncertainty into the estimate of survival gain.

Deriving the utility values is more controversial and requires some assessment of the relative desirability of various health states. Sometimes the value attached to each health state is taken from patients with actual experience of the health state but often this is not possible and so values taken from health professionals with knowledge of the health state, or members of the public to whom the health state has been described, may be used. Indeed the question of whether the perspective of the patient experiencing the health state or the perspective of the public, payers in the healthcare system is the more important and is one which remains controversial.

Often the value of the health state is obtained directly using one of three common techniques:

1. **Visual Analogue Scale** – Respondents are asked to mark a line (usually labelled 0–100) with an 'X' to indicate their valuation of the health state. The distance from 0 to X is measured and divided by 100 to give the utility value. This is a simple technique but has the disadvantage that the respondent is not asked to make any sort of trade-off or sacrifice in valuing the health state. It is therefore considered an inferior technique by economists.

2. **Time Trade Off** – In this technique individuals are asked to choose between living for a given time in a state of poor health and living for a shorter time in full health. For example, respondents are asked to imagine they have 10 years left to live and they will live these 10 years in the health state being valued. They are then asked to decide how many years they would be willing to give up in order to have full health. If a respondent indicates they would be willing to give up 2 of the 10 years to be 'cured', this would translate into a utility value of 0.8. A worse health state, in which

a respondent would give up 5 years to be free of the condition, would result in a utility value of 0.5.

3. **Standard Gamble** – Respondents are asked to imagine being in the health state being valued and are then told that there is a treatment which could restore them to full health; however the treatment also has the possibility of causing immediate death. They are asked to indicate what risk of death they would be willing to accept in order to be 'cured', a willingness to accept a higher risk of instant death leading to the value on the current health state being lower. Once again survival is being sacrificed (or at least risked) to improve quality of life.

An alternative approach to deriving utility values is an indirect method where a questionnaire is used to describe the current health state in terms of patient experience and function and then the results from the questionnaire are converted into a utility value by inviting patients or the general public to value the health states by the methods above. The EQ-5D questionnaire is commonly used – it assesses each of mobility, self-care, usual activities, pain/discomfort and anxiety/depression on a 3-point scale, and the outcomes have been converted to utility values using a survey of over 3000 members of the general public in the UK. It can be a useful method of deriving utility values though it suffers from the drawback that, with only three levels for each of the five domains, it may be relatively insensitive to changes in health state.

None of the available methods of deriving utility values is perfect but used individually or in combination some meaningful assessment of quality of life can be obtained to factor into QALY calculation. Table 25.1 shows examples of utility values for a number of common health states.

Table 25.1 Utility values from selected published studies.

Disease state	Utility value
Acute coronary syndrome (Kamon et al. 2008)	0.80
Progressive glioma (Rogers et al. 2008)	0.73
Relapse in multiple sclerosis (Gani et al. 2008)	0.50
Mild to moderate depression (Kendrick et al. 2009)	0.70
Symptomatic ulcer (Latimer et al. 2009)	0.55

Table 25.2 Cost per QALY gained figures from selected published studies.

Treatment	Cost per QALY gained
Clopidogrel in acute coronary syndrome	£2,284
Carmustine wafers in glioma	£54,500
Natalizumab in multiple sclerosis	£18,700
SSRIs in mild to moderate depression	£14,854
Addition of a proton pump inhibitor to NSAID or COX2 selective inhibitors	£1,000

With treatment A	With treatment B
Estimated survival = 12 years	Estimated survival = 10 years
Estimated quality of life = 0.7	Estimated quality of life = 0.5
QALYs = 8.4 (12 × 0.7)	QALYs = 5 (10 × 0.5)
QALY gain from treatment A over treatment B = 3.4 QALYs (8.4–5)	

If treatment A costs £10,000 more than treatment B, then the cost per QALY gained with treatment A is £2941 (£10,000(3.4). If the cost per QALY is less than a stated threshold value, it would be considered a cost-effective treatment.

How is cost-effectiveness then assessed?

As noted above, the convention in health economics is to describe the extra health gain from the more beneficial treatment and then to define the cost of this extra benefit. In CUA this leads to a measure known as the Incremental Cost Effectiveness Ratio (ICER), which can be described thus –

$$\frac{\text{QALY benefit of new treatment} - \text{QALY benefit of old treament} = \text{QALY gain}}{\text{Cost of new treatment} - \text{cost of old treatment} = \text{extra cost}}$$

From the outcome of the simple calculation above one can give a value for the ICER as the extra cost per QALY gained, commonly known as 'cost per QALY'.

To help decide if a treatment is cost-effective, the resulting 'cost per QALY' can be compared to 'costs per QALY' for other interventions already adopted by the health service or to the decision-maker's stated 'willingness-to-pay' for an additional QALY. In the UK, NICE uses a rule of thumb or 'threshold' that a cost per QALY of less than £20,000 is generally considered to be cost-effective while a cost per QALY greater than £30,000 is generally considered not to be cost-effective; decision-makers in other countries may adopt other willingness-to-pay thresholds. Table 25.2 shows the ICERs of some common healthcare interventions.

A simple example showing how such QALYs are calculated is shown in the box below.

Sensitivity analysis

As can be seen from the above, pharmacoeconomics is not an exact science and the assessment of cost-effectiveness requires a number of assumptions and/or extrapolations to be made. A good analysis should test the effect of varying these assumptions across a range of likely possibilities, showing which assumptions are the main drivers of the ICER – this is known as *sensitivity analysis*.

In a simple analysis as above, this can be done by varying assumptions one at a time (*univariate* analysis). For example, if the estimated survival with treatment A is only 10 years (i.e. we take away the survival gain) then the QALY gain falls to 2 QALYs (10 × 0.7 = 7; 10 × 0.5 = 5, QALY gain = 7–5) – the ICER is now £5000 (£10,000(2) which remains within usual cost-effectiveness limits. The survival gain, which may be based on extrapolation from the clinical trial, is not essential for the drug to be considered cost-effective. The utility values could be varied similarly.

In a more complex model involving multiple health states and more complex costs and benefits, it may be more appropriate to vary all the parameters at once across a range of likely values, giving a large number of possible ICERs reflecting different combinations of assumptions. This multivariate approach is often called *probabilistic sensitivity analysis* as it shows a range of possible ICERs with an estimate of the likelihood of the actual ICER being below any specified threshold value.

Pharmacoeconomics and decision-making

Pharmacoeconomics and cost-effectiveness assessment do not, of themselves, lead to decisions about which drug interventions a healthcare system should use. The economic assessment provides a structured, objective method to compare the costs and benefits of different possible interventions, but this may only be part of the decision-making process. While an approach based purely on economic assessment might offer the greatest efficiency in a healthcare system, other factors, such as a desire to see equality of access to treatments or a desire to favour specific patients groups (e.g. children, or patients nearing the end of their life), may lead decision-makers to adopt treatments with ICERs above the normal threshold (or reject treatments with ICERs below the normal threshold).

These difficult issues are ultimately matters of judgement rather than calculation, but the economic assessment at least provides useful background to the decision and reveals the extent to which efficiency is being sacrificed to the specific wishes of the healthcare system. While pharmacoeconomics clearly has its limitations, it offers the best available approach to underpinning the difficult decisions which scarcity and choice demand in increasingly cash-limited healthcare systems world-wide.

References

Drummond MF, Sculpher MJ, Torrance GW, O'Brien BJ, Stoddart GL. *Methods for the Economic Evaluation of Health Care Programmes*, 3rd edn, 2005. Oxford University Press: Oxford.

Gani R, Giovannoni G, Bates D, *et al.* Cost-effectiveness analyses of natalizumab compared with other disease modifying therapies for people with highly active relapsing remitting multiple sclerosis. Pharmacoeconomics 2008;26: 617–27.

Karnon J, Holmes MW, Williams R, *et al.* A cost utility analysis of clopidogrel in patients with ST elevation acute coronary syndrome. Int J Cardiol 2008;140(3):315–22.

Kendrick T, Chatwin J, Dowrick C, *et al.* Randomised controlled trial to determine the clinical effectiveness and cost-effectiveness of selective serotonin reuptake inhibitors plus supportive care for mild to moderate depression and somatic symptoms in primary care. Health Technol Ass 2009: 13:22.

Latimer N, Lord J, Grant R, *et al.* Cost-effectiveness of COX 2 selective inhibitors and traditional NSAIDs alone or in combination with a proton pump inhibitor for people with osteoarthritis. BMJ 2009;339:2538–42.

Rogers G, Garside R, Mealing S, *et al.* Carmustine implants for the treatment of newly diagnosed high grade gliomas. Pharmacoeconomics 2008;26:33–44.

Chapter 26

Poisoning and drug overdose

Clinical scenario

A 25-year-old man has been found unconscious by his friend with a suicide note in his hand. A paramedic stabilises the patient at the scene and the patient arrives in the Emergency Department with empty packets of paracetamol, paroxetine and quinine sulphate. The patient is known to have a history of depression and has been drinking heavily. How should this patient be managed?

Key points

- Most overdoses are due to impulsive actions, often in the context of alcohol ingestion, and do not result in long term sequalae
- Management of acute toxicity depends on providing general supportive measures to the patient and taking a good history (often from a bystander when the patient is unconscious), performing an appropriate physical examination and doing investigations that will determine what specific interventions are required
- If the causative agent(s) are identified information should be sought on how to manage it (them) in overdose. In the UK this information is readily available to all health care providers and Emergency Departments from the National Poisons Information Service (NPIS) via TOXBASE (http://www.toxbase.com)

Lecture Notes: Clinical Pharmacology and Therapeutics, 8th edition. By Gerard McKay, John Reid and Matthew Walters. Published 2010 by Blackwell Publishing Ltd.

Introduction

Paracelsus (1493–1541) is widely held as the father of clinical toxicology, and he observed that 'all things are poison and nothing is without poison, only the dose permits something not to be poisonous'. That is to say that all substances have the potential to cause toxic effects in people, even if they are harmless or perhaps beneficial in smaller doses. Poisoning may be considered to occur in one of five different types of exposure:

1 Intentional self-poisoning (e.g. deliberate drug overdose)

2 Accidental ingestion (e.g. drug prescription or administration error)

3 Occupational (e.g. contact with chemicals used at work)

4 Environmental (e.g. chemicals in air or water supply)

5 Covert (e.g. deliberate poisoning by third party). Intentional self-poisoning is the commonest pattern that gives rise to contact with healthcare staff, and is a manifestation of self-harm behaviour. Patients that present to hospital due to deliberate overdose often do so because of transient mood disturbance and situational stressors, and it often the only overdose presentation in a patient's lifetime. A small but significant proportion of patients have an underlying psychiatric illness or personality disorder, and the risk of further overdose episodes and suicide is much higher.

Approximately 10% of all acute hospital admissions in the UK are due to acute poisoning. The type of agent depends on what is readily accessible to the patient, and differs between countries. For example, pharmaceuticals (e.g. paracetamol) are the commonest means of self-poisoning in Westernised nations, whereas poisoning in the developing world is principally due to pesticides and other chemicals. The occurrence of exotic envenomations depends on toxicity of indigenous species and the likelihood of exposure. For example, snakebite envenomations are more common in Australasia than in the United Kingdom, and these are more likely to occur in a rural setting.

The circumstances of poisoning vary considerably with the patient's age. Poisoning in young children is normally due to accidental ingestion, for example toddlers who might inadvertently put tablets or household cleaners in their mouth. Whereas beyond age 10 years, deliberate overdose begins to emerge as the commonest pattern of poisoning, and is the predominant pattern in teenagers and young adults. Very rarely poisoning in children may be a feature of the Munchausen's Syndrome by Proxy involving a parent or guardian. Accidental poisoning may also occur in older adults due to cognitive decline and the use of increasingly complex medication patterns.

General approach to the poisoned patient

Management of patients requires detailed history, physical examination, and appropriate investigations. The route and extent of exposure should be ascertained. Studies show that there is correspondence between the type of agent the patient claims to have ingested and what is detected by laboratory investigations. Also, there is a reasonable correspondence between the stated dose ingested and measured serum concentrations, but individual patients may overestimate or underestimate the extent of exposure. Evidence of drug exposure should be sought from bystander accounts, and drug packaging should be examined if available. In certain cases it is not possible to ascertain the agent ingested, e.g. if the patient is unconscious.

Table 26.1 Ten commonest drugs associated with NPIS enquiries via TOXBASE® (April 2007 to March 2008 inclusive).

1.	Paracetamol	95,316
2.	Ibuprofen	40,197
3.	Salicylates	25,933
4.	Codeine	25,279
5.	Diazepam	16,512
6.	Citalopram	15,317
7.	Zopiclone	13,237
8.	Tramadol	13,087
9.	Fluoxetine	12,575
10.	Amitriptyline	9220

In such situations it is helpful to be aware of agents commonly ingested in self-poisoning. For example, the top 10 drugs ingested by patients that resulted in contact with the National Poisons Information Service (NPIS) in the UK from April 2007 to March 2008 are shown in Table 26.1.

In complex overdoses, where patients have ingested large quantities, multiple agents or highly unusual or toxic agents, then specialist advice should be sought. In the United Kingdom the NPIS provides advice on management of poisoning via TOXBASE, which can be found at http://www.toxbase.u5e.com. TOXBASE is provided free to healthcare professionals in the United Kingdom and is available in emergency departments. If further details on clinical management are required then enquirers can contact the NPIS via a 24-hour telephone information line is available on 0844 8920111 to discuss the case with a Specialist in Poisons Information or consultant clinical toxicologist (Table 26.2).

Many poisoning cases require only general supportive care, whilst certain patients may require specific antidote treatment and more intensive

Table 26.2 Poisons information services.

UK National database TOXBASE:
http://www.toxbase.org

UK National telephone number for more complex enquiries: 0844 892 0111

Table 26.3 Examples of symptoms associated with specific toxins.

Agitation	Anticholinergics, amphetamine, cocaine, ethanol, solvents, tricyclic antidepressants
Coma	Barbiturates, benzodiazepines, ethanol, ethylene glycol, gamma hydroxy butyrate (GBH), methanol, opiates, solvents, tricyclic antidepressants
Seizures	Amphetamine, cocaine, ecstasy, organophosphates, phenothiazines, theophylline, tricyclic antidepressants
Constricted pupils	Organophosphates, opiates, GBH
Dilated pupils	Anticholinergics, cocaine, phenothiazines, quinine, sympathomimetics, tricyclic antidepressants
Cardiac arrythmias	Anti-arrhythmics, anticholinergics, phenothiazines, quinine, sympathomimetics, tricyclic antidepressants
Pulmonary oedema	Aspirin, ethylene glycol, irritant gases, opiates, organophosphates, tricyclic antidepressants
Metabolic acidosis	Aspirin, ethanol, ethylene glycol, methanol
Hyperthermia	Anticholinergics, cocaine, ecstasy and monoamine oxidase inhibitors
Hepatic failure	Paracetamol, organic sovents, toxic mushrooms
Renal failure not related to hypotension or rhabdomyolysis	Ethylene glycol, lithium, methanol, NSAIDs, paracetamol

support. Patients that present due to intentional self-harm should receive formal psychiatric or psychological assessment to identify appropriate interventions for minimising the risk of further self-harm behaviour.

Assessment and diagnosis

Airway – ensure airway is clear and protected

Breathing – ensure ventilation is adequate

Circulation – measure pulse, blood pressure and look for signs of shock

Disability – assess level of consciousness

Exposure – look at patient for clues as to agent and route of exposure, e.g. needle track marks, transdermal patches

Appropriate resuscitation procedures may be required to be commenced before full details of the ingestion are known.

Co-morbidities, particularly cardiovascular or respiratory disease should be noted as these may affect the patient's response to both the agent or antidote treatment (e.g. greater risk of anaphylactoid reaction to acetylcysteine in patients with asthma). Accidental ingestion of small quantities of a single agent often do not require admission to hospital, whereas intentional self-harm or ingestion of large quantities or multiple agents normally require a longer period of medical and psychiatric inpatient assessment.

A number of clinical 'toxidromes' exist, which are a discrete collection of signs that indicate a specific drug effect or mechanism (Table 26.3). Conscious level is often impaired in poisoning with sedating agents, e.g. benzodiazepines and opiates. The AVPU scale may be a more appropriate measure of conscious level in poisoned patients than the more widely applied Glasgow Coma Scale (Table 26.4). The AVPU scale has the advantage

Table 26.4 The AVPU scale.

A	**A**wake
V	Responds to **V**erbal commands
P	Responds to **P**ainful stimuli
U	**U**nresponse to stimuli

Note: the more detailed Glasgow coma scale may be used in accident departments and intensive care.

of rapid application, and can identify patients at risk of respiratory obstruction that require careful monitoring and transfer to a more intensive care setting: P level (responsive only to a painful stimulus).

There is some overlap in mechanisms of adverse drug reactions and poisoning, and a good understanding of pharmacology assists in determining the likely pattern of toxicity. The onset of toxicity may vary substantially between agents depending on the route of exposure and mode of toxicity. For example, parenteral administration of opiates is likely to evoke a response within several minutes after administration whereas peak opiate toxicity may take up to 2–4 hours after oral ingestion. The toxic effects of certain agents may be delayed for many hours after exposure; for example, lithium may cause toxicity 24 hours after peak concentrations due to distribution from the circulation into tissues, and paracetamol toxicity is due to formation of a metabolite so that liver injury is often delayed by at least 24 hours after ingestion. Exposure may involve different exposure routes such as the respiratory tract (e.g. glue sniffing) or skin (e.g. paraquat, hydrofluoric acid). A careful history and clinical examination may be more valuable and certainly more readily accessible than laboratory analyses.

Examination should include not only the normal physical signs, but also the assessment of airway (burns, mouth blisters, or odour due to ethanol or volatile solvents) and the skin for needle marks or burns. In patients who have been found unconscious should be examined for pressure injury, including blistering (a non-specific marker of skin pressure injury) and rhabdomyolysis. Rarely, a compartment syndrome may occur and this requires urgent surgical decompression.

Toxicological analyses

Toxicological analyses are rarely employed in clinical practice because they often involve complex techniques that are not readily available, and there is often a poor correlation between toxicity and a drug concentration determined at a single time point. There are a number of exceptions where measurement of drug concentrations can be useful in clinical practice, e.g. paracetamol concentrations indicating a need for acetylcysteine antidote, digoxin concentrations indicating a need for Digibind® antibody fragments. The ingested agent can normally be determined from the patient history, or ascertained from bystander accounts or empty drug packaging, and the clinical features or toxidrome might indicate the specific agent. Biochemical tests may also be helpful in providing clues to likely ingested compounds, for example the presence of acid-base imbalance or altered serum potassium concentrations (Fig. 26.1). A 12-lead ECG may also be helpful for determining the agent ingested, for example prolonged QRS duration after tricyclic antidepressants, or the presence of QT prolongation indicating ingestion of selective serotonin reuptake inhibitors (SSRIs), antihistamines, and certain other psychotropic agents. The presence of QRS prolongation can indicate an increased risk of seizure and arrhythmia after tricyclic antidepressant ingestion, and indicates a need for close monitoring and consideration of sodium bicarbonate administration.

Immediate management

The term 'gastrointestinal decontamination' is used to describe methods that minimise the quantities of drug available for absorption from the gut. A variety of decontamination techniques have been described and recommendations for and against these are outlined in international position papers.

Oral activated charcoal is capable of adsorbing drugs and other substances in a non-specific manner; it is capable of adsorbing around one tenth of its own weight. It is normally administered as a suspension at a dose of 50 g to adults or 1 g/kg in children (this might be expected to adsorb up to 5 g of drug or chemical in an adult). It requires physical contact with the ingested compound to be effective, and should be given within 1 hour of ingestion (some experts consider administration up to 2 hours appropriate in patients that have ingested drugs that delay gastric motility, such as anticholinergics or opiates). It is important

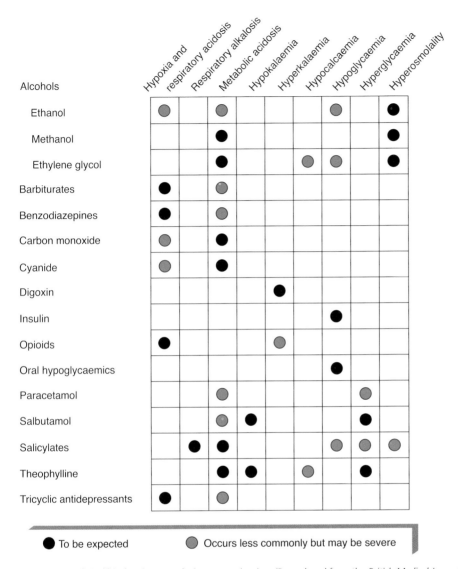

Figure 26.1 Clinical biochemistry: results in acute poisoning. (Reproduced from the *British Medical Journal*).

that the airway can be protected in view of the risk of charcoal aspiration; vomiting or suspicion of gastrointestinal obstructions are contraindications to the use of oral activated charcoal.

Induced vomiting (emesis) does not reduce drug absorption or reduce the risk of toxicity, but may be associated with potential hazards and is *not recommended* for use in poisoned patients.

Gastric lavage is associated with specific hazards, namely hypoxia, 'wash on' effect whereby there may be a paradoxical increase in the rate of drug absorption and increased toxicity, oesophageal perforation, and aspiration pneumonia. Therefore, gastric lavage is reserved only for patients that present within 1 hour of a potentially life-threatening overdose. In practice, it is rarely employed because most patients do not ingest life-threatening quantities of poison or present too late for lavage to be effective. Gastric aspiration (as opposed to lavage) should be considered

Table 26.5 Agents not adsorbed by charcoal.

Acids	Iron salts
Alcohols, e.g. ethanol, methanol	Glycols, e.g. ethylene glycol
Cyanide	Lead, mercury and other heavy metals
Lithium salts	Organic solvents

- Theophylline
Hyperkalaemia
- Ace inhibitor
- Digoxin
Hypoglycaemia
- Ethanol
- Insulin
- Salicylates
- Sulphonylureas
- Agents that cause hepatic failure (paracetamol, iron)

in patients that have ingested potentially life-threatening doses of drugs not adsorbed by oral activated charcoal, for example lithium and iron (Table 26.5).

Whole bowel irrigation may be considered for ingestions involving slow-release formulations or in drug users whole have swallowed drugs in a container or wrapping. The efficacy is uncertain.

Interpretation of investigations in poisoning of unknown cause

Blood gases
Metabolic acidosis [low pH/high H^+ with low CO_2]
Carbon monoxide
- Ecstasy
- Iron salts
- Methanol
- Paraldehyde
- Theophylline
- Cyanide
- Ethylene glycol
- Metformin
- Paracetamol
- Salicylates
- Tricyclic antidepressants
Respiratory acidosis [low pH/high H^+ with high CO_2]
- Barbiturates
- Benzodiazepines
- Opiates
- Tricyclic antidepressants
Respiratory alkalosis [high pH/low H^+ with low CO_2]
- Ecstasy
- Salicylates
- Theophylline
Hypokalaemia
- β-Agonists (e.g. salbutamol)
- Diuretics
- Insulin
- Sulphonylureas

For most ingested drugs onset of clinical features is likely to occur within 4–6 hours after ingestion, and the duration of effects will depend on the specific agent ingested. In management of poisoning, the administration of additional drugs should be avoided where possible, although specific antidotes are an exception (see later). The effect of co-prescribed medications might provoke unexpected adverse effects in poisoned patients, and may interfere with monitoring of the patient's clinical state. For example, tachycardia may be used as a marker of the extent of anticholinergic effects of tricyclic toxicity and would be masked by administration of a beta-blocker. Most patients require only supportive nursing care to allow complete recovery.

The management of specific complications

Seizures – diazepam or lorazepam (these are normally administered by IV or PR routes).

Agitation – diazepam or lorazepam, if severe consider haloperidol.

Alcohol withdrawal – although not a direct manifestation of poisoning, chronic excess ethanol consumption is common in overdose patients. In addition to controlling agitation, regular diazepam administration should be considered to prevent withdrawal seizures. Intravenous thiamine (Pabrinex®) should be considered to prevent Wernicke's encephalopathy.

Arrhythmias – correct acidosis with intravenous sodium bicarbonate to prevent tachyarrhythmia after tricyclic antidepressants. Administer magnesium in patients with drug-induced *torsades de pointes*. Note: anti-arrhythmic drugs may increase toxicity in some situations so always discuss with a senior colleague or consult TOXBASE before use.

Hypothermia – may be present in patients who have consumed vasodilators, including alcohol, and been unconscious for some time. Cautious warming should be employed, and support to prevent complications including rhabdomyolysis.

Hyperthermia – most frequently caused by drugs of abuse, particularly cocaine, amphetamine, and methylenedioxymethamphetamine (MDMA, ecstasy). Treatment of drug-induced hyperthermia requires administration of benzodiazepines (often large doses are needed), and active cooling in severe cases. Consider the possibility of co-existent infection, e.g. aspiration pneumonia in patients that have been vomiting. Malignant neuroleptic syndrome is rare in overdose.

Clinical features in poisoning (these may be complicated if more than one agent is ingested)

Tachycardia
- Anticholinergics
- Amphetamines
- β-Agonists (salbutamol)
- Cocaine
- Ecstasy
- Monoamine oxidase inhibitors
- Phenothiazines
- Theophylline
- Tricyclic antidepressants
- Sympathomimetic drugs

Bradycardia
- Beta-blockers
- Cyanide
- Digoxin
- Organophosphates

Hypertension
- Amphetamines/ecstasy
- Cocaine
- MAOIs

Hypotension
- Is common in severe poisoning from any cause, particularly with CNS depressants

---

Hypertonia and hyperreflexia
- Amphetamines
- Ecstasy
- Anticholinergics (may have upgoing plantars)
- Carbamazepine
- MAOIs
- Theophylline
- Tricyclic antidepressants (may have upgoing plantars and divergent squint)
- Carbon monoxide (may have upgoing plantars)

Hypotonia and hyporeflexia
- Alcohol
- Barbiturates
- Benzodiazepines
- Haloperidol
- Opiates
- Phenothiazines

Tachypnoea
- Amphetamines/ecstasy
- Cyanide
- Ethylene glycol
- Methanol
- Salicylates
- Theophylline

Dystonic reactions (e.g. oculogyric crisis) – these are particularly common in young adults (women more than men) and are due to central nervous system anti-dopaminergic effects of certain drugs (e.g. metoclopramide and antipsychotics). Acute dystonic reactions should be treated with diazepam or an intravenous anticholinergic.

Specific treatments

The stomach acts as a reservoir for ingested drugs, where they cause few toxicological effects (apart from corrosive agents). Clinical features occur only after absorption from the gut, and depend on the pharmacological characteristics of the specific agent. An important principle in managing a poisoned patient is that unnecessary interventions are avoided, namely those that might increase risk of toxicity or be ineffective. Unlike many areas of clinical practice, clinical toxicology suffers from a lack of robust trial data and, therefore, optimal advice on poisoning management is based on expert opinion, consensus statements and international position papers.

Toxicokinetics

Toxicokinetic characteristics (absorption, distribution, metabolism and excretion of drugs taken in overdose) are often similar to the pharmacokinetic properties seen after therapeutic doses, such that the onset and duration of effects and severity of toxicity may be predictable. However, in some situations the toxicokinetic properties differ significantly so that the effects after overdose are less predictable. For example, drug absorption may be delayed due to formation of concretions of tablets in the stomach (e.g. lithium) so that the peak effects and durations of action are prolonged compared to therapeutic doses. Certain drugs impair gastrointestinal motility such that drug absorption becomes erratic and prolonged (e.g. opiates and calcium channel blockers). Saturation of hepatic enzymes can render elimination pathways less effective for clearing large quantities of drug so that toxicity and duration of effects are greater than predicted from therapeutic doses. Drug development involves study of a range of drug dosages in people. However intentional drug overdose often involves substantially higher quantities than have been studied in clinical trials, and pharmacokinetic data from studies of therapeutic doses may not apply.

Enhanced drug elimination

Certain drugs depend on urinary excretion for elimination, and manipulation of urinary pH can alter the rate of excretion. For weakly acidic compounds, urinary alkalinisation causes drug ionisation which prevents tubular reabsorption, so that excretion is enhanced. For example, aspirin has a pKa close to physiological pH and thus ionisation is altered significantly by small changes in urinary pH. In practice it is often difficult to achieve adequate drug removal by urinary alkalisation alone, and other techniques are used to enhance elimination in severe cases of aspirin poisoning (e.g. haemodialysis).

Forced diuresis – has been attempted historically as a possible means of increasing drug elimination. However, this appears ineffective and confers the hazards of precipitating fluid overload or pulmonary edema and is no longer recommended.

Haemodialysis

For water-soluble compounds such as aspirin, ethanol, methanol, ethylene glycol and lithium, haemodialysis will effectively remove drug from the blood passing across the dialysate membrane. The rate of removal is crucially dependant upon the flow rate across this membrane, and the benefits of the treatment relate directly to the increase in clearance produced by haemodialysis. In practice only a very few drugs have their elimination effectively increased by haemodialysis. Drugs with a wide volume of distribution need prolonged haemodialysis or multiple treatments in order to adequately remove drug from tissues; short periods of treatment are followed by a rapid 'rebound' of circulating concentrations (e.g. lithium). Care should be taken to ensure that the most efficient form of dialysis is adopted, as systems designed for management of chronic haemodialysis patients such as veno–veno systems may be less effective in poisoned patients.

Haemoperfusion

Charcoal haemoperfusion is effective in removing compounds with relatively small volumes of distribution, such as theophylline, providing adequate clearances can be achieved across the charcoal column. For the vast majority of drugs, however, the modest increase in drug clearance is inadequate to warrant therapy. Patients require anticoagulation and there is significant risk of bleeding, particularly if there is behavioural disturbance and the patient might inadvertently disconnect their lines.

Physiological support systems

Occasionally cardiopulmonary resuscitation may involve direct cardiac pacing, use of aortic balloon pumps or very rarely use of heart–lung machines. Recent experimental studies suggest that albumin dialysis for the management of hepatic failure may have a role in the support of patients with established drug-induced intoxication, but for the present there is little evidence that they have a role in routine management in poisoned patients.

Features of common drug overdose

In clinical practice almost anything may be taken by a patient in emotional distress. The epidemiology of drug overdose changes with time and, at present in the United Kingdom the most common poisonings seen clinically are paracetamol, benzodiazepine and related sedatives, non-steroidal anti-inflammatories, antidepressants and antipsychotics, opioid and drugs of abuse. An outline understanding of these drugs is important, and in addition it is useful to understand clinical implications of the mechanisms of effect of a few rare poisons. A list of some antidotes that may be advised in clinical practice is shown in Table 26.6. When managing any case of poisoning it is sensible to consult TOXBASE and print off an appropriate factsheet from that database to act as an *aide-memoire* in the management of the patient during their in hospital stay.

Antidepressant drugs

Tricyclic antidepressants

These drugs inhibit the uptake of monoamines into central neurones, but also have anticholinergic (antimuscarinic), sodium channel blocking and α-adrenoceptor antagonist effects. Clinical features are due to a combination of these effects. Anticholinergic effects predominate early (dry mouth, dilated pupils, tachycardia, drowsiness and urinary retention). More severe poisoning is associated with reduced conscious level, and in these patients a prolonged QRS complex (due to sodium channel blockade) may indicate an increased risk of ventricular arrhythmias and seizures.

Activated charcoal is indicated in patients that present within 1 hour. Routine 12-lead ECG should be performed to check QRS duration, and if the patient becomes obtunded, it should be repeated. Prophylactic use of intravenous sodium bicarbonate is advised in the management of arrhythmias, particularly if the QRS duration increases beyond 110 ms. Prolonged cardiac massage is appropriate in patients with severe tricyclic poisoning, and recovery has been reported after several hours of cardiac massage. In recovery agitation often occurs, typically 24–48 hours after ingestion; acute urinary retention should be considered, and agitation should be managed by benzodiazepine administration.

Specific serotonin reuptake inhibitors

Specific serotonin reuptake inhibitors (SSRIs) are more specific than tricyclics in that they block the uptake of serotonin only. In overdose they may cause a serotonin syndrome, particularly if co-ingested with other antidepressants or drugs with serotonergic effects, e.g. ecstasy, tramadol. Features include nausea, vomiting, diarrhoea, agitation, myoclonic jerks, hyperreflexia, hyperthermia, rhabdomyolysis and in severe cases renal failure. Serotonin syndrome can be managed by using serotonin antagonists (e.g. cyproheptadine) or centrally-acting sedatives, e.g. benzodiazepines.

Other antidepressants

Venlafaxine is more closely aligned to tricyclic antidepressants, acting on reuptake of noradrenaline. It is significantly more toxic in overdose than SSRIs, and is associated with a substantially higher rate of seizures, arrhythmia, rhabdomyolysis, and prolonged hospital stay. Mirtazapine, a centrally acting pre-synaptic α2-receptor antagonist, causes drowsiness in overdose, particularly in combination with other sedative agents but is otherwise benign.

MAOIs

Monoamine oxidase inhibitors are particularly toxic in overdose and cause severe cardiovascular instability with hypertension and tachycardia. Features similar to serotonin syndrome may also develop and, in severe cases, intractable seizures.

Table 26.6 List of antidotes and their mechanism of action.

Poisons	Antidotes	Mechanism of action
Anticoagulants (Warfarin type)	Vitamin K (phytomenadione)	Cofactor for synthesis of clotting factors
β-Adrenergic blockers	Isoprenaline	Competitive agonist at β-receptor
	Glucagon	Stimulates myocardial adenyl cyclase
Carbon monoxide	Oxygen (normo or hyperbaric)	Competitive displacement of carbon monoxide from haemoglobin molecule
Cyanide	Dicobalt edetate	Chelating agent
	Sodium nitrate	Forms methaemoglobin that combines with cyanide
	Sodium thiosulphate	Accelerates detoxification of cyanide by action with rhodanase
	Hydroxocobalamin	Combines with cyanide to form cyanocobalamin
Digoxin and digitoxin	Fab antidote fragments	Antidote forms an inert complex with poison
Ethylene glycol or methanol	Ethanol	Competitive substrate for alcohol dehydrogenase, slows toxic metabolite production
	Fomepizole	Inhibitor of alcohol dehydrogenase
Benzodiazepines	Flumazenil	Competitive antagonist at benzodiazepine receptors
Heavy metals (lead, mercury, arsenic)	DMSA (2,3-dimercaptosuccinic acid)	Chelating agent
	DMPS (2,3-dimercaptopropane-1-sulphonate)	Chelating agent
	Sodium calcium edetate	Chelating agent
	Dimercaprol	Chelating agent
Hydrofluoric acid	Calcium gluconate	Forms an inert complex (calcium fluoride)
Iron salts	Desferrioxamine	Chelating agent
Narcotics (dextropropoxyphene, heroin, co-proxamol, etc.)	Naloxone	Competitive antagonist at opioid receptors
Organophosphates	Atropine	Competitive antagonist at acetylcholine receptor
	Pralidoxime	Cholinesterase reactivator
Paracetamol	Acetylcysteine	Accelerate detoxification of potentially toxic metabolite (glutathione precursor and SH donor)
Thallium	Berlin Blue	Chelating agent

Patients who have ingested significant quantities of MAOIs require specialist treatment in intensive or high dependency units.

Sedatives and benzodiazepine related compounds

Benzodiazepines, e.g. diazepam, and related drugs, such as zopiclone and zolpidem, cause drowsiness, hyporeflexia, respiratory depression and hypotension. If taken alone they are relatively safe, and patients should be treated by supportive nursing care. Dangers arise when patients vomit and are unable to protect the airway due to excessive sedation. This is a particular hazard in patients with pre-existing chronic obstructive airways disease and those that co-ingest other sedative agents, e.g. opiates.

Treatment is primarily symptomatic and supportive. Although flumazenil is a specific benzodiazepine antagonist, it should not be used as a diagnostic test or in cases of mixed overdose. In patients who are benzodiazepine-dependent it may cause seizures, and in mixed overdose involving proconvulsive agents (e.g. tricyclic antidepressants, venlafaxine, amphetamines) flumazenil may precipitate seizures making management of patients more complex. The half-life of flumazenil is shorter than most benzodiazepines.

Opioids

A wide range of drugs have opioid agonist properties, including morphine, diamorphine (heroin), pethidine, codeine, dihydrocodeine, dextropropoxyphene, buprenorphine and methadone. Features of opioid poisoning classically include drowsiness, coma and respiratory depression with pinpoint pupils. Nausea and vomiting are common particularly in opioid naïve patients. The time course of opioid poisoning depends primarily on the route of exposure. Intravenous injection and inhalation from smoking ('chasing the dragon') cause rapid clinical effects, whereas absorption from the GI tract is slower. Dextropropoxyphene (a constituent of co-proxamol) also has sodium channel blocking properties, causing cardiac arrhythmias and for this reason co-proxamol has been withdrawn in the United Kingdom. Dihydrocodeine and codeine are converted to active metabolites (dihydromorphine and morphine) and morphine itself has an active metabolite, morphine 6-glucoronide, which accumulates in renal impairment. Onset of toxicity of methadone is much slower than other agents in this category and is maximal 4–6 hours after ingestion. Tramadol is an analgesic with effects on both opioid receptors and 5HT receptors. In addition to causing the classical features of opioid poisoning it also causes seizures.

Management

The specific treatment for opioid poisoning is naloxone, a competitive antagonist. In cases with presumed opioid ingestion naloxone is titrated in doses of up to 2.4–4.8 mg (6–12 ampoules) in severe cases to match clinical response. The target is to maintain adequate respiration, rather than cause full reversal because this may provoke an acute withdrawal syndrome in addicts. The duration of action of naloxone is short, 45–90 minutes, and in patients with severe poisoning, or following ingestion of slow-release or long-acting opioids such as methadone, a naloxone infusion may be required.

Non-steroidal anti-inflammatory agents

Ibuprofen is widely available over the counter and is now frequently encountered in overdose. Non-steroidals as a class are of relatively low toxicity, with a primary toxicity being on the kidney (acute renal failure) and in patients with co-morbidity cause fluid retention. These effects are due to interaction with prostaglandin mechanisms, in the case of the kidney impairment of vascular tone affecting glomerular filtration. In severe overdose coma, seizures and hepatic damage has been reported. Mefenamic acid is a non-steroidal anti-inflammatory that is capable of provoking seizures in overdose; these should be managed conventionally with diazepam or lorazepam.

Salicylates

Aspirin is now rarely encountered as a serious overdose, and the toxicity is predictable from dose ingested, with doses of 250 mg/kg likely to lead to moderate toxicity and above 500 mg/kg severe toxicity. Clinical features include vomiting, tinnitus, deafness, sweating and hyperventilation due to direct stimulation of the respiratory centre. Respiratory alkalosis is an early features of aspirin toxicity, and progressive metabolic acidosis may also occur because at least in part because aspirin is an acidic compound. Subsequent metabolic complications include hyperpyrexia (uncoupling of oxidative phosphorylation and direct CNS effects), hypoglycaemia, thrombocytopaenia, coagulopathy and renal failure. Distribution of aspirin across the bilipid cell membranes is greatest in the unionised form, and therefore patients with acidosis are at greatest risk of CNS tissue penetration resulting in confusion, impaired consciousness, seizures and death. Consequences of salicylate poisoning are therefore dependent upon the ability to resist the metabolic acidosis, and this is particularly problematical in young children and the elderly. In severe cases (plasma concentration above 700 mg/L with metabolic complications) or in patients with renal failure, urgent haemodialysis is the treatment of choice.

Paracetamol

Paracetamol is the commonest means of overdose in Westernised nations and contributes to between 30 and 40% of acute hospital admissions due to overdose. Precise mortality figures are uncertain, but are below 0.1% for cases that reach hospital and receive appropriate treatment. Deaths attributed to paracetamol toxicity are often due to co-ingested agents, e.g. the dextropropoxyphene content of co-proxamol, which has now had its license removed in the United Kingdom.

After therapeutic doses paracetamol is metabolised in the liver to inactive conjugates. An intermediate metabolic step involves formation of *N*-acetyl benzoquinonimine (NAPQI) and this metabolite is then conjugated with glutathione. The conjugated form is inactive and non-toxic, but in the absence of adequate glutathione stores, or when the conjugation step is overwhelmed by massive paracetamol quantities, then the reactive metabolite is capable of binding to sulphydryl moieties and causing hepatic necrosis. Patients with increased susceptibility to paracetamol toxicity (so-called 'high risk' patients) are therefore those with inadequate glutathione stores such as the malnourished, patients with eating disorders and malabsorption syndromes, possibly HIV positive patients and alcoholics. Patients with hepatic enzyme induction may also be at increased risk due to rapid NAPQI formation, for example patients receiving carbamazepine, phenytoin, barbiturates, rifampicin or St John's wort.

Patients often expect paracetamol to cause symptoms, especially drowsiness early after ingestion, but this is unlikely in the absence of co-ingested drugs. Hepatic necrosis usually presents 36–72 hours after overdose with jaundice and right upper quadrant pain, and may be followed by the onset of renal failure. Note: in rare cases renal failure can occur without major hepatic impairment.

Management

Management of paracetamol poisoning depends on the time elapsed from overdose to presentation. The risk is determined from the paracetamol treatment nomogram published in the British National Formulary (BNF) and available on TOXBASE (Fig. 26.2). An urgent paracetamol concentration should be measured at 4 hours after ingestion, or as close to 4 hours as possible (concentrations taken before 4 hours are not interpretable). If the paracetamol results can be obtained within 8 hours after ingestion, then these should be used to determine the need for treatment based on the graph. Therefore, it is important to make sure paracetamol levels are done urgently, and that the results are acted upon. At 8 hours or more after ingestion the risks of hepatic injury are increasing and acetylcysteine treatment should be administered if the patient has taken a significant quantity, i.e. >12 g or

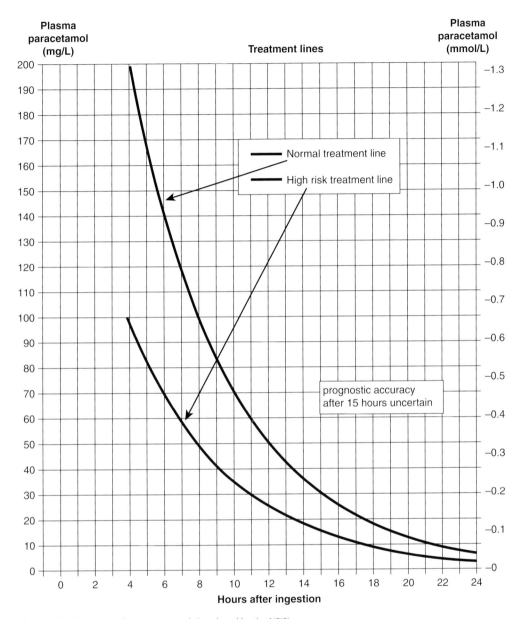

Figure 26.2 Paracetamol treatment graph (produced by the NPIS).

>150 mg/kg, whichever is less (a lower treatment threshold should be considered in high-risk patients). If acetylcysteine is commenced before paracetamol concentration is available, then treatment can be stopped if the level is subsequently found to be below the appropriate treatment line.

Beyond 20 hours evidence of efficacy in preventing liver damage is absent, and by this stage hepatic necrosis is usually well established. Use of antidotes late in the management of paracetamol poisoning may be indicated if liver function tests are abnormal, but here the treatment is to prevent hepatic encephalopathy, not liver damage itself.

Treatment

The recommended treatment of paracetamol poisoning in the United Kingdom is intravenous *N*-acetylcysteine. The dose is given in an initial loading dose, followed by two subsequent lower infusions over a period in total of 20 hours. Methionine is no longer generally recommended. Where intravenous access is impossible, then oral acetylcysteine can be considered. *N*-acetylcysteine is thought to prevent hepatic injury by replenishing glutathione that is required for detoxification of the metabolic intermediate NAPQI. *N*-acetylcysteine causes a pseudo allergic reaction (so-called anaphylactoid reaction) in around 10–20% of treated patients. Treatment should be *temporarily* discontinued, and an antihistamine or bronchodilator given if needed. Acetylcysteine can normally be safely re-introduced without provoking a further reaction. Note: the reaction is associated with histamine release but is not mediated by immunoglobulin E as in true anaphylaxis.

Assessing severity of hepatic damage

At presentation risk of hepatic damage can be predicted from the paracetamol level, although the degree of metabolic acidosis also correlates with severity of overdose. It is important to check the response to treatment, and three blood tests are necessary. Firstly, a measure of the transaminase in order to assess if liver damage has occurred (either aspartate transaminase or alanine transaminase). Secondly, prothrombin time is used as a marker of liver synthetic function and is a strong predictor of outcome. Prothrombin time that is longer in seconds (measured using Manchester reagent) than the number of hours since the overdose indicates a poor prognosis. Clotting disturbance in paracetamol poisoning should never be corrected by vitamin K or clotting factors without discussion with a specialist liver unit, as this measure is a sensitive outcome guide. Thirdly, serum creatinine should

be checked as a possible marker of paracetamol-induced renal toxicity. Changes in renal function are slower to develop than hepatic injury, and if serum creatinine increases after acetylcysteine treatment (even if only slightly) then this should be rechecked to exclude renal failure. In severe hepatic failure liver support systems, or transplantation may be indicated. Patients being considered for such treatment should be seen by a psychiatrist before they develop a hepatic coma in order that an assessment can be made.

Drugs of abuse

Common drugs of abuse include opioids (see above) and stimulants including in particular MDMA, cocaine and amphetamines. All these drugs act on central amine receptor systems to cause excitation, with the risk of tachycardia, blood pressure change and seizures. MDMA causes a syndrome similar to the serotonin syndrome (see section on SSRIs) but also stimulates antidiuretic hormone release, causing water retention. In patients who drink excess water (e.g. at raves) significant hyponatraemia may occur resulting in seizures and brain damage. Treatment is supportive with control of hyperthermia using benzodiazepines. Specific 5HT antagonists such as cyproheptadine may be considered.

Amphetamines cause seizures and cardiac arrhythmias. Management is supportive using benzodiazepines to reduce central stimulation and sympathetic outflow.

Cocaine has local anaesthetic (sodium channel blocking) activities, as well as direct and indirect amine effects. It is absorbed rapidly across the buccal and nasal mucosa causing a rapid 'high'. It causes surges in blood pressure with vasoconstriction and may result in stroke, acute myocardial infarction and gut infarcts. It also causes hyperpyrexia and seizures. Management is by use of large doses of benzodiazepines to sedate, combined in hyperpyrexia with ice baths. Myocardial infarction should be managed conventionally. Regular cocaine users are at risk of premature ischaemic heart disease due to accelerated atherosclerosis.

Other substances

Digoxin

Digoxin poisoning is uncommon, the features are vomiting and cardiac conduction abnormalities. Severe arrhythmias may require active treatment with a specific Fab antibody. As digoxin blocks sodium–potassium channels hyperkalaemia is a normal feature of severe digoxin intoxication. When taken in acute overdose the onset of digoxin poisoning may be delayed up to 12 hours. The typical features of severe poisoning include complete heart block.

Lithium

Lithium is used in the management of bipolar depression. It is excreted by the kidney and there are well-recognised interactions with NSAID's, diuretics and ACE inhibitors causing lithium retention. Presentation in chronic poisoning, in patients who develop renal impairment secondary to lithium, a recognised adverse effect of this therapy, present insidiously with confusion, nausea, vomiting, tremor, nystagmus and ataxia. As coma progresses irreversible damage to the brain occurs. In patients on lithium therapy it is therefore mandatory to monitor lithium levels regularly and avoid interacting drugs. The correlation between serum lithium concentrations and clinical outcome is generally poor, and clinical features are an important indicator of poisoning severity. Chronic lithium accumulation and acute-on-therapeutic toxicity are associated with greatest severity, and a comparatively modest increase in serum concentrations can indicate a risk of significant toxicity. In contrast, acute lithium overdose in a naïve patient may be associated with less toxicity even with high serum concentrations because these fall rapidly as lithium distributes throughout the extracellular compartment. Lithium is excreted via the kidney, and in patients with CNS features the treatment of choice is dialysis, which may be prolonged.

Iron

Iron produces toxicity as a metabolic poison, but also causes acute gastritis. It is also present with vomiting and haematemesis. Clinical features of iron poisoning reflect the onset of metabolic poisoning, particularly on mitochondrial systems, which result in metabolic acidosis, coma and death. Iron poisoning tends to come on in phases, initially presenting with vomiting, haematemesis, GI upset, drowsiness, metabolic acidosis, acute hypotension, coma and seizures. This phase lasts between 30 minutes and 6 hours. This is often followed by a short interval in which symptoms may appear to improve, but as the onset of the metabolic complications develop over 12–24 hours the patient becomes more unwell and hepatic failure with metabolic acidosis, hypoglycaemia and cardiovascular collapse, renal failure and pulmonary oedema. If patients survive this, small bowel and upper GI strictures may form in phase IV.

Assessment of iron poisoning is difficult and is based on a mixture of the clinical features seen, specifically degree of acidosis and hepatic and renal function, and the iron levels. These will often rise rapidly and then fall in the early phases of poisoning, and on their own may be only a partial index of the wider clinical prognosis. X-ray of patients who have ingested iron has been recommended, but is of doubtful benefit. The specific chelating agent desferrioxamine will bind iron, and will increase urinary excretion. In the context of severe iron poisoning large doses of desferrioxamine may be administered, and should be discussed with the NPIS.

Lead

Lead toxicity occurs from occupational exposure in industry, and occasionally environmentally, particularly in houses with lead paints. Some children develop the syndrome of pica in which they eat material containing lead. Lead causes multisystem toxicity and interacts with cations such as calcium, zinc and iron. Clinical features are only partially related to plasma concentrations following acute exposure, since lead distributes well into tissues, and assessment will therefore depend both on lead concentration and on clinical features. In young children there is some evidence that high lead levels are associated with impaired intellectual development, and in some countries screening programmes for lead concentrations are undertaken in the community. Features of chronic lead poisoning include GI disturbance, peripheral neuropathy, anaemia and wrist and ankle drop. Encephalopathy may be seen. Investigations include blood lead levels, x-rays if there is a suspicion of lead ingestion may be important. Blood films show a classical basophilic stippling and iron and calcium studies may be relevant. Chelating agents are available including DMSA, but prevention of exposure is the primary treatment of lead poisoning.

Antiepileptic agents

A number of different antiepileptic agents are used as mood stabilising agents in patients with psychiatric illness. The effects will vary between agents, but paradoxically all are thought capable of provoking seizures in overdose. Overdose involving either carbamazepine or phenytoin can be associated with significant cerebellar toxicity, and patients will have reduced conscious level, ataxia and slurred speech (understandably, such patients are often assumed to have acute ethanol intoxication). They may have significant bruising affecting the limbs and trunk and, in severe cases coma may necessitate temporary ventilatory support. Elimination of carbamazepine is enhanced by multiple dose activated charcoal (MDAC).

Sodium valproate may be associated with significant liver impairment and metabolic disturbance.

Mushrooms

A number of toxic mushrooms are present in the environment; mushrooms in the amanita family cause hepatic necrosis. There are no specific treatments for these. 'Magic mushrooms' (psylocybe) cause acute psychosis and agitation, but no long-lasting effects.

Chapter 27

Drugs you may need in a hurry

Most drugs are not given in a hurry. There is time to check facts or seek further advice. However, sometimes events move very quickly and there are some drugs, used under these circumstances, for which it is very useful to have facts and figures at your fingertips.

The purpose of this brief chapter is to provide that information for drugs used in circumstances that a newly qualified doctor might expect to encounter.

Adrenaline (epinephrine) for anaphylaxis

Why give it?

Most deaths from anaphylaxis occur in the first hour and most of these are a consequence of severe bronchospasm, increased capillary permeability or circulatory failure caused by vasodilatation. Adrenaline is given to prevent death from these causes, particularly by raising blood pressure and reversing bronchospasm.

Mechanism

Adrenaline is a potent agonist at both α- and β-adrenoceptors. It reduces bronchospasm by β_2-mediated airway smooth muscle relaxation, raises blood pressure by α_1-mediated vasoconstriction and may also reduce the release of inflammatory mediators by a β_2-mediated increase in mast cell cyclic AMP.

How to give it

Intramuscular injection – adrenaline acts quickly by this route, provided the circulation is adequate.

The adult dose is 500 μg – 0.5 mL of the 1:1000 preparation.

If there is severe shock and a serious question over absorption from muscle, adrenaline can be given intravenously – slowly, at the rate of 100 μg/minute per minute for 5 minutes or until a response is obtained, using ECG monitoring if possible. 5 mL of the 1:10,000 preparation is used.

Pitfalls

- Confusing the 1:1000 and 1:10,000 preparations.
- Ventricular arrhythmias (particularly in people taking tricyclic antidepressants.
- Adrenaline may not be effective in relieving bronchospasm in people taking non-selective

Lecture Notes: Clinical Pharmacology and Therapeutics, 8th edition. By Gerard McKay, John Reid and Matthew Walters. Published 2010 by Blackwell Publishing Ltd.

β-blockers (intravenous salbutamol will be needed under these circumstances).

• Blood pressure may rise quite dramatically – and even cause cerebral haemorrhage – in people on non-selective β-blockers because of unopposed α_1-mediated vasoconstriction.

Chlorphenamine for anaphylaxis

Why give it?

To counteract the histamine-mediated components of anaphylaxis and to help prevent a relapse.

Mechanism

Many substances are released during an anaphylactic reaction, but histamine is probably the main cause of increased capillary permeability, where histamine H_1 receptors play a significant role. Chlorphenamine is a potent H_1 receptor antagonist and is very effective at limiting the increased capillary permeability. Interestingly, it has little influence on the vascular and respiratory aspects of anaphylaxis, for which adrenaline (epinephrine) must be given.

How to give it

After adrenaline has been given and begun to work, chlorphenamine is given by intravenous injection of 10–20 mg over a minute. This drug is continued for 24–48 hours.

Pitfalls

Usually none under these circumstances, but hypotension or cerebral stimulation can occur.

Steroids also have a role in the management of anyphylactoid reactions (Chapter 17); however, their effects take hours rather than minutes to manifest themselves hence in emergency situations the delivery of adrenaline and chlorpheniramine should be prioritised.

Adrenaline (epinephrine) for cardiac arrest

Why give it?

To start the heart.

Mechanism

Adrenaline is a potent agonist at the β_1 receptor and is therefore a powerful cardiac stimulant, with effects on myocardial contractility and rate.

How to give it

100 μg intravenously – as 10 mL of 1:10,000 preparation. Preferably through a central line, or if through a peripheral line flushed with 20 mL of 0.9% sodium chloride to ensure entry to the circulation.

Pitfalls

As above.

Amiodarone for cardiac arrest

Why give it?

Amiodarone is used in cardio-pulmonary resuscitation when ventricular fibrillation or pulseless ventricular tachycardia persists despite defibrillation.

Mechanism

Amiodarone is effective against most tachyarrhythmias (Chapter 4). It has a wide spectrum of pharmacological activity and the precise mechanism(s) of its action are not known.

How to give it

Intravenous – 300 mg from a pre-filled syringe or in a glucose solution.

Pitfalls

Usually none in this context, although anaphylaxis can occur.

Atropine for cardiac arrest

Why give it?

To block vagal activity in patients with asystole or severe bradycardia.

Mechanism

Atropine is a competitive antagonist of the action of acetylcholine at muscarinic M_2 receptors on the sinoatrial and atrioventricular nodes. It therefore increases heart rate and speeds AV conduction.

How to give it

A single intravenous dose of 3 mg (the drug is quite long acting, so repeat doses are not needed).

Pitfalls

Although many of the well-described effects of atropine can occur, there are usually no serious side effects in this context.

Adenosine for supraventricular tachycardia

Why give it?

To revert supraventricular tachycardias to sinus rhythm.

Mechanism

Stimulation of adenosine A_1 receptors in the sinoatrial and atrioventricular nodes leads to a transient slowing of sinus rate; reduced AV node conduction increased AV node refractoriness (Chapter 4).

How to give it

Rapid intravenous injection of 3 mg, followed at intervals of 1–2 minutes by 6 mg and 12 mg if necessary, with cardiac monitoring. Adenosine has a very short half-life of a few seconds. Patients usually feel some chest tightness and breathlessness.

Pitfalls

- Heart block.
- Avoid in asthmatics because adenosine can cause severe bronchospasm.
- Patients with heart transplants are very sensitive to adenosine because of denervation sensitivity.
- Patients taking dipyridamole (an adenosine re-uptake inhibitor) are very sensitive to adenosine and should be give a starting dose of 0.5–1 mg

Loop diuretic for acute left ventricular failure

Why give it?

Acute left ventricular failure (LVF) is terrifying for the patient, who is dying by drowning in their own fluid, and dramatic for the doctor. The purpose of giving a loop diuretic – usually furosemide or bumetanide – is to relieve symptoms of severe breathlessness and prevent death.

Mechanism

Loop diuretics act more quickly in acute LVF than would be expected from their diuretic actions alone (Chapter 4). There are probably two mechanisms at work.

Reduction of left ventricular filling pressure by increasing systemic venous capacitance. This vascular effect has been recognised for many years but is not fully understood.

Powerful diuresis by inhibition of the $Na^+ - K^+ - 2\ Cl^-$ symporter in the ascending limb of the loop of Henle.

How to give it

Intravenously – e.g. furosemide 40 mg followed if necessary by 40 mg every 15 minutes up to a maximum of 160 mg.

Pitfalls

Usually none at this dose. Tinnitus can occur following rapid injections of high doses, but rarely seen in this context. Always consider using IV nitrate with furosemide as it acts quicker.

Morphine for acute LVF

Why give it?

Morphine is given in acute LVF for two reasons. One is to relieve distress, but the other is because it has rapid and dramatically beneficial cardiovascular effects.

Mechanism

The cardiovascular actions of morphine have been recognised for many years but are still not fully understood. Morphine causes both arteriolar and venous dilatation which is partially reversed by histamine H_1-receptor antagonists, but fully reversed by naloxone, an opioid μ-receptor antagonist (Chapter 20).

How to give it

Intravenously – 2 mg per minute up to a maximum of 10 mg.

Pitfalls

- Nausea – give an antiemetic such as metoclopramide.
- Respiratory depression – reverse with naloxone.
- Not giving adequate IV nitrate and furosemide to treat the LVF in addition to treating the symptoms.

Lorazepam for status epilepticus

Why give it?

Lorazepam has two advantages over diazepam in this condition. One is that it has a longer duration of action (diazepam enters the brain quickly, but leaves quite quickly too because of redistribution to adipose tissue). The other is that diazepam is more likely to cause thrombophlebitis.

Mechanism

All benzodiazepines limit seizure activity by GABA-mediated inhibitory effects (Chapter 7).

How to give it

Intravenous – absorption from intramuscular injection is too slow. Adult dose is 4mg into a large vein – if resuscitation equipment not readily available, give initial dose of 2 mg.

Pitfalls

Respiratory arrest

Rectal diazepam for status epilepticus

Why give it?

The rectal formulation of diazepam is useful when intravenous access is not possible.

Mechanism

As for lorazepam.

How to give it

Normal adult dose is 500 μg/kg up to a maximum of 30 mg given as diazepam rectal solution (elderly 250 μg/kg up to a maximum of 15 mg).

Pitfalls

Rectal absorption can sometimes be unpredictable.

Naloxone for opioid poisoning

Why give it?

Opioid poisoning leads to respiratory depression, hypotension and can be fatal. Naloxone is given to reverse these effects.

Mechanism

Drugs such as heroin (diamorphine) cause respiratory depression by acting on the μ opioid receptor and a significant part of their cardiovascular effects are also mediated through this receptor. Naloxone is an antagonist at this receptor and has no agonist activity (Chapter 20).

How to give it

Intravenous – the adult dose is 0.4–2 mg, repeated at intervals of 2 minutes until a maximum of 10 mg has been reached. Naloxone acts very fast, and a reversal of respiratory depression and dilation of the pupils is normally seen in about a minute.

Pitfalls

- Naloxone acts for 1–4 hours, so repeated doses may be necessary following large opioid overdoses.
- Opioid addicts may experience withdrawal reactions.
- Naloxone only partially antagonises the respiratory depression caused by pentazocine (which acts mainly at the κ opioid receptor) and buprenor-

phine (which appears to bind particularly avidly to the μ receptor).

Glucagon for hypoglycaemic coma

Why give it?

Hypoglycaemic coma can be treated either by intravenous glucose or by intravenous or intramuscular glucagon. The latter approach can be very useful if venous access is difficult.

Mechanism

Glucagon increases plasma glucose by stimulating glycogenolysis and reducing glycogen synthesis.

How to give it

One milligram by intramuscular or intravenous injection.

Pitfalls

Glucagon causes the release of catecholamines from a phaeochromocytoma.

Chapter 28

Prescribing and its pitfalls

Most doctors will prescribe drugs on a daily basis. Approximately 640 million prescriptions are written in the United Kingdom annually, equivalent to 10 prescriptions per year for each member of the UK population. Although perceived as a routine and mundane component of the work of most clinicians, the process of good prescribing requires significant skill and care and should not be undertaken without due thought and consideration. Good prescribing involves the recommendation of the correct dose and formulation of an appropriate drug, accompanied by clear instruction regarding when, how and for how long it should be taken. A prescription should be written only when in possession of adequate clinical information about the patient and the symptoms, and ideally following solicitation of the patient's preferences and discussion of alternative treatment strategies. The need for thorough training in the skill of prescribing is highlighted by the high frequency with which drugs are prescribed at the wrong dose, through the wrong route or for the wrong condition. The likelihood of patient injury occurring as a result of a drug error has been estimated at approximately 3% per inpatient stay, an error rate that would not be tolerated by major airlines handling passengers' baggage, and surely not acceptable in modern hospitals given the potential severity of the consequences. This chapter reviews the components of good prescribing practice and discusses the pitfalls inherent in the process.

Good prescribing: questions to ask yourself before picking up the pen

Is drug treatment really necessary?

It is obvious that while appropriate drug therapy can be of great benefit, inappropriate therapy is not harmless. On all occasions, there should be a positive reason for prescribing a drug. Drug treatment should never become a routine. In hospital it is still not uncommon to find 'routine' prescriptions for hypnotics, analgesics and purgatives without any consideration of individual need. Many patients may expect a consultation to result automatically in the prescription of a medicine, the provision of unnecessary antibiotic therapy for a viral illness being a common example. These situations are clearly undesirable and represent bad prescribing practice.

Which drug should I choose?

When drug treatment is indicated, it is mandatory that the most appropriate agent is given in

Lecture Notes: Clinical Pharmacology and Therapeutics, 8th edition. By Gerard McKay, John Reid and Matthew Walters. Published 2010 by Blackwell Publishing Ltd.

the correct dose and in a regimen that results in optimum treatment with minimum adverse effects. Selection of the best drug requires consideration of factors that relate not only to the range of drugs available, but also to both the patient and the condition being treated. Age and disease may influence kinetics and dynamics to a significant degree (see Chapter 23) and should be reflected in the choice of agent. Choosing the wrong drug (such as diclofenac over paracetamol for mild headache in a patient with renal impairment) may aggravate existing medical conditions. As discussed later in this chapter, concomitant therapy for co-morbid conditions may interact with any new prescription, with occasionally adverse consequences (see page 322).

By what route should it be administered?

Certain drugs (for example, the third-generation cephalosporin antibiotic cefotaxime) can only be administered intravenously. A choice of routes of administration is available for most drugs, however, and this should be considered when writing a prescription. In the context of emergencies (e.g. antibiotic treatment of severe sepsis), drug administration through the intravenous route is preferred due to the rapid, predictable delivery of treatment. Alternative routes may also be preferred in those patients unable to swallow (e.g. rectal administration of aspirin to dysphagic stroke patients).

What dose and how often?

Recommended doses and dosing intervals are given in the *British National Formulary* (BNF; see below), which should be consulted when prescribing any drug with which you are not intimately familiar. Particular care should be taken when the patient's ability to metabolise or excrete a drug may be compromised, for example patients with hepatic or renal impairment. These considerations are discussed in more detail in Chapter 22.

Writing the prescription: practical aspects

Once the choice of drug, route of administration, dose and dosing interval has been made, it must be communicated with clarity to the dispensing pharmacist. All prescriptions for medicine should be printed or handwritten clearly and in ink. Whenever a prescription is written, the following guidelines should be adhered to:

1 Specify the patient's full name, address and age, although the legal requirement is 'age if under 12'.
2 Indicate clearly the drug or medicine. As discussed below, in most cases use of the approved or generic name rather than the proprietary (brand) name is preferred.
3 Specify precisely the strength of tablets, capsules or mixtures. It is good prescribing practice to indicate these in words and figures and mandatory for prescriptions of controlled drugs.
4 Indicate the dose frequency and total quantity to be supplied or the duration of treatment. Once again it is good practice to include these in words and figures as this is a legal requirement for controlled drugs.
5 Do not leave large blank spaces on the prescription, which may be filled in by unscrupulous individuals to obtain unauthorised supplies of drugs of abuse.
6 Sign the prescription, date it and indicate your name and address. Addition of a telephone number assists the pharmacist in contacting the prescriber in the case of a prescription for an unusual drug or dose regimen.

Should generic or brand name prescribing be used?

Drugs available on prescription have approved or generic names. Individual manufacturers give their own preparations proprietary (brand or trade) names. Brand names are usually distinctive, and often easier to remember than the generic name (for example, the glycoprotein IIb/IIIa receptor antagonist abciximab is generally referred to as 'ReoPro'). When a proprietary name is used on a prescription, the pharmacist is obliged to dispense that product rather than a generic equivalent which may be cheaper and more readily available. Unlike generic names, proprietary names give no clear indication of the active constituents of the medicine. This may lead to inadvertent oversupply of a drug common to two prescribed medicines, such as Solpadeine and Panadol both of which contain paracetamol. For these reasons, in most instances, prescription by generic name is recommended. An exception to this recommendation occurs when drugs with a narrow therapeutic index (such as theophylline and lithium) are prescribed in a sustained release preparation. Clinically significant differences in absorption profiles of these drugs may exist between proprietary brands, hence brand name should be specified when these drugs are used.

The generic and proprietary names of all drugs in clinical use can be found in the BNF, a useful reference which is published every 6 months and provided free to doctors and medical students in the United Kingdom. Details of recommended doses together with brief notes on adverse effects, contraindications and interactions are provided. It is widely used as a reference by doctors and pharmacists, and is particularly practical when used in conjunction with formularies compiled and published at a local hospital or general practice level. These formularies are now very common and essentially serve to indicate which drugs will be readily available to prescribers in a particular locality or hospital.

General pointers on good prescribing

The ability to prescribe drugs in a safe, effective and thoughtful manner is one of the defining characteristics of a good clinician. It can be a deceptively difficult skill to acquire, and requires constant maintenance as the range of drugs available expands. The following advice is distilled from many years of experience of prescribing and is offered to provide some general principles applicable to most situations.

1 Wherever possible, minimise the number of drugs and total number of doses to be given. Always satisfy yourself that a prescription is necessary before considering a pharmacological solution to the problem. Compound preparations are helpful in achieving this goal when there is an established therapeutic need for all the constituents, and where the combination of two or more drugs aids adherence.

2 Make an effort to ensure that the patient understands the reason for the prescription, and is aware of how it should be taken.

3 Familiarise yourself with a limited number of well-established drugs with known effects and side effects. Do not chop and change amongst equivalent preparations on whim or fancy. Avoid trying out new preparations simply because of novelty or extensive commercial promotion.

4 Check the dose carefully each time you prescribe. Do not trust to memory and be particularly careful when doses are in the microgram range or when prescribing for children and the elderly.

5 Finally, always review drug prescriptions regularly: every day in hospital patients or weekly or monthly as appropriate in outpatients or general practice. When reviewing prescriptions ask the following questions:

- Is the drug treatment still necessary?
- Is the optimum dose regimen being followed?
- Is the desired effect being achieved?
- Are there any symptoms or adverse effects that could be secondary to drug treatment?
- In general practice, has a maximum of one month's supply been prescribed?

Do not continue treatment by repeating prescriptions over long periods of time without assessing the response in the patient, or worse still, without seeing the patient.

Comment. The basis of good prescribing is a sound training in clinical methods and pathophysiology, which, together with an understanding of pharmacodynamic and pharmacokinetic properties of the drugs being used, permits maximum benefit to be achieved with the minimum risk of adverse effects. Prescriptions are legal documents. They should consist of clear, legible instructions to the pharmacist. Illegible, incomplete or ambiguous prescriptions are not only bad medicine, but they are also illegal.

When prescribing goes wrong

Any drug can be harmful if used improperly. The mechanisms through which drugs may injure patients are many and varied: problems may arise solely as a result of one drug (adverse drug reactions) or as a consequence of prescription of combinations of agents (drug interactions). This section reviews the more commonly encountered problems in this area and discusses methods of reducing the burden of adverse events related to drug prescribing.

Adverse drug reactions

Adverse drug reactions comprise any unwanted effect of a drug. They are best considered in two broad groups: *predictable* (and usually dose-related) effects and *unpredictable* (or idiosyncratic) effects. Predictable effects are relatively common and usually seen shortly after the drug is initiated, dose increased or in some cases discontinued. Conversely, unpredictable effects occur less frequently and need not necessarily be dose-dependent.

Predictable effects

Predictable adverse drug effects are due to excessive pharmacological activity of the drug in question. This arises particularly with central nervous system depressants, cardioactive, hypotensive and hypoglycaemic agents. Specific examples of this type of reaction are:

1 Respiratory depression in patients given morphine or benzodiazepine hypnotics

2 Hypotension resulting in stroke, myocardial infarction or renal failure in patients receiving excessive doses of antihypertensive drugs

3 Bradyarrhythmias in patients receiving excessive digoxin doses

Less obvious but equally important are predictable adverse effects where the particular pharmacological effect involved is not the one for which the drug was initially administered. For example, a patient receiving an antihistamine for the prevention of motion sickness may become drowsy.

All patients are at risk of developing this type of reaction if high enough doses are given. However, certain subgroups are particularly susceptible and include those with renal disease, liver disease, the very young and the elderly. Specific considerations relating to these more vulnerable groups are discussed in Chapters 22 and 23.

Withdrawal symptoms or rebound responses after discontinuation of treatment

This type of reaction is unusual in that it occurs in the absence of the causative agent. The abrupt interruption of therapy is followed by a characteristic withdrawal syndrome:

1 Extreme agitation, tachycardia, confusion, delirium and convulsions may occur following the discontinuation of long-term central nervous system depressants such as barbiturates, benzodiazepines and alcohol.

2 Acute Addisonian crisis may be precipitated by the abrupt cessation of corticosteroid therapy.

3 Withdrawal symptoms may be characterised by agitation and autonomic overactivity after discontinuation of narcotic analgesics.

Unpredictable effects

The most frequently encountered unpredictable effects relate to drug allergy and hypersensitivity. They occur only in a small proportion of the population exposed to the drug, and it is usually impossible to determine in advance which patients may experience this response. The reactions may vary from a mild erythematous skin rash to a major anaphylactoid reaction which carries significant risk of death. An allergic adverse effect of a drug is characterised by the fact that:

1 The reaction does not resemble the expected pharmacological drug effect.

2 There is delay between first exposure to the drug and the development of a reaction.

3 The reaction recurs upon repeated exposure even to traces of the drug.

The drugs most frequently associated with allergic skin reactions are the penicillins, the sulphonamides and the blood products.

Genetic factors

Adverse drug reactions may arise in certain individuals with a particular genotype or genetic make-up. Hereditary disorders such as pseudocholinesterase deficiency prevent affected individuals from metabolising the muscle relaxant succinylcholine, causing a potentially fatal syndrome of prolonged paralysis and apnoea following its use (Chapter 20). A further example is glucose-6-phosphate dehydrogenase deficiency, a disorder particularly prevalent in Sephardic Jews and Black populations, which predisposes to acute haemolysis after exposure to a wide variety of drugs, including the antimalarial drug primaquine and antibiotics such as the sulphonamides and nitrofurantion.

Genetically, variability in activity of the enzyme N-acetyl transferase causes clinically significant differences in response to a number of drugs metabolised by this enzyme. In contrast to the genetic factors described above, this polymorphism causes delayed adverse effects that may not be immediately apparent to the patient or treating physician. Drugs such as isoniazid, hydralazine and procainamide are metabolised in the liver by the enzyme. There is a bimodal distribution of acetylator capacity in the population, with some individuals being slow and others fast acetylators. Slow acetylators of isoniazid given standard doses are much more likely than fast acetylators to suffer from peripheral neuropathy. The drug-induced lupus syndrome is much more common in slow acetylators receiving hydralazine or procainamide. In the future, tissue typing may help to predict susceptibility to these genetically determined adverse effect of drugs.

Idiosyncratic drug reactions

The term idiosyncrasy is used primarily to cover unusual, unexpected or bizarre drug effects that cannot readily be explained or predicted in individual recipients.

Also included in this type of reaction are drug-induced fetal abnormalities such as phocomelia (limb deformity), which develop in the offspring of mothers receiving thalidomide in early pregnancy.

Drug-induced malignant disease is fortunately rare and may be considered an idiosyncratic drug effect:

1 Analgesic abuse may rarely cause cancer of the renal pelvis.
2 Long-term oestrogens without coincidental progestogens may induce uterine cancer.
3 Immunosuppressive drugs may induce lymphoid tumours.
4 Intramuscular iron preparations may cause sarcomata at the site of injection.
5 Thyroid cancer may develop in patients who have received ^{131}I-therapy in the past.

Drug interactions

When administration of one drug influences the effect of another, the term 'drug interaction' is used. Interactions account for approximately one quarter of all adverse drug reactions, and are most commonly seen in elderly people taking a variety of drugs for multiple problems. Many hundreds of interactions have been described, and this section focuses upon the general principles involved, using more commonly encountered interactions as illustrative examples. Drug interactions commonly involve interference with any of the pharmacokinetic or pharmacodynamic processes described in Chapter 1. More rarely they may arise as a consequence of a direct chemical reaction between two agents, for example precipitation of chalk following administration of sodium bicarbonate and calcium salts through the same intravenous catheter. A further, more recent concern is the potential for 'herbal remedies' purchased over the counter to interact with prescribed drugs. St. John's Wort, a substance sometimes taken without prescription for depressive symptoms, may cause failure of the oral contraceptive pill.

Table 28.1 Examples of pharmacokinetic interactions.

Absorption interactions

Tetracyclines chelate calcium and magnesium salts leading to reduced antibiotic absorption.

Cholestyramine reduces warfarin absorption by binding to it.

Distribution interactions

Aspirin displaces warfarin from plasma proteins, potentiating the anti-coagulant effect.

Valproate displaces phenytoin from plasma proteins, increasing plasma-free phenytoin.

Metabolism interactions

Induction

Carbamazepine induces enzymes which metabolise phenytoin, necessitating larger doses of phenytoin.

Phenytoin induces enzymes responsible for metabolism of estrogens and progestogens in the oral contraceptive pill, so increasing the risk of unplanned pregnancy.

Inhibition

Warfarin may be potentiated by metronidazole, which inhibits metabolism of the warfarin molecule.

Allopurinol potentates the cytotoxic effect of azathioprine by inhibiting xanthine oxidase, the enzyme responsible for its enzymatic degradation.

The most commonly encountered drug interaction causing the need for hospital admission involves warfarin and antibiotic treatment. Antibiotics may influence warfarin's effects through a number of mechanisms, including disturbance of intestinal flora with subsquent reduction in vitamin K production, malabsorbtion of vitamin K or direct inhibition or potentiation of warfarin metabolism. Caution should always be used when prescribing antibiotic treatment for a patient already on warfarin, and careful monitoring of INR in this circumstance is mandatory.

Pharmacodynamic interactions

These tend to involve the administration of two drugs with similar effects. Such interactions may involve two agents acting at one receptor (attenuation of salbutamol's bronchodilatory effect by non-specific beta-blockers) or through a less specific effect upon particular tissues (potentiation of the sedative effect of benzodiazepines by alcohol). Pharmacodynamic interactions at one receptor may have therapeutic use, such as the reversal of opiate toxicity by naloxone. The clinical effects are largely predictable and can be prevented by thoughtful prescribing.

Pharmacokinetic interactions

These interactions involve interference with absorption, distribution or metabolism of one drug as a consequence of the administration of another. They tend to be less easy to predict than pharmacodynamic interactions, although the consequences may be no less severe. Some commonly encountered pharmacokinetic interactions are summarised in Table 28.1.

An exhaustive list of all potential interactions lies outwith the scope of this text. Appendix 1 of the BNF provides a useful reference, and should be consulted whenever the question of a potential interaction arises.

What can we do to minimise drug-related harm to patients?

Although the age of the patient is often cited as a determinant of the frequency of adverse drug reactions, the total number of drugs taken by the patient is a more important factor. Many studies have demonstrated a rise in frequency of adverse drug reactions as the number of drugs increases, and significantly the frequency of these interactions falls following rationalisation of drug therapy. As a ballpark figure, long-term treatment with two drugs will lead to drug-related adverse effects in 10–15% of patients: this figure rises to more than 50% in patients taking five drugs on a regular basis. Careful prescribing and the application of the principles described above will minimise the problems caused by predictable adverse reactions; however, other idiosyncratic, unpredictable or rare adverse effects may be encountered even following the most assiduous prescribing. These effects are particularly prevalent in new drugs, as despite the extensive evaluation which occurs before a drug is marketed, some adverse drug effects only become apparent when the drug is used in clinical practice. A framework for the detection, analysis and reporting of these less common effects is necessary. The system used in the UK is described in Chapter 2.

Compliance, concordance and adherence

Clinical scenario

A 74-year-old man with high blood pressure is admitted to hospital for a routine operation (transurethral resection of prostate). The admitting doctor writes up his drug chart for the 3 different blood pressure tablets he is normally prescribed. The day after his operation he is given the three drugs by the nurse doing the drug round. The patient then complains of dizziness on standing and is noted to have a low blood pressure with postural drop. Is there a problem with adherence?

Compliance, concordance and adherence are terms that have been and are used to describe whether or not patients take the medications prescribed for them. The term compliance, to act in accordance with a direction (prescription), was felt by some to betray a paternalistic attitude to the patient on the part of the prescriber; excluding the patient from any decisions regarding their treatment regimen and the prescriber from any responsibility if the patient chose not to take the medications prescribed. As a result many chose to use the term concordance. This implies that the prescriber and patient come to an agreement about the regimen they will take. Although it is important that prescribers spend time with the patient explaining the treatment recommended

and agreeing on the treatment regime, this term assumes that patients have a reasonable understanding of the treatment recommended and does not capture whether patients actually follow the agreed regimen. Perhaps the best terminology to use is adherence which means, 'persistence in a practice', better reflecting whether patients take the recommended treatment or not. For practical purposes compliance and adherence are more or less interchangeable terms. Many patients do not adhere to treatment regimens that they are prescribed even when there has been concordance with the prescriber.

Is good adherence important?

Adherence to beneficial drug therapy is associated with lower mortality than poor adherence and good adherence to harmful drug therapy is associated with increased mortality. Interestingly good adherence to placebo has been shown to be beneficial suggesting that adherence is a surrogate marker for healthy behaviour. The ability of physicians to recognise non adherence is poor, and interventions to improve adherence have had mixed results.

Methods of measuring adherence

Direct – this can be by direct observation of treatment being taken or by measuring the drug level (e.g. anti-convulsant) or biological marker (e.g. cholesterol when patient on a treatment to lower it).

Indirect – this can be done by patient questionnaires/diaries, pill counts/electronic medication monitoring, rates of repeat prescription requests.

Factors that reduce adherence

Many factors may influence adherence including psychological problems or coginitive impairment, patients' beliefs, polypharmacy, treatment of asymptomatic disease, side effects and treatment costs. Many of these barriers to adherence can be improved by the clinician through good communication.

Means of improving adherence

The problem needs to be identified in the first instance. It is important to spend time explaining the need for the medications in a language that the patient understands and where possible provide written instructions. Sometimes the help of a family member or community services can be invaluable, and particularly for those on many different medications the use of a medication aid such as a blister pack may help.

Prescribers should always regularly review the medications of their patients on repeat prescriptions. This includes asking patients nonjudgmentally about medication taking behaviour. Whilst there is scant evidence for specific interventions that improve adherence it is likely that a multifaceted approach will help including clearly explaining to the patient the recommended regimen, in language they understand, and customising the treatment in accordance with the their wishes.

Index

Note: Page numbers in *italics* indicate figures and those in **bold** indicate tables.